THE AFRICAN STATE AND THE AIDS CRISIS

Global Health

Series Editors: Nana K. Poku and Robert L. Ostergard, Jr.

The benefits of globalization are potentially enormous, as a result of the increased sharing of ideas, cultures, life-saving technologies and efficient production processes. Yet globalization is under trial, partly because these benefits are not yet reaching hundreds of millions of the world's poor and partly because globalization has introduced new kinds of international problems and conflicts. Turmoil in one part of the world now spreads rapidly to others, through terrorism, armed conflict, environmental degradation or disease.

This timely series provides a robust and multi-disciplinary assessment of the asymmetrical nature of globalization. Books in the series encompass a variety of areas, including global health and the politics of governance, poverty and insecurity, gender and health and the implications of global pandemics.

Also in the series

International Public Health
Patients' Rights vs. the Protection of Patents
Yves Beigbeder
ISBN 07546 3621 6

The Political Economy of AIDS in Africa
Edited by Nana K. Poku and Alan Whiteside
ISBN 0 7546 3897 9

Health as International Politics
Combating Communicable Diseases in the Baltic Sea Region
Geir Hønneland and Lars Rowe
ISBN 0 7546 4256 9

Global Population Policy
From Population Control to Reproductive Rights
Paige Whaley Eager
ISBN 0 7546 4162 7

The African State and the AIDS Crisis

Edited by
AMY S. PATTERSON
Calvin College, USA

Routledge
Taylor & Francis Group
LONDON AND NEW YORK

First published 2005 by Ashgate Publishing

Published 2018 by Routledge
2 Park Square, Milton Park, Abingdon, Oxon OX14 4RN
605 Third Avenue, New York, NY 10017

Routledge is an imprint of the Taylor & Francis Group, an informa business

Typeset in Times New Roman by Saxon Graphics Ltd, Derby

A Library of Congress record exists under LC control number: 2004025011

ISBN 13: 978-0-815-39742-7 (hbk)
ISBN 13: 978-1-351-14788-0 (ebk)

Contents

List of Figures

List of Tables

List of Contributors

Karen Ball is Associate Professor of Exercise and Health Science at Alma College in Michigan. She has published articles in *Biochemistry* and the *Journal of Molecular and Cellular Cardiology*. Her recent research, funded by the National Institutes of Health, examines the effect of diabetes on the heart.

Crystal Barcelo is a student in the Department of Political Science, Binghamton University, State University of New York.

Jake Batsell received a Master's degree in Government from the University of Texas in 2001. While there, he was awarded grants from the Institute for International Education and the University Co-operative Society to conduct research on Zimbabwean politics. He is now a journalist and journalism instructor in the Dallas area.

David Cieminis is a 2004 graduate of Calvin College in Grand Rapids, Michigan. He was awarded a McGregor Fellowship in 2002 to conduct research on global AIDS policies. He works with the Christian Reformed World Relief Committee on AIDS programs for Africa.

Fred Eboko is a research fellow with the Institut de Recherche pour le Développement and Associate Researcher at the Centre d'Etude d'Afrique Noire, Institut d'Etudes Politiques de Bordeaux in France. He has published in journals and edited volumes, including *Travaux et Documents*, *Politique africaine, Autrepart-Cahier des sciences humaines*, and *Le désarroi camerounais: L'épreuve de l'économie-monde*.

Patrick Furlong is Professor of History at Alma College in Michigan. A native of South Africa, he is the author of *The Mixed Marriages Act: A historical and theological study* and *Between crown and swastika: The impact of the radical right on the Afrikaner nationalist movement in the fascist era*. He has published articles in *Ufahamu*, *African Affairs*, the *South African Historical Journal*, and *New Contree*.

Debora Halbert is Associate Professor of Political Science at Otterbein College in Westerville, Ohio. She is the author of *Intellectual property in the information age: The politics of expanding property rights*, as well as numerous articles on copyright law.

Bernard Haven is a 2004 graduate of Calvin College in Grand Rapids, Michigan. He was awarded a McGregor Fellowship to conduct research on AIDS policies in Ghana and he completed field research in Accra in 2003. In 2004 he began graduate study in International Development at the London School of Economics.

Maite Irurzun-Lopez is an Economic Affairs officer at the United Nations Commission on HIV/AIDS and Governance in Africa in Addis Ababa. Since October 2001 she has worked as a health economist with the United Nations Economic Commission for Africa. Previously she worked for the Asian Development Bank, the Universidad Javeriana of Cali, Colombia, and the Institute of Development Studies in the United Kingdom.

Christopher May is Reader in International Political Economy at the University of the West of England in Bristol. His recent books include *The information society: A skeptical view* and *Authority and markets: Susan Strange's writing on IPE.* He has also published in *Global Society, New Political Economy, Urban Studies,* and the *European Intellectual Property Review.*

Babacar Mbengue received his Ph.D. from Cheikh Anta Diop University in Dakar, Senegal. A former Fulbright scholar, he wrote his dissertation on the legal implications of the contemporary Islamic financial system. He currently teaches in Chicago.

Robert L. Ostergard, Jr. is Associate Director of the Institute of Global Cultural Studies and Assistant Professor of Political Science, Binghamton University, State University of New York. His books include *The development dilemma: The political economy of intellectual property rights in the international system* and the forthcoming *HIV/AIDS and the threat to national and international security*. He also has published in the *Journal of World Intellectual Property* and *Third World Quarterly.*

Amy S. Patterson is Assistant Professor of Political Science at Calvin College in Grand Rapids, Michigan. She has published in several journals and edited volumes, including the *Journal of Modern African Studies*, *Africa Today*, *African Studies Review*, the *Canadian Journal of African Studies, PS: Political Science and Politics, The redistribution of authority,* and *The children of Africa confront AIDS: From vulnerability to possibility.*

Nana Poku is Research Director at the United Nations Commission on HIV/AIDS and Governance in Africa in Addis Ababa. His recent works include *Redefining security: Population movements and national security, Security and development in southern Africa, Global health and governance: HIV/AIDS*, and *Migration, globalisation and human security.*

Patricia Siplon is Associate Professor of Political Science at Saint Michael's College in Colchester, Vermont. She is the author of *AIDS and the policy struggle in the United States* and numerous publications on national and global AIDS policy. She was a Rotary International Teaching Fellow at the University of Dar es Salaam in Tanzania.

Alan Whiteside is Director of the Health Economics and HIV/AIDS Research Division and Professor at the University of KwaZulu-Natal. He has written widely on AIDS in Africa. His recent books include *AIDS: The challenge for South Africa* (with Clem Sunter) and *AIDS in the twenty-first century: Disease and globalisation* (with Tony Barnett).

Acknowledgements

Ku am kudu du làkk. The person with a spoon does not burn herself. In my years living in Senegal, I often reminded myself of the truth of this Wolof proverb. That is, if I used the tools available to me, I would be better off. Indeed, I have been very fortunate to have many people guide and support the process of editing this book. Without their help, I could not have completed this project.

I first must express my gratitude to the contributors to this volume, who rewrote chapters, pleasantly accepted my editorial changes, and endured what must have at times seemed like incessant emails. I am particularly grateful to Nana Poku and Robert Ostergard for including this book in the Ashgate series on Global Health. Catherine Boone also provided encouragement as I approached possible contributors. The work has benefited from the comments of external reviewers and editors at Ashgate.

I have been fortunate to receive immense support from Calvin College. Joel Carpenter provided funding, Lorrie Menninga thoroughly copyedited the book, and my colleagues, particularly Corwin Smidt, Doug Koopman, and Simona Goi, shared invaluable insights about publishing edited volumes. Calvin College also provided release time and student researchers for me through a Calvin Research Fellowship, two McGregor Fellowships, and a grant from the Center for Social Research. Two students – Bernard Haven and David Cieminis – worked diligently on summer research, never arguing when I made them 'find out more' or challenged their conclusions. I am grateful to work at such a generous institution with colleagues who support me and students who make teaching a joy.

Most important, I thank my husband Neil and my three year old daughter Sophia. They never doubted my ability to complete this project and they did not question the hours I put into it. Through her laughter, songs, and play, Sophia helped me put the project into perspective. Their love and compassion for others continue to remind me why I choose to study the politics of AIDS in Africa.

Amy Patterson

Acknowledgements

[illegible]

Chapter 1

Introduction: The African State and the AIDS Crisis

Amy S. Patterson

In July 2004, the Joint United Nations Program on HIV/AIDS (UNAIDS) reported that over the previous year, roughly five million adults and children were newly infected with the human immunodeficiency virus (HIV) that causes the acquired immunodeficiency syndrome (AIDS). An estimated 25 million adults and children are thought to be living with HIV/AIDS in sub-Saharan Africa. In the same period, over two million adults and children in the region died because of AIDS (UNAIDS 2004). This volume examines the role of the African state in addressing this crisis. Through the chapters, the book questions how the African state, which is usually seen to be institutionally weak, limited in resources, and lacking in international power, has responded to AIDS. The work broadly defines a state to include institutions, territory, laws, bureaucratic and military apparatus, and ideology (Englebert 2000, 4).

As Boone and Batsell (2001) argue, political scientists have been noticeably absent from much of the analysis of AIDS in Africa.[1] Yet, because power, resources, ideology, and institutions shape policy making on HIV/AIDS, any responses to the epidemic are intensely political. Through the contributions of African, American, and European scholars, this book examines the nexus between the African state and the AIDS epidemic. It questions how African state power in the international system, state dependence on donor resources, democratic and economic transitions, ideology, political culture, and state-civil society relations shape Africa's fight against HIV/AIDS. The chapters draw on several case studies to demonstrate the complexity and diversity of variables shaping the interface between AIDS and the African state.

The AIDS Epidemic in sub-Saharan Africa

The AIDS epidemic in Africa is characterized by its magnitude and its potential long-term impact on society, politics, and economics. With over 30 per cent of the people living with HIV/AIDS globally, southern Africa is the region most affected. As of 2004, HIV prevalence rates were approximately 37 per cent in Botswana and Swaziland, roughly 21 per cent in South Africa, and 24 per cent in Zimbabwe (UNAIDS 2004). The prevalence rates in East and Central Africa were not as horrendous, but roughly 13 per cent of citizens in the Central African Republic were estimated to be HIV positive. In West Africa, AIDS has manifested itself in a variety of ways. Senegal's HIV rate remains approximately 1 per cent, reflecting the country's early HIV-prevention and awareness programs. However, in an alarming trend, HIV prevalence among sex workers in Dakar and small cities has risen recently. In 2004, HIV prevalence rates were between 3 per cent and 4 per cent in Burkina Faso and Ghana, while the situation in Côte d'Ivoire and Nigeria was graver, with rates over 10 per cent in some parts of those two countries (UNAIDS 2003a, 8–12; UNAIDS 2004). In a hopeful sign, prevalence rates among 15 to 24 year old pregnant women in some cities have declined. For example, HIV rates fell to 8 per cent in Kampala in 2002 from 30 per cent a decade earlier; prevalence in Addis Ababa declined from 24 per cent in 1995 to 11 per cent in 2003. Despite the variation in HIV prevalence rates and some signs that the epidemic has reached its peak in some countries, 'The epidemic in sub-Saharan Africa … remains rampant' (UNAIDS 2003a, 4).

However, these statistics only tell part of the story. In most countries, HIV rates in urban areas are higher than in rural areas, reflecting the migration of individuals into areas where they may lack social connections and often face economic insecurity. Without networks of family and friends to discourage risky sexual behavior, individuals are more vulnerable to contracting HIV. Yet, there are exceptions to the urban concentration of AIDS, such as the rise of HIV prevalence in small southern Nigerian cities and the similar urban and rural HIV prevalence rates in Swaziland (UNAIDS 2003a, 12). Additionally, areas with high cross-border trade and migration (and sex workers to serve these traders and migrants) often have higher HIV prevalence rates. For example, HIV prevalence is highest along Ghana's eastern border (GAC 2003). AIDS also has a gender bias in sub-Saharan Africa, where women are at least 1.3 times more likely to be infected with HIV than men. In 2004, UNAIDS reported that 57 per cent of those infected in sub-Saharan Africa were women (UNAIDS 2004).

AIDS is closely linked to inequality and poverty. Over 95 per cent of the HIV-positive individuals globally live in the developing world, with over two-thirds of these individuals living in sub-Saharan Africa. With an average life expectancy of 46 years, a gross national income per capita of \$460, and a mortality rate of 171 deaths per 1,000 children under five years old, sub-Saharan Africa is the most impoverished region of the world. Poverty has led to reliance on foreign aid and indebtedness. In 2001, the region received \$13.9 billion in foreign development assistance, while it owed \$202 billion to bilateral and multilateral lenders. In the majority of sub-Saharan African countries, at least 50 per cent of the population lives below the national poverty line (World Bank 2003). These factors contribute to what Barnett and Whiteside (2002, 73) term 'risk environments', or social and economic environments in which an infectious disease can rapidly develop into an epidemic.

Poverty increases an individual's vulnerability to HIV infection by decreasing access to good nutrition; by limiting access to health care such as prenatal care, HIV testing, and treatment for sexually transmitted infections (STIs); and by necessitating migration for employment. Poverty also makes it more likely that women will engage in survival sex to provide for their children and themselves (Whiteside 2002).

The neoliberal economic policies encouraged by the World Bank and International Monetary Fund have compounded the link between AIDS and poverty. By requiring a reduction in state employment and privatization of national industries, these policies contributed to unemployment. Unemployment is one factor in the risk environments for HIV, if men are forced to migrate far from their families to find jobs and women must turn to survival sex to feed their children. Neoliberal policies also have encouraged the introduction of user fees for education and health services, a factor which has made it more expensive for citizens to access these services. Yet primary health care is essential for preventing the spread of HIV, through HIV testing, prenatal care, and treatment for STIs.

Another consequence of the decline in state spending on health and education is that African states must rely more on international donors and nongovernmental organizations (NGOs) to provide basic human services. Reliance on these external actors has two consequences. First, the development of comprehensive AIDS policies has been made more complex, because NGOs and donors are outside the control of the state and may challenge state policies. For example, Médecins sans Frontières (Doctors without Borders) began to import generic drugs for AIDS patients into South Africa, despite state objections to the plan. While such actions are certainly important for providing individuals with access to needed medicines, they do illustrate the lack of coordination in AIDS programs and policies in Africa. Second, because of the large amount of funding they provide for AIDS programs, international organizations have played a key role in designing many state AIDS programs and decision-making institutions throughout Africa. For example, as Chapter 5 demonstrates, the Ghana AIDS Commission developed from consultations among UNAIDS, the UN Development Fund, and the US Agency for International Development; its initial funding came from the World Bank and the UK Department for International Development.

Neoliberal policies have sought to incorporate Africa into the global economy by liberalizing trade and encouraging foreign investment in the continent. Donors have increasingly focused on 'trade not aid' through legislation such as the US African Growth and Opportunity Act of 2000. To get the lower tariffs on textiles, agricultural products, and clothing that the legislation promises, African states have had to join the World Trade Organization and accept its related treaties. Though Africa's share of global trade is minimal, these trade agreements have had a disproportionate impact on the continent's ability to fight AIDS; the ability of African states to provide access to patented medications to treat AIDS and the opportunistic infections that accompany it has been hampered. Likewise, because of the focus on trade, African states have had to court international investment through promises of cheap, non-unionized labor. As Whiteside points out in Chapter 6, this type of foreign investment may increase the risk environments for the spread of HIV/AIDS.

The AIDS epidemic directly threatens African states. Without comprehensive, well-organized efforts, the epidemic will decrease life expectancy, decimate military forces, and challenge state efficiency. Economically, the epidemic threatens the advances in development that the continent has made since independence. The illness affects households, as families must sell assets such as land and livestock or use savings to pay for the increased costs of medicines and funerals. In the long term, households may be unable to recover because of these losses (Rugalema 2000). As the southern African humanitarian crisis illustrates, AIDS kills farmers, prevents adults from passing down knowledge on food production to future generations, and leaves families without labor, seeds, or savings which will carry them through periods of drought (*New York Times*, 19 November 2002). In several southern African countries, 60 per cent to 70 per cent of farms have suffered labor losses as a result of HIV/AIDS (UNAIDS 2003b). The outcome is that six million people in southern Africa needed food aid in 2003. Since 2002, food shortages have affected 14 million people in Lesotho, Swaziland, Malawi, Zambia, Mozambique, and Zimbabwe (UN Integrated Regional Information Network, 1 December 2003).

Because of the loss of productive labor in society, many scholars believe that AIDS will have a detrimental macroeconomic impact. For example, Botswana's economy may be 24 per cent to 38 per cent smaller in the next 25 years because of HIV/AIDS (Whiteside 2002). AIDS will cause governments to divert state expenditures from poverty alleviation and other social services to health care, and more specifically, to hospitalization of those with AIDS. The long-term cost of this diversion may negatively affect education, teacher training, and primary health care, at just the time when these services are most needed for African countries to prepare for the future and to prevent new HIV infections (Brown 2004). In 2003, economists at the World Bank and Heidelberg University predicted that because of HIV/AIDS, incomes in South Africa will halve over the next three generations and child labor will be ubiquitous by 2080. Because of the erosion of the country's intellectual capacity, South Africa faces an inescapable descent into economic backwardness (Bell, Gersbach, and Devarajan 2003).

Furthermore, the AIDS epidemic threatens to erode the ability of the state to provide order and security in society. Though admitting that data on HIV prevalence rates in African militaries is fraught with problems, Elbe (2002) illustrates the high levels of HIV infection among African militaries, with Angola and Malawi near 50 per cent; Zambia, 60 per cent; Zimbabwe, 55 per cent; and South Africa, 15 per cent to 20 per cent. AIDS is the primary cause of death among Congolese soldiers. These rates will have implications for staffing decisions and military preparedness, and they will necessitate additional military resources for recruiting and training soldiers to replace those dying of AIDS. In Chapter 8, Ostergard and Barcelo illustrate that the realization that AIDS may decimate the Ugandan military caused President Yoweri Museveni to reframe AIDS as a security issue. Likewise, the estimated 11 million African children under 15 years old who have lost at least one parent to AIDS will challenge the state's ability to promote security. By 2005, nearly one million South African children will be AIDS orphans. AIDS orphans are more likely to be depressed, to use drugs, and to be involved in crime (Schötenich 1999; Segendo and Nambi 1997). Lacking positive socialization experiences, these young people may contribute to societal instability; they may challenge the state's legitimacy, if it cannot address this growing problem. In 2001, the United Nations General Assembly Special Session on HIV/AIDS agreed that by 2005 all countries should work to implement comprehensive national programs to protect and support children affected by AIDS. Despite this pledge, almost no African country has a national orphan policy in place (UNAIDS 2003a).

State Actions on HIV/AIDS

Given the potential economic, social, and political challenges of the epidemic, what have African states done to fight HIV/AIDS? For many state leaders, the initial response to the news that AIDS existed inside their territories was denial. For example, Kenya's President Daniel arap Moi stated that the foreign press was conducting a hate campaign against his country when it reported in 1985 that Kenya had 20 AIDS victims (Fortin 1987). The King of Swaziland only declared the HIV/AIDS epidemic a national disaster in 1999, after the UN Children's Fund published a report in the *Times of Swaziland* on the likely long-term negative impact of AIDS on the society (Daly 2001). As Furlong and Ball illustrate in Chapter 7, the apartheid regime in South Africa tried to downplay AIDS by portraying it as a disease that only infected 'deviant homosexuals'. On the other hand, President Museveni of Uganda admitted the presence of HIV/AIDS in his country when he came to power in 1986. He cooperated with the World Health Organization's Global Program on AIDS to develop comprehensive prevention programs. He also publicly discussed the disease, urging abstinence and monogamy. Low-Beer and Stoneburner (2004) maintain that part of the reason that Uganda's anti-AIDS efforts were effective was because the government provided a space in which local groups, faith-based organizations, neighbors, and friends could discuss the disease and educate one another.

Policy responses to HIV/AIDS can fit into three overall categories: prevention, care and support, and treatment. Most African states, international donors, and NGOs have focused on prevention, through messages about abstinence, monogamy, healthy living, and compassion for those with HIV/AIDS. Prevention also encompasses setting up centers for voluntary counseling and testing, providing treatment for STIs, providing drugs that decrease the transmission of HIV from mother to child, and developing peer education programs for sex workers, young people, and others at risk. Care and support activities include orphan care, food and housing support for family members affected by HIV/AIDS, school fee support for AIDS orphans and other family members affected by the disease, and palliative care. In 2002, the *Lancet* reported that through the implementation of a variety of prevention, care, and support efforts, by 2010, 45 million new infections globally could be averted (Stover et al. 2002). However, on a continent with high levels of poverty and underdeveloped health-care services, such programs are conspicuously absent. UNAIDS (2003a, 4) reports that a mere 1 per cent of pregnant women in heavily affected countries have access to services for prevention of mother-to-child transmission. In 2004, UNAIDS found that only 8 per cent of out-of-school youth have access to education on prevention in sub-Saharan Africa (UNAIDS 2004, 11).

African states also have been unable to provide their citizens with antiretroviral (ARV) treatment, the combination therapies that directly attack the virus in the body. Of the roughly 25 million HIV-positive Africans, only about 50,000 had access to ARVs in 2003. The first ARV (AZT or zidovudine) was developed in 1987 and belongs to a group of drugs termed nucleoside reverse transcriptase inhibitors. These drugs slow down production of the reverse transcriptase enzyme and make HIV unable to infect new cells and duplicate itself. The more powerful class of drugs termed protease inhibitors was discovered in 1995 and made widely available in 1996. They break down the protein that HIV uses to reproduce itself. These drugs can slow the reproduction of the virus and the process of noninfectious virus cells becoming mature and infectious. The protease inhibitors have been extremely successful in reducing AIDS deaths in the United States and West Europe. In 2001, combination therapies involving protease inhibitors cost approximately $10,000 to $12,000 per year per patient. By 2004, the price for certain generic combinations had declined to $300 per year per patient. Though prices have decreased, drug access remains limited because of the lack of health-care infrastructure and shortages of health-care personnel in many African countries. As Halbert and May demonstrate in Chapter 10, some generic producers have begun to develop simple ARV regimens through combination dosages. Yet, problems with drug distribution, drug storage, and ample personnel to educate patients on drug adherence remain (UNAIDS 2004).

Constraints and Opportunities: The African State and the Fight against HIV/AIDS

What aspects of the African state have shaped its ability to respond to AIDS with prevention, care, support, and treatment efforts? While this volume acknowledges the variations in governance across the continent, there are some commonalities among African states. First, the state has a hybrid nature; it mixes informal, and sometimes traditional, institutions with the legal-rational structures found in the modern state (van de Walle 2001, 127). Because of colonialism, bureaucratic institutions with formal rules such as planning administrations and budgeting offices coexist with governance based on informal networks and prebendal rewards. Customary law still has sway over issues such as land ownership, marriage, and the rights of women and girl children. Personal rule from presidents to village chiefs influences resource allocation, while parliaments may pass laws on some of these same issues.

The constant negotiating between informal and formal institutions creates both challenges and opportunities for the state to address AIDS. Green (2003) maintains that the incorporation of Muslim leaders into AIDS awareness and prevention programs has contributed to the low level of HIV prevalence in Senegal. Since before independence, the Senegalese state had a long-standing relationship with Muslim leaders, which was based on informal networks of patronage and personal rule. Muslim leaders also have a close relationship with their followers, though their electoral influence and their ability to mobilize their disciples to vote for certain candidates has waned in recent elections (Villalón 1995; Patterson 1999; Cruise O'Brien 1971). Throughout urban and rural Senegal, elders, chiefs, and leaders of civil society groups demonstrate explicit knowledge about AIDS prevention (Ndoulo village elder, interview with author, 2 May 1995).[2] The informal networks among state officials, Muslim leaders, and citizens facilitated prevention efforts so much that despite the low prevalence of HIV in the country, Senegalese citizens feel personally at risk of HIV infection. The result is a low percentage of citizens who engage in risky behaviors (Green 2003, 11).

In Chapter 2, Siplon examines how traditional institutions such as customary law affect women's vulnerability to HIV. She argues that some practices deprive women of autonomy, resources, and decision-making power. Women often must rely on their husbands, fathers, boyfriends, and employers, a fact which may increase their exposure to HIV. Because patriarchy shapes the formal institutions of the state, even laws intended to decrease women's vulnerability are often not enforced. Likewise, patriarchal attitudes that discourage women's participation in politics cause women to be underrepresented in AIDS policy making. Several of these same themes are evident in Chapter 6. Whiteside demonstrates the direct role that the state plays in fostering patriarchy, through an explicit recognition of women's unequal legal status. Whiteside also provides an important insight into AIDS in a country that is still ruled primarily through a traditional leader, the Swazi king. Though Swaziland has a parliament, there have been no multiparty elections since 1973 when the constitution was suspended. On the positive side, this centralization of power has allowed the king to begin a discussion of AIDS without concern for the political ramifications. On the other hand, the king's autocratic rule has meant that AIDS policies have been made with limited input from society and minimal transparency.

A second aspect of the African state that is apparent in this volume is the state's overall lack of legitimacy (Englebert 2000, 5). For state officials to maintain support, they may resort to patronage, corruption, and nepotism, even as international financial institutions have demanded good governance and transparency. As Chapter 5 on Ghana illustrates, AIDS projects and policies are not immune from these neopatrimonial practices. In another example, a 2002 audit of the National AIDS Control Council of Kenya discovered that council funds were missing. The Kenya Medical Association alleged that the council gave money to sham AIDS groups and political figures instead of real AIDS organizations (*Nation*, 30 May 2002; *East African Standard*, 25 September 2002). In 2003, the news media reported that only 6 per cent of the council's funding had ever been spent on AIDS-related activities (*East African Standard*, 27 June 2003). The theme of misuse of AIDS funds is apparent in Chapter 4, in which Batsell demonstrates that corruption under President Robert Mugabe has led to the disappearance of needed resources from the Zimbabwe AIDS levy.

The African state's limited legitimacy also means that it is protective of its role in the development process. While international donors and NGOs can provide needed resources, the presence of these organizations can challenge the state. Chapter 9 illustrates that in the international realm, African states have sought to preserve this development role through representation on AIDS decision-making bodies, such as the Country Coordinating Mechanisms (CCMs). The Global Fund to Fight AIDS, Tuberculosis, and Malaria requires that a country form a CCM composed of NGOs, state officials, and international donors before it applies for a grant. Though intended to be a public-private partnership, the CCM has preserved the central role of the state and international donors in designing AIDS programs and allocating funding; civil society groups have had limited input on the CCMs. Since many of the CCMs only recently emerged, it is difficult to determine if they might provide resources for the neopatrimonial state. But, in one example, Ghana's CCM received $378,000 for administrative costs from its successful 2002 Global Fund grant.

Several of the chapters highlight a third aspect of the African state: the tension between the state and civil society. The Declaration of Commitment on HIV/AIDS that was signed at the 2001 United Nations General Assembly Special Session on HIV/AIDS calls for leadership from government and civil society to fight AIDS. Chapters 2, 3, 4, 5, and 7 illustrate various patterns of state-civil society interactions and the impact these patterns have on AIDS policies. These contributions demonstrate that African states are fairly autonomous from societal pressures for policy changes, often not because of the strength of the state, but because of the weakness of civil society. Groups in civil society may lack resources, leadership, and connections, and associations may become co-opted by the state in return for not challenging state policies (Patterson 1998; Fatton 1995; Ndegwa 1996; Chabal and Daloz 1999). In Chapter 4, Batsell illustrates that the state in Zimbabwe has been able to remain relatively impervious to civil society pressures for AIDS policies. When such policies have been developed (such as the AIDS levy), they have been poorly implemented. Lack of coordination among NGOs, their meager resources, and their concern about state repression have limited the effectiveness of these groups. Similarly, because of constraints on women's time, labor, and resources, women's associations are necessary, but insufficient, organizations to address the link between patriarchy and AIDS. Chapter 2 argues that women's representation in AIDS policy-making bodies must complement the prevention, care, and support roles that women's associations perform.

In Chapter 3, Eboko moves beyond a narrow focus on particular civil society organizations to demonstrate how political culture shapes state actions on AIDS. He asserts that political culture – a society's attitudes, political experiences, and patterns of mobilization – explains the variety of state responses to AIDS found on the continent. He maintains that the Cameroonian state has been able to ignore AIDS because the state is relatively isolated from the people; its interrupted democratization process and citizens' focus on survival have allowed the state to be apathetic about AIDS. In the case of South Africa, he asserts that President Thabo Mbeki's questioning of the link between HIV and AIDS must be understood in the context of a larger political culture that is struggling to assert its autonomy from its white colonial past. In contrast, the maintenance of close political and scientific ties with France has shaped the political culture of Senegalese elites. When the first AIDS cases emerged in the country, Senegalese scientists and public-health officials were already part of an international network of researchers examining the disease. The international and domestic scientific community, and the emergence of a body of internationally accepted knowledge on AIDS, encouraged Senegalese policy makers to proactively address the disease (Haas 1980).

In Chapter 7, Furlong and Ball further highlight the role of civil society in the development of AIDS policies in South Africa. In their analysis of AIDS policies during the apartheid and post-apartheid periods, they demonstrate that both governments have relied on rhetoric to appease supporters, while neglecting the development of coherent AIDS policies. The chapter also illustrates that recently, the post-apartheid state has responded to civil society pressure to provide free universal access to ARVs. They argue that civil society organizations were successful, because this movement incorporated the alliance partners of the ruling African National Congress, namely the Congress of South African Trade Unions and the South African Communist Party. In contrast to the AIDS organizations of Zimbabwe that Batsell analyzes, the South African organizations have utilized the militant tactics of the liberation movement and they have capitalized on the political experience, leadership skills, and institutions that they developed during the apartheid struggle.

Given the global nature of the AIDS epidemic, it is important to expand the concept of civil society beyond national borders. The globalization of trade, communication, and transportation have empowered AIDS activists to build cross-national networks to lobby governments, shape media coverage of the disease, and influence national and international policy-making agendas. For example, Siplon's chapter argues that the Greater Involvement of People with AIDS (GIPA) initiative can be a model for increasing women's involvement in AIDS decision making. GIPA is a global initiative which western AIDS activists articulated in the 1980s, national delegations accepted in 1990s, and international organizations such as UNAIDS now use to encourage representation on national AIDS councils and CCMs. GIPA illustrates the power of nonstate actors working across state borders to shape AIDS programs.

Chapters 9 and 10 also highlight the role of an international civil society in the AIDS struggle. Chapter 9 shows how many AIDS organizations, alongside western scientists and public-health workers, have challenged the views of policy makers on ARV treatment in Africa. Before 2000, treatment was not thought possible on the continent. In contrast, UN Special Envoy on HIV/AIDS in Africa Stephen Lewis (2003) stated in 2003, 'Suddenly there is a recognition … that treatment is possible, that it should be affordable, that lives are prolonged, and that treatment brings hope. It is not just an idea whose time has come; it is a reality whose time is now.' In Chapter 10, Halbert and May illustrate how international civil society organizations have resisted international trade regimes, such as the Trade-Related Intellectual Property Rights (TRIPS) Agreement. Through lobbying first-world governments, protesting pharmaceutical companies, publicizing high drug prices, and developing often illegal programs to import generic ARVs, these organizations have challenged western understandings of intellectual property rights. Their effectiveness has been heightened through the use of the internet for communication, information dissemination, fundraising, and mobilization. These chapters show that the relationship between African states and civil society is complex. At times, African states have benefited from the political activities of international and domestic NGOs. At other times, domestic and international civil society associations have revealed the weakness and illegitimacy of the African state.

A fourth aspect of the African state that is apparent in some of the chapters is its recent experience with democratic transitions. In 2004, Freedom House rated 11 countries in Africa as 'free', 20 as 'partly free', and 17 as 'not free'. In comparison, only two countries were free in 1989, while 28 were not free (Freedom House 2004). In many countries, democracy has not been consolidated, in that all political elites have not come to value civil liberties, alternation of power, and the rule of law (Diamond and Plattner 2001, xv). However, in African countries where democracy is being consolidated, it is possible to examine how political liberalization has influenced AIDS policies. In Ghana, for example, the state did not develop high-level institutions to address AIDS until after the historic 2000 election. Likewise, Kenya's 2002 election in which Mwai Kibaki's Rainbow Coalition defeated Daniel arap Moi's handpicked successor provided new opportunities to discuss the

AIDS issue and to develop long-needed government policies on AIDS. President Kibaki formed a cabinet-level committee which he chaired to address AIDS in March 2003 and he starred in new anti-AIDS advertisements for television, billboards, and posters (*East African Standard*, 24 March 2003; *Nation*, 31 May 2003). UN Representative Stephen Lewis commented about Kibaki's commitment to HIV/AIDS:

> He's providing very open and public leadership on the issue of AIDS. ... It's hard to convey the startlingly changed atmosphere in the political precincts of Nairobi and by extension, in the population overall. If ever there was a time to turn the pandemic around in Kenya that time is now. There is no reason in the world, given the commitment of the new Government to tackle HIV/AIDS, why Kenya cannot become the next Uganda (*AllAfrica.com*, 2 May 2003).

While new governments may use the goodwill that accompanies democratic transitions to enhance the fight against AIDS, Chapter 5 on Ghana illustrates that merely discussing the disease may not lead to a deep political commitment to AIDS. Rather, officials must be concerned about the political ramifications of ignoring AIDS, something that has yet to occur in most African states.

The South Africa case in Chapter 7 provides another view of the impact of democracy on AIDS policies. South Africa exemplifies the fact that democratic transitions are periods of uncertainty and often, continuity, in terms of AIDS policies. The chapter illustrates the difficulties that former nationalist movements such as the African National Congress face in addressing economic and social problems, while also learning how to govern. In some ways, the post-apartheid government has resembled the apartheid regime in its tendency to centralize AIDS policy making and to use inflammatory rhetoric to deflect criticisms. Despite the fact that South Africa has a very liberal constitution, an active, independent media, and a history of civil society activism, post-apartheid policies on AIDS have lacked consistency, resources, and high-level political commitment. In the years immediately after the end of apartheid, AIDS policies did not benefit from political liberalization to the extent that many South Africans and AIDS activists believed they should. Yet, despite the government's foot-dragging, recent AIDS policies in the country have been more in keeping with public opinion, especially in the area of ARV treatment. Unlike Ghana, the AIDS issue has become politicized in South Africa.

A fifth aspect of the African state that is illustrated in this volume is its lack of developmental capacity, or its inability to design and implement long-term development policies. State capacity involves investments in infrastructure, human capital, and institutions of good governance. Capacity has declined since independence, with states lacking well-trained personnel, access to equipment, and well-maintained roads, airports, and ports. In areas such as the rule of law, institutions to protect private property, laws to protect vulnerable groups in society such as women and children, and oversight bodies to check government expenditures remain either nonexistent or not enforced (van de Walle 2001, 92, 182). The low level of state capacity directly relates to the AIDS epidemic. Even if African states develop comprehensive prevention, care, support, and treatment policies, the lack of capacity makes it more difficult to implement and sustain such programs. As illustrated above, many African states have been unable to develop needed prevention activities in the fight against AIDS.

Morgan (2004) demonstrates the negative impact that limited state capacity can have on the World Bank Multi-Country AIDS Program, a project to provide money to local committees to oversee grassroots AIDS prevention and care efforts. The requirements for applying for and reporting on this money have been so detailed that many local officials lack the skills and education to acquire these needed resources. The same situation has existed in Ghana, where rural community groups and district assembly members have had more difficulty accessing available resources from the Ghana AIDS Commission (Patterson and Haven n.d.). In Chapter 6, Whiteside provides another angle on the relationship between AIDS and state capacity. Because of AIDS, the Swazi state will lose personnel, will need to hire and train more workers, and will face declining state revenues. The Swazi state's lack of transparency and accountability will exacerbate these challenges to state capacity.

A final aspect of the African state that this book illustrates in the context of the AIDS fight is the continent's dependence on international donors. Despite structural adjustment policies, some African states have increasingly relied on foreign aid and loans to survive. Between 1990 and 1995, foreign aid represented the equivalent of over 50 per cent of African government revenues and 71 per cent of government public investments. 'Donors captured parts of the state to which they directed projects,' relieving pressure on the state to address those problems and dictating policies in those arenas (van de Walle 2001, 207). Dependence on donors is manifested in funding for AIDS programs. In the six countries of Lesotho, Swaziland, Botswana, Mozambique, South Africa, and Zimbabwe, 72 per cent of spending on HIV/AIDS comes from external sources: multilateral and bilateral donors, NGOs, and businesses. In three countries – Mozambique, Swaziland, and Lesotho – external actors provide over 80 per cent of total AIDS funds (Martin 2003).

Botswana illustrates some of the dynamics of international funding of AIDS programs. With a population of 1.6 million and a per capita gross domestic product of $3,300, the country is one of the wealthiest in sub-Saharan Africa. Yet, it also has the second highest HIV prevalence rate in the world, with 37.3 per cent of citizens estimated to be HIV positive. AIDS has already led to a decline in life expectancy from roughly 60 years in 1987 to approximately 39 years in 2001 (World Bank 2003). Of the $113 million spent in Botswana on HIV/AIDS in 2001, $96 million came from external donors. Botswana has collaborated with the African Comprehensive HIV/AIDS Partnership, a group composed of the Bill and Melinda Gates

Foundation, Bristol-Myers Squibb, and Merck Pharmaceutical Company. This public-private partnership will provide $100 million over five years for treatment, care, support, and prevention activities. Additionally, the Gates Foundation has promised $50 million over a five-year period and Harvard University has given $1 million to assist with a new HIV laboratory and to train new health-care workers (*Economist* 2002; Martin 2003, 10–11).

External actors have been attracted to Botswana because of its political stability and the recent attention that President Festus Mogae has given to HIV/AIDS. The president chairs the country's AIDS council and was the first African leader to promise free ARVs to all citizens with AIDS. Yet, the Botswana case raises questions about the role of the African state in such donor-funded AIDS programs. State capacity has limited the ability of the Botswana government to provide ARVs to the 110,000 people estimated to need them. Botswana has faced difficulty recruiting doctors, nurses, and social workers to participate in the ARV distribution program; government officials reported that Britain alone had recruited 120 of its nurses (*New York Times*, 13 November 2003). Although the donor-financed programs are supposed to be integrated with the government's priorities on HIV/AIDS, it is unclear if dependence on donors will give these international actors inordinate influence in AIDS policy making. The overall effectiveness of AIDS efforts in countries with high donor funding may be shaped less by government efficiency and more by donor efficiency. The *Washington Post* (14 October 2003) wrote about the Gates Foundation: 'The group is pumping money out the door so fast that spending it effectively could prove to be a huge challenge.' Finally, what does dependence on external donor resources mean for African state sovereignty? Barnett and Whiteside (2002, 355) assert that traditional notions of the state have diminished in importance with the AIDS epidemic. As donors design, fund, and implement AIDS programs, this may become increasingly true.

Several chapters in the volume highlight the complex role of donors in AIDS policy making and implementation. In Chapter 8, for example, Ostergard and Barcelo argue that outside funding has enabled the Ugandan government to both fight AIDS and to increase military spending for more immediate security threats. Chapter 9 illustrates how African state dependence on donor resources shaped the diplomatic process for a global agreement on HIV/AIDS. Before the United Nations General Assembly Special Session on HIV/AIDS in 2001, many African states were reluctant to publicly discuss the disease. Yet, once faced with the fact that political commitment was essential to gain donor resources to combat the disease, African political leaders began to develop AIDS policies and high-level decision-making bodies. However, the robustness of these donor-directed institutions and programs may actually enable the African state to become less, not more, committed to AIDS.

Overall, as Chapters 8, 9, and 10 maintain, the weakness of the African state in the international system has limited its ability to influence international actions on HIV/AIDS and trade treaties on pharmaceutical products. In the process of building consensus for the Declaration of Commitment on HIV/AIDS, African states relied on international civil servants at UNAIDS, the UN Secretary General, more powerful UN member-states, and international NGOs to influence aspects of the agreement. Likewise, African states had little sway in the 1995 negotiations that led to the World Trade Organization and the accompanying TRIPS Agreement. Though the implications of the TRIPS Agreement for the African AIDS crisis may have not been clear in 1995, by the end of the decade, it was apparent that Africa's acceptance of the TRIPS Agreement harmed its ability to acquire cheap ARVs. As Chapter 10 argues, with only recent opposition from the developing world, the European Union and the United States have pushed the view that the patent rights of pharmaceutical companies are superior to global public health.

Yet, the volume also demonstrates that the power of the African state in the international area is more complex than it initially may appear. For example, African states have found ways to resist the TRIPS Agreement through developing their own generic drug manufacturing plants or making plans to import medicines from generic producers. Likewise, while African states did not proactively build support for the Declaration of Commitment on HIV/AIDS, they were able to build coalitions with other developing countries to get their ideas included in the document. More generally, African states have benefited from the increasing realization among policy makers that in this era of globalization, disease, poverty, and instability in poor countries can impact the security, economies, and way of life of citizens in wealthy countries. As the human cost of AIDS becomes more profound, African states can benefit from a perspective on public health that looks beyond national-level policies to include the activities of states, international organizations, and nonstate actors.

The chapters in this book illustrate the above-mentioned aspects of the African state. Though several of the themes are woven throughout the chapters, the book starts at the sub-national level with an examination of the effect of patriarchy (Chapter 2), political culture (Chapter 3), and civil society (Chapter 4) on state actions to address AIDS. Next, the book investigates anti-AIDS efforts at the national level. It questions the impact of economic and political transitions on the AIDS epidemic and the ability of states to address AIDS, using the case studies of Ghana (Chapter 5), Swaziland (Chapter 6), and South Africa (Chapter 7). Chapter 8 situates a national-level analysis of AIDS policies in Uganda in the larger context of national and international security concerns, particularly in light of the weakness of the African state. Finally, the book turns to the international level. Chapter 9 illustrates the role of African states in the development of the Declaration of Commitment on HIV/AIDS and the Global Fund to Fight HIV/AIDS, Tuberculosis, and Malaria and Chapter 10 demonstrates the impact of the TRIPS Agreement on the ability of African states to fight AIDS. The conclusion raises questions about the future role of the African state in combating AIDS. It maintains that in a changing international environment African states must adopt AIDS governance to sustain current efforts to combat the disease.

Notes

1 For a notable exception, see de Waal (2003).

2 This information emerged during an interview while I was conducting research on the role of rural civil society associations in Senegal's democracy. The interviewee, a very elderly, well-respected village leader, proceeded to tell me about how a rural health leader and Muslim official had visited the community to discuss how AIDS is spread, how citizens can protect themselves, and how men can use condoms.

References

Barnett, Tony, and Alan Whiteside. 2002. *AIDS in the twenty-first century: Disease and globalisation*. Basingstoke: Palgrave Macmillan.

Bell, Clive, Hans Gersbach, and Shantayana Devarajan. 2003. *The long-run economic costs of AIDS: Theory and an application to South Africa*. Report for the World Bank. http://www1.worldbank.org/hiv_aids/docs/BeDeGe_BP_total2.pdf.

Boone, Catherine, and Jake Batsell. 2001. Politics and AIDS in Africa: Research agendas in political science and international relations. *Africa Today* 48 (2): 2–33.

Brown, Lynn. 2004. Economic growth rates in Africa: The potential impact of HIV/AIDS. In *HIV & AIDS in Africa: Beyond epidemiology*, ed. Ezekiel Kalipeni, Susan Craddock, Joseph Oppong, and Jayati Ghosh, 291–303. Malden, MA: Blackwell Publishing.

Chabal, Patrick, and Jean-Pascal Daloz. 1999. *Africa works: Disorder as political instrument*. Bloomington, IN: Indiana Univ. Press.

Cruise O'Brien, Donal. 1971. *The Mourides of Senegal*. Oxford: Clarendon Press.

Daly, John. 2001. AIDS in Swaziland: The battle from within. *African Studies Review* 44 (1): 21–35.

de Waal, Alex. 2003. How will HIV/AIDS transform African governance? *African Affairs* 102: 1–23.

Diamond, Larry, and Marc Plattner, eds. 2001. *The global divergence of democracies*. Baltimore: Johns Hopkins Univ. Press.

Economist. 2002. Fighting back – AIDS in southern Africa, 11 May.

Elbe, Stefan. 2002. HIV/AIDS and the changing landscape of war in Africa. *International Security* 27 (2): 159–77.

Englebert, Pierre. 2000. *State legitimacy and development in Africa*. Boulder, CO: Lynne Rienner Publishers.

Fatton, Robert. 1995. Africa in the age of democratization: The civic limitations of civil society. *African Studies Review* 38 (2): 67–110.

Fortin, Alfred. 1987. The politics of AIDS in Kenya. *Third World Quarterly* 9 (3): 906–19.

Freedom House. 2004. Freedom in the world. http://www.freedomhouse.org/research/index.htm.

Ghana AIDS Commission (GAC). 2003. *Annual report*. http://wwwghanaids.gov/gh/about/annualreport.asp?subnav=annualreport.

Green, Edward. 2003. Faith-based organizations: Contributions to HIV prevention. Paper for US Agency for International Development. Washington, DC: USAID.

Haas, Ernst. 1980. Why collaborate? Issue-linkage and international regimes. *World Politics* 32 (3): 357–405.

Joint United Nations Program on HIV/AIDS (UNAIDS). 2003a. *AIDS epidemic update: December 2003.* http://www.unaids.org.

——. 2003b. HIV/AIDS and food security. Fact sheet for UNAIDS. http://www.unaids.org.

——. 2004. *Report on the global AIDS epidemic.* http://www.unaids.org/bangkok2004.html.

Lewis, Stephen. 2003. Speech at the Conference of the Center for AIDS Program of Research in South Africa, Durban, South Africa, 3 August.

Low-Beer, Daniel, and Rand Stoneburner. 2004. Uganda and the challenge of HIV/AIDS. In *The political economy of AIDS in Africa*, ed. Nana Poku and Alan Whiteside, 165–90. Aldershot: Ashgate Publishers.

Martin, Gayle. 2003. *A comparative analysis of the financing of HIV/AIDS programmes*. Report for the Human Sciences Research Council. http://www.hsrcpublishers.co.za/index.html?finance.html~content.

Morgan, E. Philip. 2004. The multilateral HIV/AIDS regime and the African state. Paper presented at the International Studies Association conference, Montreal, 18 March.

Ndegwa, Stephen. 1996. *The two faces of civil society: NGOs and politics in Africa.* Westport, CT: Kumarian Press.

Patterson, Amy. 1998. A reappraisal of democracy in civil society: Evidence from rural Senegal. *Journal of Modern African Studies* 36 (3): 423–41.

——. 1999. The dynamic nature of citizenship and participation: Lessons from three rural Senegalese case studies. *Africa Today* 46 (1): 3–27.

Patterson, Amy, and Bernard Haven. n.d. AIDS policy in Ghana: A disconnect between government and NGOs. Unpublished paper.

Rugalema, Gabriel. 2000. Coping or struggling? A journey into the impact of HIV/AIDS in southern Africa. *Review of African Political Economy* 86: 537–45.

Schötenich, Martin. 1999. AIDS and age: South Africa's crime time bomb. *AIDS Analysis Africa* 10 (2): 1–4.

Segendo, James, and Janet Nambi. 1997. The psychological effect of orphanhood: A study of orphans in Rakai district. *Health Transition Review: The Cultural, Social, and Behavioral Determinants of Health* 7 (supplement): 105–24.

Stover, John, Neff Walker, Geoff P. Garnett, Joshua A. Salomon, Karen A. Stanecki, Peter D. Ghys, Nicholas C. Grassly, Roy M. Anderson, and Bernhard Schwartländer. 2002. Can we reverse the HIV/AIDS pandemic with an expanded response? *Lancet* 360 (July 6): 73–77.

van de Walle, Nicolas. 2001. *African economies and the politics of permanent crisis, 1979–1999.* New York: Cambridge Univ. Press.

Villalón, Leonardo. 1995. *Islamic society and state power in Senegal.* New York: Cambridge Univ. Press.

Whiteside, Alan. 2002. Poverty and HIV/AIDS in Africa. *Third World Quarterly* 23 (2): 313–32.

World Bank. 2003. *World development indicators.* Washington, DC: World Bank.

Chapter 2

AIDS and Patriarchy: Ideological Obstacles to Effective Policy Making

Patricia Siplon

The global catastrophe that is the HIV/AIDS pandemic has exposed the dangers of many of the institutions and practices that societies have developed over time. Patriarchy, with its attendant denial of resources, respect, and decision-making ability for women, represents one such form of managing power and relationships that has become deadly in the era of AIDS. The disproportionate burden of infection rates on women and the differential impacts felt by women in AIDS-affected households are not coincidental. Rather, these aspects of the epidemic can be understood by closely examining the interaction of HIV/AIDS with the institution of patriarchy. Such an examination leads to an exploration of poverty and the denial of human rights. These serve as manifestations of patriarchal systems and as factors that contribute to the spread of HIV and the severity of its consequences for women and girl children.

The link between human rights abuses and HIV/AIDS was first forcefully articulated by the late Jonathan Mann, founding director of the World Health Organization Global Program on AIDS. He understood the relationship between human rights and HIV/AIDS to be reciprocal, in that HIV/AIDS not only has created conditions of discrimination, stigma, and marginalization for those infected and affected, but also that those belonging to groups which are discriminated against, stigmatized, and marginalized are made vulnerable to infection (Mann 1999). The dynamic around poverty works in a similar fashion. The lack of financial resources, like the lack of respect for human rights, deprives individuals of agency and autonomy in their lives. The concept of 'choice' becomes meaningless in a context where one must engage in risky behavior as a survival strategy (Irwin, Millen, and Fallows 2003, 20–24). The fact that poverty is a risk factor for becoming HIV positive has been demonstrated within and among countries (Stine 2001, 12). Given this relationship, it is predictable that Africa, and particularly sub-Saharan Africa, bears most of the global AIDS burden. Sub-Saharan Africa has 38 countries that the World Bank classifies as 'low income', and of all global regions, sub-Saharan Africa has the highest share (50.5 per cent) of people living at less than one-third of average national consumption (World Bank 2001, 24, 334).[1] Poverty in sub-Saharan Africa has gotten worse, with the number of Africans living on less than $1 a day increasing from 217 million in 1987 to 291 million in 1998 (World Bank 2001, 23). Thus, the magnitude of the AIDS epidemic in sub-Saharan Africa sketched in the introduction of this book should come as no surprise.

Although patriarchy is literally 'rule of the fathers', in this chapter, I start with Tadesse's description of patriarchal family systems as being 'guided by the principles of domination of old over young and male over female' (1982, 211; See also Abunzwa 1997, 27). But patriarchy occurs at the state level as well. As Tsai (2002, 50) notes, the state and the household may be seen as 'interactive rather than as parallel institutions in generating, perpetuating and actualizing gender biases'. This understanding of the interaction of institutions leads me to adopt a working definition that describes patriarchy as 'a system of interrelated social structures which allow men to exploit women' (Gordon 1996, 17–18).

The current patriarchal systems of African states were strongly reinforced by colonial events. Schraeder (2004, 66–67) notes that in much of precolonial Africa, there were parallel gender-segregated systems of governance that allowed women to make decisions in at least some spheres. But colonial powers, by refusing to recognize any but male authorities, destroyed the authority and capacity of such women-controlled decision-making bodies, and also ensured that the occasional emergence of women as national leaders could not occur. Similarly, the imposition of a patriarchal form of Christianity by missionaries meant both that men would dominate church hierarchies and that patriarchal interpretations of the Bible would be used (Mbilinyi and Kaihula 2000, 81). The resulting legacy of patriarchal structures that directly or indirectly deny women economic resources and decision-making capacities is deadly in the age of AIDS.

The importance of the contribution of women to the functioning of families and economies of sub-Saharan Africa is difficult to overstate. Women are 50 per cent of the population, but are responsible for much of the labor needed to grow cash crops, and provide an even higher proportion of the work necessary for growing food to feed families. In Senegal, for instance, women account for 81 per cent of agricultural labor and 70 per cent of agricultural production, and in Uganda the numbers are even higher, with women accounting for 80 per cent of agricultural labor and 90 per cent of food production (Wanyeki 2003, 19, 21). Women are often excluded from salaried employment, and if not, they are paid less than men in comparable positions (Elson 1995, 76). Women make up a very large sector of the informal economy as traders, domestic servants, and agricultural laborers on the land of others (Gordon 1996, 86–87). Additionally, the responsibility (but not decision-making power) for the domestic sphere is seen as almost entirely within the realm of women, which means that they are required to do agricultural and other 'outside' work in addition to child care, medical and nursing care, cooking, cleaning, and gathering water and cooking fuel. This inequity in work expectations accounts for the difference in working hours between men and women. One study in Uganda found that women averaged 16 hours a day of work, compared to five hours for men (Tripp 2000, 142). The disproportionately high HIV infection rate among women will mean that much work will go undone when women become sick and die and that more work will fall on the shoulders of other women who are not yet ill. Women also are solely responsible for bearing children and breast-feeding, reproductive roles which have important implications for the disproportionate labor burden on women and women's vulnerability to HIV.

The following pages explore the relations between AIDS, the African state, and patriarchy. The next section begins with an examination of the ways patriarchy is expressed in the institutions and laws of African states. The outcomes of these state expressions of patriarchy are surveyed in the third section, which examines how patriarchy and HIV/AIDS have combined to the detriment of the health and well-being of women and girls in sub-Saharan Africa. From there, the chapter examines a possible new approach for addressing these patterns and their effects, namely the Greater Involvement of People Living with HIV/AIDS (GIPA) initiative and self-empowerment strategies that have been embraced by many AIDS activists and United Nations (UN) agencies. Finally, the chapter returns to the opening theme of patriarchy and the African state by concluding with some ideas about the role of the state, and of actors influencing the state, in overcoming the HIV/AIDS crisis.

Patriarchy and the African State

The expression of patriarchy in African states is pervasive. At the official government level, patriarchy exists in government institutions, where women are underrepresented and constrained by sexism and stereotyping, and where women's groups are purposely subverted. At perhaps the most easily measurable level, women's representation in government, the gender gap does not seem particularly notable, at least in a comparative sense. There are no women heads of state, but the same is true of North America. In 2004, the percentage of women serving in African parliaments (14.6 per cent) was not much lower than the percentage of women in other region's legislatures (16.1 per cent in Europe excluding the Nordic countries and 18.6 per cent in the Americas). The exception is Nordic countries, where women represent 39.7 per cent of parliamentarians (Inter-Parliamentary Union 2004). These numbers, however, mask certain practices that limit women's power. Women are rarely appointed to the most powerful ministries, such as finance, defense, foreign affairs, or industry. Instead, women are relegated to secondary ministries such as culture, social welfare, and community development. Such relegation, Beck finds in her study of Senegal, has an additional consequence: in less powerful ministries, women have fewer political resources at their disposal to dispense to constituents to maintain their support. Consequently, they have proportionally higher turnover rates in office than their male counterparts, often disappearing 'into political oblivion after a brief stint in government' (2003, 164). A number of African countries have reserved legislative seats for women, a policy that facilitates gender balance but also allows leaders to hand pick women who can be reliably expected to support the regime and its practices. Additionally, these women are often excluded from informal networks that have powerful political influence (Tripp 2000, 19; Beck 2003). Finally, gender stereotypes and expectations continue to constrain women in government positions. For example, in March 2002 former Ugandan Vice President Specioza Kazibwe came forward publicly as a victim of domestic violence and sought a divorce from her husband. Rather than being hailed for her leadership in helping to publicize and destigmatize the problem of domestic violence, she was heavily criticized in the press and by many of her colleagues (Nankinga 2002; Human Rights Watch 2003b).

At the level of civil society, Tripp (2000, 8–10) suggests that African states employ a number of tactics to render women's organizations ineffectual. These include the outright banning of organizations viewed as threatening to the state, the creation of new mass organizations (often as an auxiliary wing of the ruling party), and the co-optation of existing groups. Once created or co-opted, these organizations mirror their parent parties in their leadership selection (usually through patronage, as exemplified by the 'first lady syndrome') and undemocratic structures (Tripp 2000, 9). An example of such co-optation is the 31st December Women's Movement of Ghana, which was so closely tied to the government that it could not exert pressure on it. In turn, this association absorbed grassroots-level women's groups, rendering them equally voiceless (Tripp 2000, 16). Additionally, the state may use its power to control or destroy less-dependent organizations through registration requirements and regulations for fund usage. This appears to have been the strategy used by the government against the Tanzanian women's group Baraza wa Wanawake wa Tanzania (the National Women's Council), whose registration it withdrew in 1997 (Kelsall 2001, 145).When all else fails, governments may use harassment, as in the famous case of the Greenbelt Movement of Kenya. The regime of Daniel arap Moi used imprisonment, threats, and physical attacks on demonstrators to quash the women-led movement when it moved from its originally apolitical tree-planting goals to actively opposing policy decisions of the regime (Ndegwa 1996).

Laws formally passed by government institutions represent another way that the state perpetuates patriarchy. Hamblin and Reid (1991) identify four ways in which law may impact women affected by HIV/AIDS. First, they note the relationship between law and economic dependency. Gender-biased laws governing land ownership, marital property laws, credit regulations, and inheritance keep women economically dependent on men, and ultimately leave women with only two primary means of economic support – marriage or some form of transactional sex work (1991, 14). In Kenya, for instance, women are only 5 per cent of registered landholders nationally, although they account for over 80 per cent of the agricultural labor force (Human Rights Watch 2003a, 9). Although the Kenyan constitution outlaws discrimination based on gender in Article 70, it makes a wide range of exemptions in Article 82 in the areas of adoption, marriage, divorce, devolution of property, and 'gazetted' land areas (a distinction that includes most rural areas). This has the practical consequence of rendering the gender protection of Article 70 inapplicable to virtually any situation regarding women's access to and ownership of land.

Hamblin and Reid (1991) point to a second role of law in regulating the status of women, both within marriage and in other sexual relationships. Recognizing or not recognizing the rights of women to make reproductive decisions, and more fundamentally, to make decisions about whether and when sexual intercourse occurs, may powerfully affect the ability of women to control their risk for contracting HIV. For example, the existence and enforcement of rape and domestic violence laws, particularly ones that recognize rape within marriage, could potentially bring the force of the state onto the side of women seeking to empower themselves in their relationships. In most African countries, such laws either do not exist or are not enforced. With the sole exception of South Africa, marital rape is not recognized as a crime by African states, and only Senegal, South Africa, and Zimbabwe have laws and penalties against domestic violence (Human Rights Watch 2003c, 80).

In a few other countries, including Zambia and Malawi, women's groups have successfully lobbied for laws and/or constitutional reforms that address marital rights, domestic violence, and inheritance rights (Tripp n.d., 19–21). Unfortunately, the state has failed to provide resources needed to enforce the changes. Zambia is an instructive case. On paper, its penal code prohibits many of the rights violations previously discussed, and it even created a victim support unit of the police force in 1997. But because of clashes with customary law, unwillingness to acknowledge widespread disregard for the law, and ineffectual performance of the victim support unit, statutory changes have not translated into meaningful changes in the circumstances of women and girls.

The third potential role of law is to serve as policy responses to activities affecting the transmission of HIV/AIDS. Such policy responses to certain activities, Hamblin and Reid (1991) note, may have a desired effect on behavior, particularly male behavior. For example, they find that in some southern African states men have responded to laws that require them to provide financial support for children they father by having fewer children.

Finally, law may be used to distribute positive incentives, such as tax concessions or government goods and services. For example, funding may be used to achieve certain policy objectives, such as broader access of women to AIDS-related goods and services. This role of law will become increasingly important in future years as prevention measures, such as mother-to-child transmission programs, and treatment, including antiretroviral drugs, become more prevalent in sub-Saharan Africa. Ideally, such programs will alleviate not only the immense human suffering of people living with HIV/AIDS, but also will address many of the societal problems wrought by the pandemic, such as the orphan crisis and the shortage of productive agricultural labor. Similarly, law could require governments either to pay for girls to attend secondary school or to provide funding to schools which show progress in the number of female students they enroll and retain.

Although formal statutory law has often failed to protect women and their rights, an even larger obstacle for most women is customary law, which in many sub-Saharan African countries is formally or informally permitted to trump statutory law in local and domestic matters. Since 2002, Human Rights Watch has issued three in-depth reports on aspects of HIV and human rights violations relating to women and girl children in Kenya, Uganda, and Zambia (Human Rights Watch 2002, 2003a, 2003b). Human Rights Watch (2003c) also released a more general report on the same topic covering all of Africa. All cite customary law as a major source of patriarchal practices that strip women and girl children of property, autonomy, and safety. Customary law is typically unwritten, and therefore is fluid and open to interpretation. As one Kenyan chief put it, 'Customary law is what I describe' (Human Rights Watch 2003a, 11). It is usually applied by traditional leaders such as elders, and local authorities such as government-appointed chiefs, although judges and magistrates may also apply customary law in some court settings (Human Rights Watch 2003a, 11).

In many areas, the practices permitted by customary law may include: polygamy (men having more than one wife); payment of bride price by a groom to a bride's family; wife inheritance (by a brother of the deceased husband); ritual sexual cleansing (sexual intercourse with a man paid to have sex with a widow); 'ownership' of children no longer breast-feeding by the father and father's family; discriminatory inheritance practices including no inheritance for married daughters and inheritance of a dead husband's property by his parents and brothers; and loss of all property by the wife (and usually return of the bride price by the bride's family) in the case of divorce or separation. As with the practices previously discussed, these customs keep women economically dependent on men, especially their husbands, and make women unable to exercise autonomy in their decisions regarding their own actions. Additionally, the interaction between statutory and customary law means that in those cases where a state has made laws protecting and empowering women that are actually enforced, there is usually still a way to ignore the law through the application of customary law. One study examining seven African countries points out that in Nigeria, for example, while the 1978 Land Use Act reinforces some contextual inequality of land ownership, customary law is the primary determinant of women's access to and control of land. On a broader scale, the study finds that in all seven countries in the area of land regulation 'without exception, customary law is accommodated by statutory law, also to women's detriment' (Wanyeki 2003, 31). Taken together, the combined manifestations of patriarchy in both the institutions and the laws of sub-Saharan African states create a wall of mutually reinforcing exclusionary mechanisms for women. The laws keep women from access to economic and political power, which in turn makes it very difficult for them to access the tools, institutions, and resources they need to change the laws.

The Intersection of HIV/AIDS and Patriarchy

On World AIDS Day 2002, the Executive Director of the Joint United Nations Program on HIV/AIDS (UNAIDS), Peter Piot, announced that 'this year, for the first time in the epidemic's history, the number of women living with HIV has risen to 50 per cent of the global total' (Piot 2002, 1). This shift in demographic is largely because of the gender imbalance in HIV infection occurring in sub-Saharan Africa; UNAIDS estimated in 2004 that 'there are on average 13 infected women for every 10 infected men' (UNAIDS 2004, 6). The gender imbalance is because of both biological and socioeconomic factors. The dominant mode of transmission in sub-Saharan Africa is heterosexual intercourse, and within this mode of transmission women are biologically more vulnerable to infection than men are (Baylies 2000, 5). This is particularly true for young women and girls, whose vulnerability is heightened because their vaginal tissues and cervices are not yet fully developed (UNAIDS 2002, 18; Human Rights Watch 2003c, 9).

The social and economic sources of female vulnerability to HIV relate to the above-discussed effects of patriarchy on law and politics. Political, economic, and social systems that rob women of their power to make decisions regarding sexuality, reproduction, and resource allocation and that place control of these decisions with husbands and elder male family members increase women's vulnerability to HIV. The array of life 'choices' under such constraints – marriage, formal or informal employment, commercial sex work, or taking sponsors or 'sugar daddies' – often lead to risky behavior dictated by men. The pages below explore the strategies and choices that women use in an attempt to secure economic security for themselves and their children. This security usually comes at the expense of autonomy and respect for their rights. It is also often transitory, in that this security is almost always lost when women become HIV infected or when the households in which they live are affected by any HIV-positive member.

Given the cultural importance of women's roles as wives and mothers, as well as the economic importance of having an adult male provider, marriage is highly valued. Yet marriage is no guarantee against HIV infection. Among many African ethnic groups, the practice of paying a bride price is still common. Unlike a dowry, which usually represents a transfer of wealth from the bride's family to the groom's, bride price is given to the parents of the bride, and among many groups, represents an acknowledgement that the bride now 'belongs' to the groom and his family. The wife is responsible for all household work (whether or not she is employed or does other work outside of the home), and for bearing and raising children. Since having children is valued within marriage, there is a very strong incentive for women to submit to unprotected sex, even if they know their husbands are not monogamous. But even without the incentive of children, most women have little choice about marital sex. It is the husband who will dictate when, where, and under what circumstances intercourse will take place. As Joyce Kasolo, Director of the Women and Children's Crisis Center in Kampala, Uganda, explained, 'When you say, "I do" you have consented to sex anytime, anyplace, anyhow' (Human Rights Watch 2003b, 22). A wife who asks her husband to use a condom may be subject to physical violence and charges of unfaithfulness. Paradoxically, all these factors mean that marriage has become a risk factor for many women. Baylies (2000, 11) points out that this may be particularly true for young women because of the social need to have children, the tendency of men to have most of their outside sexual partners in the early years of the marriage, and the risk of male 'straying' during the wife's pregnancy or early postpartum period. Joyce Namulondo from the Uganda AIDS Commission offered a similar observation, 'A woman properly married in the home is at greater risk as far as HIV/AIDS is concerned, the reason being power relations. … The single woman does not have a contract' (Human Rights Watch 2003b, 23).

The power imbalance within marriage is so great that even AIDS advocacy organizations admit that they do not openly challenge it. A description of Walio katika Mapambano ya AIDS, Tanzania (Those in the struggle against AIDS in Tanzania), a prominent AIDS service organization in Tanzania, notes that the group specifically avoids confronting men's behavior, even if that behavior puts women at risk. This avoidance also means that men who abandon infected wives, partners, and children are not pursued, and women are not informed when they are known to be at risk (Bujra and Mokake 2000, 169).

Another strategy women may employ is to attempt to become economically self-sufficient either within or outside of marriage. But again, patriarchal practices that place decision making and preferential treatment with men generally, and with elder men within families particularly, make this a very difficult option. High levels of unemployment translate to very high levels of competition for skilled jobs. Women are further disadvantaged by generally lower education levels (a problem that is currently accelerating because of the HIV/AIDS crisis), the competing demands of their domestic responsibilities, lack of access to patronage networks, and pervasive sexism. Women must find work in low-skilled and low-paying occupations. The few jobs available to young women who migrate to the cities, such as working as housemaids or bar attendants, often require sexual work as a condition of keeping the job or as a means of supplementing inadequate income. A study of girls aged nine to 16 who were employed as housemaids in Nyanza province, Kenya found that 18 of the 25 interviewed were HIV positive. Of the 18, 15 reported that their first sexual experiences were forced, and that they occurred with their employer or someone in his family or circle of friends. Most of the 18 had worked in several places and reported being sexually abused in all or most of them (TEMAK 2000). The goal of achieving economic autonomy comes at the expense of sacrificing autonomy in decision making about risk behavior, a dilemma not lost on advocates for gender equity:

> Bar workers prefer their economic independence compared to the alternatives of an abusive marriage, dependence on elders, or being overworked in a village; but they are hardly 'independent' when they are unable to negotiate condom use with regular partners, though some claim to demand this with casual partners (Keller et al. 1999, 28).

For some women, especially young women, a third strategy may involve finding one or more sponsors or 'sugar daddies'. In his South African study of this practice, Hunter (2002, 100) differentiates what he terms 'transactional sex' from prostitution in two ways: first, partners are constructed as 'girlfriend' and 'boyfriend' (as opposed to 'prostitute' and 'client'); and second, the gifts received for sex are part of a broader set of obligations that may not be predetermined. He sees three major contributing factors that lead to these arrangements. First, there is the privileged economic position of men; second, the high societal value for men having multiple sexual partners; and finally, the agency of women themselves, in that they consciously use these arrangements to access power and resources (Hunter 2002, 100). Hunter looks at the dynamics of these relationships in an informal setting and a township and finds that in the first case, women's extreme poverty and vulnerability caused them to use these relationships to meet basic subsistence needs. But in the township, cultural premiums on fashion and consumption goods (such as cell phones) fueled the propensity of young women to take on sugar daddies. In both cases, it may take more than one man to provide for the women's material needs: 'a comment often made in Isithebe [the informal settlement], reflecting the concern with subsistence, is that women *qoma* (choose a man) "one for rent, one for food, one for clothes"' (Hunter 2002, 111). A *New York Times* article on 18 August 2003 illustrates how sugar daddies have undermined Uganda's HIV prevention efforts among teenage girls. Uganda has started many well-attended, school-based clubs that promote abstinence. But those same club members are propositioned 'just about every day by older men who offer them a chance of a better life in exchange for sex'. Ironically, many girls, including those who have been orphaned or impoverished by AIDS, must accept such propositions to provide the school fees to attend the same schools with the abstinence clubs.

The result of this sexual partnering of younger women with older men is a key to understanding one of the starkest numerical discrepancies in African AIDS statistics: approximately twice as many young women as men between 15 and 24 years old are infected with HIV in sub-Saharan Africa (UNAIDS

2002, 18). For example, in 1999 in Kisumu, Kenya and Ndola, Zambia, 15 per cent and 23 per cent of teenage girls aged 15 to 19 were HIV positive, compared to only 4 per cent of males in the same age group. The findings also indicated that the young women contracted the virus from men over age 25, of whom 26 per cent in Kisumu and 40 per cent in Ndola were HIV positive (Kaiser Daily Reports 1999). As the devastating dynamics of HIV/AIDS continue to deprive children and young adults of parental support, and as patriarchal systems continue to deny women adequate ways to provide for themselves, it becomes increasingly likely that girls and teenagers will enter into these intergenerational relationships at younger ages.

Some women are forced into relying on transactional sex on a more frequent basis with more partners and become commercial sex workers. As Irwin, Millen, and Fallows note, 'for the majority of women, commercial sex work is not a "lifestyle choice" but a last-ditch survival strategy in a situation where other possible escape routes have been shut down' (2003, 23). While it may be an act of desperation, an increasingly large number of nongovernmental organizations (NGOs) are reporting that, particularly among girls and young women, the structural constraints of their situations make both the decision and the subsequent health risks inevitable. An analysis conducted in Kenya, Uganda, Tanzania, and Ethiopia by Save the Children-Sweden concludes that homeless orphan girls will almost always end up working as prostitutes (Savenstedt, Savenstedt, and Haggstrom 2000). A Human Rights Watch report on HIV among girls in Zambia quotes Clemire Karamira of Movement of Community Action for the Prevention and Protection of Young People Against Poverty, Destitution, Diseases and Exploitation: 'Girls die in a very short time – that's the bottom line. STDs, HIV/AIDS, violence, mental abuse, physical abuse. They don't have time to make money.' Karamira also notes that the majority of the prostitutes she has worked with are very young – 12 to 18 years old (Human Rights Watch 2002, 40–41). The danger of sex work is also reflected in the very high HIV prevalence rate among Zambian sex workers, which was estimated to be 68 per cent in 1998 (Human Rights Watch 2002, 38).

The tragic irony of these strategies is that, in the context of patriarchal societies, they facilitate the spread of HIV, either indirectly within the family unit or directly to women and girls. And when that happens, women's original goal of economic security, as well as the rights and autonomy they sacrificed for economic security, diminish greatly. Though it is overwhelmingly men who bring HIV into marriage, it is women who are commonly blamed. The plight of many widows who survive their husbands is an extreme example of the ways in which patriarchy can undermine human rights. The title of one Human Rights Watch report, 'Just die quietly', summarizes the collective impact of a host of practices. Some involve violations of economic rights, such as property grabbing. Interviews with 13 HIV-positive widows in Tanzania indicated that all but one had been victims of property grabbing by their husbands' families. (In the exceptional case, the husband's family lived in South Africa.) In many cases, however, the women were expected to continue to support not only themselves and their own children but also other children left by their deceased husband and other family members (Siplon and Novotny 2002). Often a widow is forced off the property she has lived on and is left with no belongings and nowhere to go. Other human rights violations occur when widows are forced to be 'cleansed' by a man paid to have sexual intercourse with them, or are required to become an additional wife of the deceased husband's brother. Although some argue that wife inheritance was designed to ensure that the widow and her children were provided for, the practice can often become predatory by allowing the inheritor to profit from the free labor of another woman and to inherit the property of his brother (Human Rights Watch 2003a, 12). Given that widows have often been infected by their husbands before they died, the practice is also a vector for introducing HIV into another family group. As for sexual cleansing, it is not only often a violent act of rape, but it also carries an inherently high risk of HIV transmission and/or reinfection, since the men who are paid to perform the cleansing often have done so multiple times. Human Rights Watch interviewed a man who had cleansed at least 75 widows in the previous two years, but had never been tested for HIV and had never used condoms (Human Rights Watch 2003a, 12).

Even when they are not infected, women and girls suffer disproportionately from the effects of HIV/AIDS because of the patriarchal systems in which they live. This is mainly because of two prominent effects of patriarchy. First, because patriarchal systems limit women's access to resources, including wealth, land, education, and opportunity, the resource-depleting effects of AIDS are disproportionately borne by women. This is true not only when male members of a household die and women lose their property as discussed above, but also when males are still alive but ill. When a household head becomes ill, income declines, while costs for medicine, nutritious food, linens, and other home-care necessities increase. Such constraints on resources will almost inevitably result in deprivation that will fall disproportionately on women and girl children, who will have less access to school fees, health care, and food when rationing decisions are made. In the Tanzanian context, Omari and Mbilinyi (2000) note that the resource-limiting impacts of both economic crisis and structural adjustment programs are disproportionately borne by women and girls. An example of the same impact from HIV/AIDS is suggested by Human Rights Watch, which notes that in Kenya's Eastern province, the region least affected by HIV/AIDS, 42 per cent of grade-five primary-school students were girls, but in the heavily AIDS-affected province of Nyanza, only 6 per cent of children in the same grade were girls (Human Rights Watch 2003c, 17).

Second, because patriarchy creates divisions of labor that make women responsible for the health and well-being of the family, women and girls overwhelmingly bear the burden of caregiving for any sick family member. The additional child care needed for children with sick parents and for orphans will also fall to women, as, in many cases, will additional farming work necessary for feeding their families. A study of 51 AIDS patients in Mwanza, Tanzania found that only six were being cared for by a male relative and in all these cases, it was because there was no surviving female available (Nnoko et al. 2000, 552). The study also detailed both the drudgery and the time required for such work. It notes, for instance, that many home-care providers were forced to deal with the soiling effects of 15 to 20 bouts of diarrhea daily, sometimes in situations where bed linen was extremely scarce and water sources a long distance away. Ultimately, at the terminal stage of AIDS, caregivers were found to reach a point where they had no time to give to any other daily activities (Nnoko et al. 2000). The cumulative tragic impact of these burdens on women, and especially young women and girls, was described by the head of the UN Development Fund for Women (UNIFEM), Noreen Heyzer, in a speech addressing the 2001 UN General Assembly Special Session on HIV/AIDS. She discussed the 'story of women sacrificing their lives to fill the gap left by government and the global community because of their genderblindness.' The cost of such blindness, she contended, is that 'Fields go untended. Sick and well go hungry. Development is postponed. Girls are pulled out of school. Women remain at home, outside the public sphere, excluded from decision-making, deprived of opportunities to become self-reliant, economically-independent, full citizens with power and authority over their own lives, and participatory roles in the world they inhabit' (Heyzer 2001, 2).

GIPA: A Potential Way Forward

Analyses of the global HIV/AIDS pandemic have increasingly recognized the link between patriarchy and HIV/AIDS in sub-Saharan Africa. For example, both the Statement of Concern on Women and HIV/AIDS issued at the International Conference on HIV/AIDS in Durban, South Africa and the UN General Assembly's Declaration of Commitment on HIV/AIDS that member-states signed at the special session on HIV/AIDS in June 2001 highlight the significance of gender inequality and the need for women's empowerment for dealing with HIV/AIDS. Although these statements are a positive development, much less progress has been made in thinking through specific empowerment strategies to help women gain the necessary autonomy and resources to protect themselves and their families.

One strategy that has been used by sub-Saharan African women predating the recognition of HIV/AIDS has been organizing local women's groups. Despite considerable obstacles including poverty, the heavy demands of work on their time, and, in many cases, the disapproval of husbands and other male relatives, women in sub-Saharan Africa have displayed formidable talents since colonial times in organizing to collectively pursue their goals. This organizational capacity has been the subject of some controversy, however, based on a dichotomy that has emerged among scholars about the goals of women's organizations. Molyneaux (1985) distinguished between practical gender interests and strategic gender interests. According to this typology, women pursue practical gender interests when they organize to better provide for their basic needs or to improve conditions for themselves, as for example in achieving new sources of income generation or local services. But organizing for such goals does not include organizing to transform the power structures or decision-making processes that subjugate them. This transformative work is the goal of strategic gender interests, which are achieved when women come together specifically to challenge the subordination, discrimination, and labor divisions that are institutionalized in societies. The distinction has been criticized for, among other things, being overly rigid and missing the point that many practically-based struggles inherently come to involve larger gender-based power struggles and consciousness raising (Tripp 2000, 164–66). But it has also been specifically applied to women's AIDS-related organizing as a useful tool for evaluating short-term interventions to ensure that they 'are consistent with and permit progress toward long term objectives' (Baylies 2000, 18). The organizational skills and inclinations of African women, therefore, represent a powerful tool that has not yet been fully maximized in dealing with the HIV/AIDS crisis.

The political response to the AIDS pandemic has a unique history, and this history may offer a model to help direct these organizational efforts of at-risk women and their advocates. When recognition of the immune deficiency that would come to be known as AIDS happened in the United States, early surveillance suggested that four identifiable groups would be most at risk. This so-called 'AIDS 4-H' club consisted of homosexual men (among whom the first cases were identified), hemophiliacs, Haitians, and heroin users. Of these groups, it was homosexual men, together with the larger gay and lesbian political community, that came to be strongly identified with AIDS in the United States (Siplon 2002). While this identification initially had costs in the form of stigmatization and discrimination, it also ultimately was crucial in creating the political space for the gay and lesbian community to redefine issues of AIDS prevention and treatment and to help dictate the United States' HIV/AIDS policies.

A key event in this self-empowerment process occurred in 1983 at the second annual AIDS Forum held in Denver, Colorado. About a dozen people with AIDS (PWAs) had individually decided to attend the conference to ensure that their ideas and interests were directly represented.[2] When they assembled in a hospitality suite and compared notes, they discovered that all felt they had been treated in a patronizing way. This in turn prompted them to produce a manifesto, which they unveiled with a dramatic banner drop which disrupted the closing session. After unfurling the banner which read 'Fighting for Our Lives', the PWAs took turns reading aloud the 17 principles they had written (Nussbaum 1990, 108–110). These principles, which came to be known as the Denver Principles, strongly resemble ideas from the US women's health movement of previous decades.[3] They promoted self-empowerment, beginning with the idea that people who had AIDS should be known as neither 'victims' (because the term implies defeat) nor 'patients' (because the word implies passivity, helplessness, and dependence), but rather as 'people with AIDS'. Additionally, the principles enumerate five rights of PWAs and offer recommendations for all people and for PWAs. Particularly key in the activist struggle since the 1980s have been three self-empowerment recommendations: PWAs should choose their own agendas, representatives, and strategies; they should be involved at all levels of decision making and serve on the boards of directors of service organizations; and they should be included in all AIDS forums with credibility equal to that of other participants (Campbell and Callen 1983).

A few years later, PWAs operationalized these principles at an organizational level by banding together with members of the larger, primarily gay and lesbian, activist community to form a new and highly successful direct-action group, the AIDS Coalition to Unleash Power (ACT UP). Beginning with a successful action in New York City in 1987 which targeted the drug company then known as Burroughs Wellcome, ACT UP's use of dramatic demonstrations and direct actions, together with fact-filled, widely distributed information, forged a new model for activism that inspired other organizations throughout the 1990s. Other ACT UP chapters formed in the United States and internationally in cities such as London, Paris, and Sydney. A key feature of ACT UP's work was its embrace of the ideas within the Denver Principles, including the active participation and leadership of people living with HIV/AIDS (Siplon 2002).

Two of the other most successful AIDS activist movements in the world, those of Brazil and South Africa, also adopted this strategy of relying heavily on the talent, leadership, and expertise of individuals who are from highly vulnerable and/or HIV-positive communities. In the case of Brazil, which is often pointed out as an outstanding success story for the state's accomplishments in both the prevention and treatment arenas, the gay community, which suffered the first heavy losses from AIDS, led the fight to make AIDS a political priority (Rosenberg 2001). South Africa has seen the development of a world famous treatment activist movement, the Treatment Action Campaign, which started in 1998. Its most famous leader, Zackie Achmat, is HIV positive, as are many other leaders and participants in the organization, which now numbers in the thousands. Working to lobby a government that until late 2003 was openly opposed to the provision of antiretroviral treatment, it has had major successes in, for example, pushing for the administration of the drug nevirapine to prevent mother-to-child transmission. As highlighted in other chapters in this volume, the organization has also taken on the global pharmaceutical industry in court. In August 2002, it was a key actor in launching a Pan-African HIV/AIDS Treatment Access Movement (Achmat 2003, xi–xvi).

On 1 December 1994, 42 national governments formally accepted the Denver Principles by signing the Declaration of the Paris AIDS Summit.

These governments committed to support 'greater involvement of people living with or affected by HIV/AIDS' in participating at all levels in 'the creation of supportive political, legal and social environments' (UNAIDS 1999, 1). UNAIDS also has strongly endorsed GIPA, and has sponsored consultations and provided materials to demonstrate best practices and ideas of how GIPA can be implemented. As UNAIDS explains, GIPA is not the tokenism that occurs when programs and organizations allow people living with HIV/AIDS (PLHAs) to participate marginally as speakers or symbols. Even involving PLHAs at the policy-implementation stage to work as peer educators, caregivers, or outreach workers may not fully utilize GIPA, if the implementers do not have a say in program design and decision making. Rather, GIPA is realized when PLHAs are called on as experts and decision makers in addition to their roles as implementers and speakers (UNAIDS 1999, 3).

Although GIPA remains a rhetorical commitment in much of the world, it is an approach that holds much promise for the empowerment of women in sub-Saharan Africa. Methods of conceptualizing people living with and affected by HIV/AIDS have changed over time, from simply labeling 'people with AIDS' to realizing the active role that 'people living with HIV/AIDS' play in addressing the disease. Most recent is the decision in some contexts to broaden the concept of GIPA to refer to 'the Greater Involvement of People Living with *or Affected by* HIV/AIDS' (UNAIDS 2000, 3). This somewhat controversial decision expands the scope of women's potential involvement since, as this chapter points out, women are disproportionately affected by HIV/AIDS even when they are not infected. GIPA, which has been credited as a successful AIDS intervention model in the United States, Brazil, and South Africa, may challenge patriarchy by putting decision-making power in the hands of infected and affected women. The model also may combat HIV/AIDS, by allowing those with valuable experience and inputs to design appropriate responses to the problems they face. Anecdotal evidence suggests that affected women voice the need to address both immediate conditions (i.e., practical gender needs) and power relations (i.e., strategic gender needs). Similarly, the work of the earlier PWA movement from which GIPA is drawn also focused on immediate concerns (e.g., access to experimental treatments) and power relations with state and corporate actors. When asked about their own goals and needs, for example, Tanzanian widows identified specific needs such as school fees for their children, medical treatment, and money for income-generating projects. But they also identified the need for larger societal changes, as in their statement that AIDS needs to be seen as a societal problem rather than an individual misfortune (Siplon and Novotny 2002). Similarly, a recent UNIFEM consultation with women's groups from South Africa, Lesotho, Swaziland, Namibia, and Zimbabwe called for not only provision of women's basic needs, but also for a fundamental redefinition of women's roles within their marriages and families. Specifically, women called for an end to sexual harassment and abuse if they do not wish to engage in sex because they are sick, and they asked that men assume a share of traditional women's work such as cooking, cleaning, and caregiving (UNIFEM 2003).

Conclusion

As the differential impact of HIV/AIDS on women in sub-Saharan Africa continues to increase, it will become increasingly difficult for the global community to ignore the need to address both the disparity that is occurring and the devastating impact of this disparity. The Denver Principles, from which GIPA derives much inspiration, was an invention of a group of people with a specific orientation and talents. They had the advantages of money, skills, and access to mass communication venues that do not readily translate to the situation of sub-Saharan African women. Despite these differences and limitations, the Denver Principles may still hold out potential that has until now remained unrealized by GIPA. For example, a crucial component of the Western self-empowerment model is an attempt to apply it at all levels – individual, family, societal, and international. There are good reasons to believe such a multilevel application will be more challenging in an African context. For one thing, the whole concept of self-empowerment may be viewed as inherently individualistic. This is a characteristic much more strongly associated with Western cultures, particularly that of the United States, whereas African cultures are usually seen as more communitarian. It is possible, however, to overstate this difference. Many, if not most, of the behaviors such self-empowerment would seek to alter, such as male dictatorship of the circumstances of sex between men and women, are neither motivated by the well-being of the community nor do they advance communitarian goals. But self-empowerment for women can foster communitarian well-being. At the family level, for instance, there is ample documentation that women, when they are able to control resources, are much more inclined to spend them on the nutritional, health, and educational needs of the household, whereas men tend to emphasize spending on personal consumption including entertainment and recreation (Elson 1995, 73; Kapunda 2000, 229). Economic self-empowerment for women in such a scenario would not only afford them more autonomy, but would simultaneously improve the well-being of the rest of the family.

At the societal level, a second objection might be made around the specific source of agency for women's empowerment. The PWA movement in the United States was led and organized primarily (though not exclusively) by skilled, middle-class gay white men, who were able to demand a seat at decision-making tables. African women lack most of these advantages. To overcome these obstacles, well-established indigenous NGOs, international NGOs, and donor nations most likely will need to initiate change at two levels. First, they must examine their own methods of operation and programs. They must seek out women living with, vulnerable to, and affected by HIV/AIDS not only as clients, but more importantly, as staff, consultants, and partners. They must examine and alter their own policies regarding discrimination, confidentiality, provision of medical treatment for staff, and other benefits. Second, they must look at their programming and seek to provide options for women to exercise financial and relational autonomy. Such options should cover immediate needs, such as emergency shelter and food, as well as long-term autonomy needs, such as income-generating programs and provision of medical care for women seeking economic self-sufficiency.

Through a variety of mechanisms, African states can play a major role in determining whether women and girl children will continue to bear the ever-escalating burden brought on by HIV/AIDS. Here again, NGOs may play a necessary catalyzing role in lobbying African states to get involved in the provision of the goods and services listed above, as well as promoting representation of women infected and affected by HIV in positions of authority. Such positions include seats on national AIDS commissions and in the leadership of planning bodies, such as the Country Coordinating Mechanisms that submit proposals to the Global Fund for AIDS, Tuberculosis and Malaria. Currently, this representation is occurring on only a minimal level, but the global AIDS activist movement may play a central role in pushing for fuller inclusion of women, if countries wish to see their proposals funded or renewed. Autonomous women's organizations must be encouraged and listened to, and their calls for reform in both statutory and customary laws must be heeded.

In the United States, the AIDS movement had transformative impacts that went beyond the goals of the movement itself. PWAs were empowered at the policy level, as when they were able to successfully challenge the standard operating procedures of government bureaucracies, pharmaceutical companies, the health care industry, and the media. At the personal level, they redefined power relationships within their own lives, like those with their doctors and their families. As with all societal changes, particularly ones that challenge existing power relationships, the changes will be resisted and continuously renegotiated. But the cost of inaction is unacceptably high. It will be measured in the millions of women's and girls' lives lost or saved – and in the death or survival of the families and societies that depend on them.

Notes

1 The World Bank defines a low-income country as having a per capita gross national product of $755 or less.

2 This acronym has been modified with time and geography. Currently, the accepted terminology is people *living with* HIV/AIDS, which is variously abbreviated as PLHA, PLWA, and PLWHA. In this chapter, I use the acronym PLHA except when discussing the US-based self-described PWA movement in historical context.

3 The women's health movement of the 1970s was predicated on the idea that women should not be passive recipients of health care from (usually male) doctors, but rather should view themselves as qualified participants in decision making about their own lives and bodies. Prominent members of the PWA movement, especially Michael Callen, credit lesbian activists who were veterans of this earlier movement for communicating these ideas to PWAs (Nussbaum 1990, 108).

References

Abunzwa, Judith. 1997. *Women's voices, women's power: Dialogues of resistance from East Africa.* Peterborough, Ontario: Broadview Press.

Achmat, Zackie. 2003. Preface. In *Global AIDS: Myths and facts,* ed. Alexander Irwin, Joyce Millen, and Dorothy Fallows, xiii–xvi. Boston: South End Press.

Baylies, Carolyn. 2000. Perspectives on gender and AIDS in Africa. In *AIDS, sexuality and gender in Africa: Collective strategies and struggles in Tanzania and Zambia,* ed. Carolyn Baylies and Janet Bujra, 1–24. London: Routledge.

Beck, Linda J. 2003. Democratization and the hidden public: The impact of patronage networks on Senegalese women. *Comparative Politics* 35 (2): 147–67.

Bujra, Janet, and Scholastica Mokake. 2000. AIDS activism in Dar es Salaam: Many struggles, a single goal. In *AIDS, sexuality and gender in Africa: Collective strategies and struggles in Tanzania and Zambia,* ed. Carolyn Baylies and Janet Bujra, 153–73. London: Routledge.

Campbell, Bobbi, and Michael Callen. 1983. The Denver principles.
http://wwwactupny.org/documents/Denver.html.

Elson, Diane. 1995. Gender-aware analysis and development economics. In *The political economy of development and underdevelopment,* 6th ed., ed. Kenneth Jameson and Charles Wilber, 70–80. New York: McGraw-Hill/Irwin.

Gordon, April. 1996. *Transforming capitalism and patriarchy: Gender and development in Africa.* Boulder, CO: Lynne Rienner.

Hamblin, Julie, and Elizabeth Reid. 1991. Women, the HIV epidemic and human rights: A tragic imperative. United Nations Development Program issues paper 8. http://www.undp.org/hiv/publications/issues/english/issue08e.htm.

Heyzer, Noleen. 2001. Address to the United Nations General Assembly Special Session on HIV/AIDS, New York.
http://www.un.org/ga/aids/statements/docs/unifemE.html.

Human Rights Watch. 2002. *Suffering in silence: Human rights abuses and HIV transmission among girls in Zambia.*
http://www.hrw.org/reports/2003/zambia/zambia1202.pdf.

——. 2003a. *Double standards: Women's property rights violations in Kenya.*
http://www.hrw.org/reports/2003/kenya0303/kenya0303.pdf.

——. 2003b. *Just die quietly: Domestic violence and women's vulnerability to HIV in Uganda.*
http://www.hrw.org/reports/2003/uganda0803/uganda0803.pdf.

——. 2003c. *Policy paralysis: A call for action on HIV/AIDS-related human rights abuses against women and girls in Africa.*
http://www.hrw.org/reports/2003/africa1203.pdf.

Hunter, Mark. 2002. The materiality of everyday sex: Thinking beyond 'prostitution.' *African Studies* 61 (1): 99–120.

Inter-Parliamentary Union. 2004. Women in national parliaments. http://www.ipu.org/wmn-e/world.htm.

Irwin, Alexander, Joyce Millen, and Dorothy Fallows. 2003. *Global AIDS: Myths and facts.* Boston: South End Press.

Joint United Nations Program on HIV/AIDS (UNAIDS). 1999. *From principles to practice: Greater involvement of people living with or affected by HIV/AIDS.* http://www.unaids.org/publications/documents/persons/una9943e.pdf.

——. 2000. *Report of the Nairobi consultation on GIPA.* http://www.unaids.org/publications/documents/persons/nborep.doc.

——. 2002. *AIDS epidemic update.* http://www.unaids.org/worldaidsday/2002/press/update/epiupdate2002_en.doc.

——. 2004. *Report on the global AIDS epidemic.* http://www.unaids.org/bangkok2004.html.

Kaiser Daily Reports. 1999. *11th international conference on AIDS: Epidemic 'exploding' among teen girls in Africa.* http://www.kaisernetwork.org/aids/1999/09/kh990915.3html.

Kapunda, S. M. 2000. Gender inequality, poverty and food insecurity in Tanzania. In *Gender, family and work in Tanzania*, ed. Colin Creighton and C. K. Omari, 220–36. Aldershot: Ashgate Publishers.

Keller, Bonnie, Demere Kitange, and the Tanzania Gender Networking Programme (TGNP). 1999. *Toward gender equity in Tanzania: A profile in gender relations.* Dar es Salaam: TGNP.

Kelsall, Tim. 2001. Donors, NGOs and the state: Governance and 'civil society' in Tanzania. In *The charitable impulse: NGOs and development in East and North-East Africa*, ed. Ondine Barrow and Michael Jennings, 133–48. West Hartford, CT: Kumarian Press.

Mann, Jonathan. 1999. Human rights and AIDS: The future of the pandemic. In *Health and human rights: A reader,* ed. Jonathan Mann, Sofia Gruskin, Michael Grodin, and George Annas, 216–26. London: Routledge.

Mbilinyi, Margaret, and Naomi Kaihula. 2000. Sinners and outsiders: The drama of AIDS in Rungwe. In *AIDS sexuality and gender in Africa: Collective strategies and struggles in Tanzania and Zambia*, ed. Carolyn Baylies and Janet Bujra, 76–94. London: Routledge.

Molyneaux, Maxine. 1985. Mobilization without emancipation? Women's interests, the state and revolution in Nicaragua. *Feminist Studies* 11: 227–54.

Nankinga, Margaret. 2002. Hide in the kitchen if your man beats you. *Africawoman.* http://www.africawoman.net/files/20nov02/AW7P07.pdf.

Ndegwa, Stephen. 1996. *The two faces of civil society: NGOs and politics in Africa.* West Hartford, CT: Kumarian Press.

Nnoko, Soori, Betty Chidou, Flora Wilson, Wences Msuya, and Gabriel Mwaluko. 2000. Tanzania: AIDS care – learning from experience. *Review of African Political Economy* 86: 547–57.

Nussbaum, Bruce. 1990. *Good intentions: How big business and the medical establishment are corrupting the fight against AIDS.* New York: Penguin Books.

Omari, C. K., and D. A. S. Mbilinyi. 2000. Born to be less equal: The predicament of the girl child in Tanzania. In *Gender, family and work in Tanzania*, ed. Colin Creighton and C. K. Omari, 292–313. Aldershot: Ashgate Publishers.

Piot, Peter. 2002. World AIDS day message. http://www.unaids.org/worldaidsday/2002/press.

Rosenberg, Tina. 2001. Look at Brazil. *New York Times Magazine*. 28 January.

Savenstadt, Stefan, Gerd Savenstadt, and Terrtu Haggstrom. 2000. *East African children of the streets – A question of health.* Stockholm: Save the Children – Sweden.

Schraeder, Peter. 2004. *African politics and society: A mosaic in transformation.* 2nd ed. Belmont, CA: Thompson/Wadworth.

Siplon, Patricia. 2002. *AIDS and the policy struggle in the United States.* Washington, DC: Georgetown Univ. Press.

Siplon, Patricia, and Kristin Novotny. 2002. Women, AIDS and autonomy in sub-Saharan Africa. Poster presentation at the annual meeting of the American Political Science Association, Boston.

Stine, Gerald. 2001. *AIDS update 2001.* Upper Saddle River, NJ: Prentice Hall.

Tadesse, Zenebeworke. 1982. The impact of land reform on women: The case of Ethiopia. In *Women and development: The sexual division of labor in rural societies*, ed. Lourdes Beneria, 203–22. New York: Praeger.

Teenage Mothers Association of Kenya (TEMAK). 2000. *Violation of basic needs and basic rights of domestic workers in Kisumu: Report of a rapid study*. Kisumu: TEMAK.

Tripp, Aili. 2000. *Women and politics in Uganda.* Madison: Univ. of Wisconsin Press.

——. n.d. New trends in women's political participation in Africa. http://www.democracy.stanford.edu/Seminar/AiliTripp.pdf.

Tsai, Kellee S. 2002. State, ideology and women in rural China. In *Women in developing countries: Assessing strategies for empowerment*, ed. Rekha Datta and Judith Kornberg, 47–74. Boulder, CO: Lynne Rienner.

United Nations Development Fund for Women (UNIFEM). 2003. Southern African women living with HIV/AIDS voice concerns to UNIFEM. Press Release. http://www.unifem.org/pressreleases.pho?f_page_pid=6&f_pritem_pid=1.

Wanyeki, L. Muthoni. 2003. Introduction. In *Women and land in Africa: Culture, religion and realizing women's rights*, ed. L. Muthoni Wanyeki, 1–28. London: Zed Books.

World Bank. 2001. *World development report 2000/2001: Attacking poverty.* New York: Oxford University Press.

Chapter 3

Patterns of Mobilization: Political Culture in the Fight Against AIDS

Fred Eboko; translated by Babacar Mbengue

As the AIDS pandemic enters its third decade, there is an abundance of scientific research on the disease in sub-Saharan Africa. More than ever, the biomedical and social sciences have sought to inform each other's analysis of AIDS on the continent. Now the prevailing belief is that interdisciplinary perspectives yield a better understanding of AIDS and facilitate more effective action against one of the worst trials that Africa has ever faced. Yet, the balance of power between different scientific perspectives has helped enshrine some discourses at the expense of, or in opposition to, others. Knowledge about AIDS in Africa is very dependent on the efforts of the involved actors, from global institutions to international scientific teams. AIDS research, including that involving epidemiologists and social scientists, needs to be qualified and questioned to better assess the relevance of African states and societies in addressing the AIDS challenge. Political scientists can and should play a more important role in the study of the pandemic, alongside anthropologists who for two decades have increased our understanding of the rapid and deadly spread of HIV/AIDS on the continent (Boone and Batsell 2001). The social sciences have benefited from anthropologists, who have challenged the idea that African cultures facilitated the spread of HIV.

This chapter is rooted in the anthropological study of the failure and success of various patterns of social and political mobilization to combat AIDS (Schoepf 2001; Becker et al. 1999; Kerouedan and Eboko 1999). This chapter examines different theoretical models for analyzing the political and social situations shaping actions on AIDS in Africa.[1] The work elucidates the meanings of the political commitments and/or 'passivity' of African states facing the epidemic. The chapter illustrates how the concept of 'political culture' explains how the different historical paths of African states conditioned their political responses to AIDS, despite the overall spread of the disease on the continent.

These themes of international involvement and political culture help explain unpredictable aspects of AIDS in Africa. For example, during the first decade of the AIDS epidemic, international actors presented Cameroon and Nigeria as 'miracles', whereas they viewed Uganda as the embodiment of 'African demise'. In the third decade of endemic AIDS, international actors present Uganda as a model because of its reversal in infection rate, particularly among female teenagers, while they report that Cameroon has one of the highest rates of HIV prevalence in central and western Africa. At the time of the early predictions, whoever asserted that in 2003 Cameroon (with 6.9 per cent prevalence) would have a higher rate of infection than Uganda (with 4.1 per cent prevalence) would have been considered a maverick epidemiological forecaster (UNAIDS 2004). The Ugandan achievement is the result of two decades of collective mobilization in all sectors of society, including the highest ranks of the state, individuals living with HIV/AIDS, and state partnerships with international governmental and nongovernmental organizations. In contrast, Cameroon pays the price of a politics of passive adhesion to international rules, officially and artificially adopted during the 1980s and the 1990s. Another unpredictable case in the politics of AIDS is Botswana, which challenges often-repeated assumptions about the relationship between economic development and public health. With nearly 40 per cent of its population between 15 and 49 years old HIV positive, Botswana had the second highest HIV prevalence rate in the world in 2003 (UNAIDS 2004). Yet, Botswana belies the common belief that there is a simple causal link between poverty and HIV. The country's gross domestic product per capita of $3,080 in 2002 remains one of the highest in sub-Saharan Africa, and its health-care system is one of the best on the continent (UNDP 2004).

These examples illustrate that the generic term 'Africa' insufficiently reflects the broad spectrum of societal phenomena on the continent, and specifically those relating to AIDS. Political scientists need to examine AIDS policies in sub-Saharan Africa in the context of particular time periods and dynamic political cultures. Political scientists can highlight relationships between, on the one hand, the unprecedented political changes in Africa since the 1990s, and on the other hand, past political events and the appearance of AIDS in the 1980s. This chapter asserts that political commitment or lack thereof is crucial to explain the trends of the epidemic since the early 1980s. Metaphorically, the chapter views the AIDS pandemic in Africa to be an 'Acquired Political Immune Deficiency Syndrome' (Eboko 2000, 235). The nature of the African state further shapes an understanding of state activity or inactivity in addressing HIV/AIDS. In that perspective, I present three models of political mobilization against AIDS found in one or more countries: (1) the model of active dissidence seen in South Africa; (2) the model of active participation illustrated in Uganda and Senegal; and (3) the model of passive adhesion exemplified by Côte d'Ivoire and Cameroon. It is important to note, though, that none of these cases is immutable and that there may be overlap across categories, depending on a country's history and the social and political changes it has experienced.

Mobilization and Political Cultures: Modeling Political Action

I define political culture to be the dynamic and heterogeneous ground of collective identities, ideologies, and historical pathways of different political forces. The possibilities for political mobilization are rooted within the configuration of these forces. The political cultures that explain the on-going social and political dynamics in the fight against AIDS are never fixed. They are rooted in the social and historical evolution of a particular country and the epidemiological, economic, political, social, and health situation of a country in which AIDS exists. Political cultures give meaning to the discourses and actions of leaders. This study considers and illustrates the political cultures within which leaders choose to formulate their 'political grammar' on AIDS.

The concept of political culture has evolved. The original idea posited that attitudes differ from one locality, country, or global region to another. The simplest example comes from Italy where two relatively different attitudes toward politics could be identified between the North and the South: a parochial attitude in the South including Sicily and a culture inclined toward participation in the North (Almond and Verba 1963). Today, this understanding of political culture draws criticisms for its lack of analytical potency. It has been criticized for ignoring historical factors shaping culture and for assuming political cultures are immutable. It portrays 'the disembodied *homo politicus* devoid of any anthropological consistency and any historical depth' (Cefaï 2001a, 9). Otayek considers political culture through a wide range of political repertoires from different periods like a 'by-product of the ever-changing history.' His approach is 'a case for the consideration of African political cultures as part of history' (1997, 803). This view runs counter to the ethnocentrism which Otayek finds so pervasive in some concepts of political culture, particularly those implying that some cultural attitudes and behaviors are antithetical to development. The concept of political culture can be viewed from a host of vantage points, as demonstrated by the numerous studies about the concept. However, these studies increasingly concur on the changing nature of political culture in contemporary societies.[2]

A more useful view of political culture is that it should be understood 'through the notions of experience, sensitivity, imagination, emotionality, and sociability' (Cefaï 2001a, 17). African leaders whose countries are challenged by AIDS act according to a host of criteria that may reflect this view of political culture. For example, the actions of leaders may stem from their experience with the epidemic, their personal sensitivity, the collective imagination regarding the AIDS etiology, the emotions displayed by political actors in public communication, collective identities, and their sustaining ideologies. Social norms shaping the balance of power between men and women, the relations between leaders and citizens, power between elders and young people, and the attitude toward those perceived as 'the other' also affect state actions on AIDS. Political culture constitutes a heterogeneous set of values and identities. As the next section illustrates, such identity-based ideologies are particularly vivacious in South Africa. Martin (2001) explains the power of political culture to affect state actions: 'The political culture would refer, within a determined group, to the prevailing representations of politics, therefore to the representation of symbolic organizations reminiscent of it, and to some cultural practices where some mechanisms of symbolism come into play. ... [I]t would imply that ... these cultural practices represent some stakes due to their "thought-inducing" capability and their great ability to move and mobilize' (Martin 2001, 135).

The following case studies help increase our knowledge of some major trends in political mobilization against AIDS in Africa, using the analytical lens of the political cultures that sustain these mobilizations. Cefaï (2001b, 95) writes: 'Political cultures cannot be studied as mere symbolic or functional systems. ... They need to be approached through case studies that set forth the analyses of the logic of action and situation, and show *in vivo* and *in situ* how some actors [interpret political culture]... to express and support some crises and conflicts, to criticize or justify some discourses or actions, to lay out some world views and problematic situations'. This logic informs the following cases.

Southern Africa under Shock: Active Dissidence in the Epidemiological Crisis

Since the late 1990s, southern Africa has been the African region most affected by AIDS. In 2003, 38.8 per cent of citizens in Swaziland were HIV positive; in Botswana, this percentage was 37.3 per cent (UNAIDS 2004). These were the two highest HIV prevalence rates in the world that year. This section focuses on the case of South Africa, though Chapter 6 in this volume further illustrates some of the political and social variables shaping state reactions to AIDS in Swaziland. South Africa has one of the highest numbers of infected people in the world: 4.8 million South Africans are HIV positive. One of every nine South Africans is HIV positive and one of every eight new cases of HIV infection in Africa occurs in South Africa (UNAIDS 2000a, 2000b, 2001, 2004). As the country faces predictions of a high death toll from AIDS, political and ideological factors cannot be overlooked in an analysis of state responses to the disease.

AIDS in South Africa

AIDS is situated within the context of a profoundly changing South Africa, in which the official end of apartheid led to the implosion of society into violence (Benatar 2001).[3] Fifty years of apartheid divided society, created distrust among citizens, and led to grossly unequal economic development (Barbier 1991; Darbon 1993, 1999). The spread of HIV/AIDS challenges a country searching for direction and power in the face of social and economic shock and the 'disenchantment of freedom' (Hermet 1993). AIDS is merely one of the many competing priorities the country faces. Initiated by Nelson Mandela and continued by Thabo Mbeki, the process of political change has been coupled with the ideology of 'African renaissance'. President Mbeki seeks to impose this ideology on his country and the world, and he has actively sought to advance this ideology through the regional and continental recognition of his country's power. The much-publicized international clashes between Mbeki and the scientific community in 2000 concerning AIDS are situated within this political agenda. Mbeki's dissenting declarations on the link between HIV and AIDS indicate the challenges of fighting AIDS in a country whose reconstruction is dependent on finding new social references (Fassin 2000). AIDS seems to be a reflection of South Africa's social change and a window by which the country can become both a leader on the continent and a leader from Africa on the world stage.

In a society full of damaging contradictions that are the legacy of apartheid, AIDS policies also seem contradictory. For example, though the government has challenged drug producers, high-level political leaders have questioned the effectiveness or even the usefulness of antiretroviral (ARV) therapies. Additionally, South Africa's international tussle with pharmaceutical companies is emblematic of the symbolic willingness of the president to put South Africa among the countries 'to be reckoned with'. In 1997, the country passed the Medicines Act, which allowed domestic production of generic medicines for those with HIV/AIDS. Coupled with Brazil's action to produce its own generic drugs, the South African legislation challenged the control that Western pharmaceutical companies have over AIDS medications. After suing the South African government for breech of international trade laws, 39 drug companies then dropped the suit in 2001. The legislation and legal victory seemed to illustrate Mbeki's desire to stand against Western science, corporations, and ideology.

Yet, while the Mbeki government has challenged Western institutions, his government has been criticized by civic associations for its complacency in developing AIDS policies, especially for universal access to ARVs. The anti-AIDS organizations in South Africa are pioneers when it comes to collective mobilization in Africa. They were a crucial link in the international mobilization that caused the pharmaceutical companies to back down from the aforementioned lawsuit. These organizations have also opposed Mbeki and his minister of health's questioning of the efficacy and safety of ARVs, and they deem such official statements on AIDS and ARVs to be counterproductive (Irvin, Millen, and Fallows 2003). These organizations are involved in both South African and international civil society; on both levels, these groups have sought to pressure the state to provide ARVs. South Africa's anti-AIDS organizations contrast with groups in other African countries, particularly in French-speaking Africa, that have merely followed the lead of nongovernmental organizations from industrialized countries on the issue of access to ARVs (Fassin 2002).

President Mbeki's 2000 letter to world leaders

President Mbeki's famous letter of 3 April 2000 to world leaders provides insight into how the country's reactions to AIDS reflect both a participatory political culture and a political culture that rejects international injunctions. Covered extensively in the international press, the letter asserted that the nature of the HIV/AIDS epidemic in Africa requires uniquely African solutions to the crisis. The letter raised vehement outcries concerning its public health ideas. But its political meaning needs further analysis.[4] From the perspective of political sociology, an analysis of the South African president's discourse falls between an analysis of political culture and a cognitive approach to public policy making. Mbeki's controversial attitude must be viewed in a wider context of a political culture that is being reformulated, a process that represents a vehicle for Mbeki's ideological objectives.

The letter appeared a few months before the first-ever global AIDS conference held in Africa, the International AIDS Conference hosted from 9 to 14 July 2000 in Durban. Given the timing of the letter, Mbeki's contradictory reasoning seemed surprising. To understand the political and ideological stakes in the letter, one must go back to apartheid and its abolition, to Mandela's accession to power in 1994, and to his succession by Mbeki. The apartheid system was built on a model of racial separation supported by the ideology of the superiority of the white minority over the black and colored populations. The apartheid regime founded its segregationist practices on differences believed to be insuperable; that is, on the belief in the absolute inferiority of all nonwhites, especially the black majority. From 1948 until roughly 1990, the ethical struggle of the black majority clashed with the silence of some democratic Western powers toward the regime of Pretoria. In fact, the South African white elite regarded that passive response to 'white power' as tacit support for the ideology of apartheid. This historical experience sheds light on the possible resentment of South African officials to the dominant position of Western opinions on health issues in debates among political personalities who are supposed to be on equal footing.

Because of the long liberation battle against apartheid, the political culture of post-apartheid leaders, including those of the African National Congress, is shaped by the concepts of refusal and struggle. The contemporary history of divisions in South Africa, in which the black community was defined by skin color and its 'Africanness', represents a fundamental element for understanding the president's letter. Mbeki's letter is also situated in the larger global context and in the letter, Mbeki positions his own country as part of the international community. Far from being a paradox, Mbeki's protests are consistent with a historical attempt to secure a 'place' for those previously lacking representation and to demand some evenhandedness in the treatment of different points of views. Mbeki asserts that even the most extreme scientific ideas about HIV/AIDS must have a place in the discourse, and the president himself admits that even his letter might be extreme: 'It may be that these comments are extravagant' (Mbeki 2000).

In the letter, Mbeki sets forth two elements in his questions on the science about HIV/AIDS in Africa. First, he uses the following syllogism: the major modes of HIV transmission are homosexual and masculine in the West, while they are heterosexual in Africa. He argues that responses to AIDS in Africa should be different than those used in the West because the epidemiological dynamics of the two epidemics are dissimilar. Second, Mbeki deals with the scientific studies of the harmful nature of ARVs. He compares the 'casting aside' of some scientists whose views Mbeki embraces to the worst human tragedies, using rhetoric and daring analogies that go far beyond the framework of the scientific debate on HIV/AIDS. He writes: 'It is suggested, for instance, that there are some scientists who are "dangerous and discredited" with whom nobody, including ourselves, should communicate or interact. In an earlier period of human history, these would be heretics that would be burnt at the stake!' (Mbeki 2000, 20).

Mbeki's intention seems to be to affirm that Africans are entitled to hold different views and to have different experiences from those of the former champions of apartheid. Since these champions were wrong during apartheid, why would they not be now? By sending the letter to global leaders, Mbeki implicates not only former apartheid leaders in South Africa, but also their direct and indirect defenders in Western, industrialized countries.[5] He asserts: 'Not long ago, in our country, people were killed, tortured, imprisoned and prohibited from being quoted in private and in public because the established authority believed that their views were dangerous and discredited. We are now being asked to do precisely the same thing that the racist apartheid tyranny we opposed did, because, it is said, there exists a scientific view that is supported by the majority, against which dissent is prohibited' (Mbeki 2000, 20).

The president's rationale is primarily ideological and aims to reject everything that may nurture a 'single thought' system that excludes those who do not agree with what he calls 'the established authority'. The letter's political thought and discourse are inspired by the anti-apartheid struggle to which he clearly refers: 'We are now being asked to do precisely the same thing that the racist apartheid tyranny we opposed did.' The president shifts the focus from the scientific opponents of those who question established findings on HIV/AIDS to the historical enemies of the freedom of the African people. This shift supports the president's incriminating, vehement, aggressive, and witty discourse: 'Some agitate for these extraordinary propositions with a religious fervour born by a degree of fanaticism, which is truly frightening' (Mbeki 2000, 20).

Beyond the letter's official purpose, Mbeki invites his readers to join a struggle that is redolent of past fights for freedom of thought and expression. In that dynamic, the president expands the struggle beyond South Africa to the global realm, so that Africans can form an alliance with Westerners to refuse the imposition of a (Western) worldview on Africa. Do the issues raised in Mbeki's letter relate solely to scientific debates about HIV/AIDS or are they about the formation of a broader identity-based opposition? That question stands out in the last sentence of the letter: 'I am greatly encouraged that all of us, as Africans, can count on your unwavering support in the common fight to save our continent and its people from deaths from AIDS' (Mbeki 2000, 20).

Some aspects of Mbeki's biography help explain his desire to move the debate from more than a narrow focus on AIDS in South Africa to an international focus. Fassin (2002, 16) writes: 'Thabo Mbeki is, unwillingly, a product of transnationalism which is, sociologically speaking, viewed as the most characteristic feature of globalization. After spending a short time in prison, he left South Africa to get his training in Great Britain, in the Soviet Union and particularly in the leadership circles of the exiled ANC throughout Africa. By turning some discussions on AIDS in South Africa into a "global controversy," he is less naïve than some aspects of his rhetoric might suggest.'

Mbeki's letter is situated in a dissident political culture inherited from the past struggle against apartheid. The current AIDS situation on the continent revitalizes the notion of dissidence to the potential benefit of South Africa, which can gain recognition as a sub-regional economic and political power. Since South Africa's power could not be expressed in the ideological terms of the abolished regime, a new slogan with the advantage of a new political meaning has been coined to reclaim the economic status of South African power. 'The topic of the "African renaissance" identifies and legitimizes different forms of international "power" ... It is to be reviewed within the particular context of a tradition of blaming that the countries of the region assimilate to the internal oppression or the external aggression. Therefore, taking into account the imbalances of power, the South African leaders hesitate to explicitly summon up a repertoire of legitimacy founded on that power' (Sindjoun and Vennesson 2000, 917).

In this context, AIDS is an element and an indication of the dynamics of social change in Africa, as well as in the global arena (Raynaut and Muhongayire 1993). The prominence of a media-covered event such as the 2000 Durban conference on AIDS was an opportunity for the South African president not only to connect AIDS and poverty, but also to remind the world about the indirect and direct involvement of external actors in Africa's underdevelopment. The AIDS epidemic in South Africa highlights a political culture that simultaneously expresses powerlessness in the global arena and that desires a renaissance. The political model of active dissidence suggests more than state reactions to international policies and opinions on AIDS; it also reflects a larger definition of South Africa's role on the global stage. As Fassin and Kazatchkine write on 16 May 2000 in *Le Monde*: 'Observations from different parts of the world, including from countries of the former Soviet bloc, indicate that long periods of social and political contention end with some drastic changes in the societies and an accrued sensitivity to epidemic situations. This is apparent in M. Mbeki's letter when he writes about the memory of apartheid in recalling the epidemiological specificity of the infection in southern Africa.'

In the same token, one needs to be cautious enough to draw the line between the provocation and the political meaning of Mbeki's letter. Fassin provides important insights: 'More than a protest against globalization *per se*, it is the way that the rules are imposed to the nations and peoples under domination that he questions. The resentment ... of those who notice the world political disorder and the hegemony of the western worldview represent a powerful leverage for heterodoxy. The controversy about AIDS in South Africa indicates that the perception of injustice can undermine the construction of the truth and blur the poorly-thought-through distinction between the global and the universal' (2002, 17).

The ideological issues raised in Mbeki's letter are both new and old. The dramatic and specific nature of the AIDS epidemic in southern Africa raises new issues. In contrast, questions about the 'ideological magnitude' of scientific knowledge are not new. The sociologist Colette Moreux was referring to Max Weber, not to Mbeki, when she wrote that 'according to Weber, the so-called "rationality" and superiority that the West is claiming and by which it justifies its domination over the physical world and over the other cultures is nothing more than a "belief in rationality", an ideology. Like Weber, at the same period, Durkheim already understood that the appreciation of truth or error does merely proceed from a collective definition and that there was no difference in nature between the scientific "faith" and the religious, political and, more broadly, the cultural convictions' (Moreux 1982, 11).

In summary, it is difficult to measure the cost of the controversy triggered by Mbeki's letter, as well as his other statements on AIDS.[6] It is important to remember that Mbeki is not the only actor in the fight against AIDS in South Africa. As other chapters in this volume illustrate, active civic organizations have challenged government policies and developed their own AIDS programs. Additionally, Mbeki has to some extent tempered his rhetoric and, in late 2003, his administration agreed to provide universal access to ARVs for South Africans. AIDS has been a means for Mbeki to voice a different and original African view on the world stage. But, the controversy surrounding Mbeki's words also indicates the powerlessness that state officials feel toward the AIDS tragedy in southern Africa.

The Model of Active Participation: Uganda and Senegal

Unlike South Africa, Uganda and Senegal have had more success in the fight against AIDS. International actors and Western political leaders have praised the commitment of these countries' officials in addressing HIV/AIDS. The experiences of these two countries contrast with the ideological struggle surrounding the epidemic in South Africa.

Uganda: Political courage and collective mobilization in a dramatic epidemiological situation

When Yoweri Museveni became president of Uganda in 1986, he inherited a country devastated by 20 years of military ethnocracy, which included a decade of Idi Amin-led violence (Prunier and Calas 1994; Perrot 1999). Uganda's HIV prevalence rates in the mid-1980s were alarming. In Kampala, the most important economic city, the infection rate among the sexually active population – the population between 15 and 49 years old – was 30 per cent. Even the rural areas, yet untouched in other countries, were paying the heavy cost of social disruption and family dissolution because of AIDS. For example, within a short period the agricultural area of Rakai near Lake Victoria became a symbol of the negative impact of AIDS on individuals, families, and communities. In Rakai, the population pyramid took on an unprecedented shape, dominated by an inordinate number of children and elderly people; the most productive members of society were struck down by the 'slim disease', the dismal name given to AIDS (Verboud 1994).

Soon after becoming president, Museveni took the lead in the mobilization against HIV/AIDS. Despite some considerable economic problems in the mid-1980s that made providing care for those with HIV/AIDS difficult, Museveni has actively supported AIDS awareness campaigns. These campaigns have been run and financed largely by British and American nongovernmental organizations and aid agencies, and they have used various media throughout the country (Dicklitch 1998). Meanwhile the spread of the disease itself has caused so much damage that having to face the disease – either directly or indirectly – has been enough to trigger awareness among citizens.

Unlike other countries, in Uganda the authorities made it easy for people infected with HIV/AIDS to speak out and get involved in the fight against the disease. This attitude of openness helped to remove the deadly feelings of guilt, shame, and dereliction that often accompany AIDS (Low-Beer and Stoneburner 2004). One of the unique outcomes of Uganda's political commitment to AIDS has been that the country developed a multidimensional approach to fighting AIDS, at a time when AIDS tended to be viewed solely as a health issue. The political commitment has been decisive insofar as 'in being the first African head of State to publicly admit the AIDS impact on his country, President Museveni has displayed some political courage' (Verboud 1994, 277). Verboud aptly points out that the Ugandan president 'has some flair because by rejecting the impossible silence, he veers clear from some of the political responsibility for an epidemic that, in hindsight, proves to be one of the most damning legacies of the previous governments' (1994, 277).

In addition to presidential leadership, the support and mobilization of local communities has been decisive in curtailing the spread of HIV/AIDS. In her capacity as the head of The AIDS Support Organization (TASO) since 1987, Noerine Kaleeba has developed a broad initiative geared toward providing care to patients and she has invented new techniques for counseling before, during, and after an HIV test. TASO works closely with international partners and has developed a circle of reliable people in an environment of collective awareness about the epidemic. The organization has a team of 150 full-time staff and 2,000 volunteers who work throughout the country. As a result of

TASO's efforts, Uganda became the African country with the highest number of citizens being voluntary tested for HIV/AIDS. HIV-positive herself, Kaleeba has become one of the icons in the fight against AIDS and an important relay between Ugandan citizens and the larger international community. TASO manages a multi-million dollar budget, much of it used to finance the schooling of children under 14 years old and to care for roughly 1,500 orphans (Verboud 1994, 277; Fabing 1998; TASO 2004).

In 1998, the infection rate among Uganda's teenagers dropped by 130 per cent and the country experienced a decline in the epidemic. The HIV infection rate among pregnant women under 20 years old was 28 per cent in 1991. That rate dropped to 6 per cent in 1998 (UNAIDS 2002). Uganda is the first African country where the decline in HIV prevalence has been recognized by international organizations, the media, AIDS activists, and scientists. The combination of political commitment and community-based mobilization such as exemplified by TASO must be credited for Uganda's success. The Ugandan example establishes a link between the spread of the epidemic on the one hand, and the social, political, economic, and cultural changes occurring in a country, on the other. Not long ago, forecasters predicted that AIDS would decimate the then hard-hit country. The country has challenged epidemiological predictions and has become a model for the fight against HIV/AIDS in Africa. For example, President Museveni's 'A-B-C' policy of 'Abstinence, Be Faithful, Use a Condom' has become the basis of donor approaches to AIDS in other African countries. This has been particularly true of the US government's prevention efforts under the 2003 President's Emergency Plan for AIDS Relief (*New York Times*, 14 July 2004).

Nonetheless, it is essential not to confuse the Ugandan struggle to combat HIV/AIDS with the issues uncovered by that struggle, particularly poverty, social inequalities, and international cooperation. Poverty and inequality are still pervasive in Uganda, and for some communities, have been exacerbated by the AIDS epidemic (UNDP 2004). As Chapter 8 by Ostergard and Barcelo indicates, interactions with international organizations continue to shape the fight against AIDS. The Uganda government has cooperated with the Joint United Nations Program on HIV/AIDS (UNAIDS) and the World Health Organization (WHO) to gain more access to ARV therapies and in June 2004, the government began to distribute free ARVs to approximately 3,000 HIV-positive people (*Boston Herald*, 14 June 2004). One must keep in mind that the drop in the HIV infection rate, although linked to broad collective mobilization and political commitment, also has been prompted by the carnage that struck Uganda in the early 1980s. The extremely high AIDS-induced mortality rates, particularly in Rakai, have encouraged prevention efforts (Barnett and Blaikie 1992).

Since the decline of HIV prevalence in Uganda, concern among AIDS activists and international actors has shifted to other countries, particularly those in southern Africa. Yet, as a model of active participation, the Uganda case illustrates important points about the interaction of political culture and

HIV/AIDS. First, the case demonstrates the vibrant nature of Ugandan communities, which, when given the political space in which to develop AIDS messages and programs, used the opportunity to create organizations to educate society about the epidemic. Second, Uganda illustrates the importance placed on centralized leadership in rebuilding the country after the war and in guiding the fight against AIDS. Third, the Uganda case shows how a society's experiences with AIDS shape the ways that individuals, as well as the state, seek to combat the disease. Finally, Uganda illustrates a desire on the part of the country and particularly Museveni to turn from the destructive and isolationist aspects of Uganda's past to incorporation into the global arena. Active engagement with international organizations in the fight against HIV/AIDS has facilitated this process.

Senegal: International scientific hub, epidemiological advantages, and political commitment

Senegal also has actively addressed the AIDS epidemic, though its responses have been shaped by different aspects of its political culture. Senegal became involved in the international fight against AIDS through cooperation in international scientific research. In 1984, while virologists had begun to question the existence of additional strains of HIV beyond HIV-1, Senegalese scientist Souleymane Mboup of LeDantec Hospital, Dakar, and two of his French colleagues, Francis Denis of the University of Limoges Hospital and Francis Barin of the University of Tours Hospital, sensed something new in their research. From samples taken from some prostitutes in Dakar, Mboup's research team discovered a new virus which has physiopathological and clinical effects that are different from those of HIV-1. For example, none of Mboup's patients fell ill at that time. Based on these findings, researchers including Mboup discovered HIV-2 and in 1986, published in the *Lancet* conclusions of primary importance: HIV-2 is less pathogenic than HIV-1, the form of the virus which is prevalent in Europe, the United States, and central Africa (Seytre and Rozenbaum 1993).[7] Part of the Senegalese reaction to AIDS has centered around this discovery and the continued involvement of African, specifically Senegalese, scientists in research on AIDS. The priority given to scientific research explains why Senegal has become one of the African centers for French cooperation in the study of AIDS. Along with Bobo Dioulasso and Abidjan, Senegal has become a crucial site under the aegis of the National Agency for Research on AIDS.

The prominent role of Senegalese scientists contrasts with the larger situation of a country with limited experience with the disease. While HIV/AIDS has spread throughout central and southern Africa, the HIV prevalence rate in Senegal has remained between 1 per cent and 2 per cent (UNAIDS 2002). Senegal's initial success in addressing HIV/AIDS has provided a continuous incentive for state authorities to remain active in the struggle. During the 1992 Summit of African Heads of States in Dakar, for example, President Abdou

Diouf invited his counterparts to take the lead in the fight against AIDS in their respective countries. The combination of strong community socialization, links to scientific networks, state openness to cooperation with international organizations, political commitment, and the presence of the less pathogenic and virulent HIV-2 have enabled Senegal to become a model in the fight against HIV/AIDS.

Senegal's actions against AIDS are set within a larger political culture that has been characterized as relatively stable. This stability has been strengthened over time through political competition. The country has experienced limited civil strife, except for the violence in the Casamance region. However, even the Casamance crisis has been framed as a situation in which the military serves to guarantee the territorial integrity of a sovereign state. From its independence to the pluralist competitions of the 1990s, the country has enjoyed international legitimacy, a fact which was heightened by the 2000 presidential election and the defeat of the ruling party (Galvan 2001). The domestic popularity of the country's first leader, Léopold Sédar Senghor, also advanced state legitimacy (Coulon 1988). The democratic transition in Senegal illustrates the country's capacity to address legitimate political conflicts in a relatively peaceful manner through the institutions of elections and an increasingly independent judiciary. These democratic foundations have facilitated state action on AIDS in Senegal. Based on the international success of their scientists, community norms which limit risky behaviors, the AIDS education efforts of the Islamic brotherhoods, and the mobilization of people living with HIV/AIDS, the Senegalese authorities successfully addressed AIDS, long before the international community exerted any pressure on African states to commit to the issue (UNAIDS 1999). The model of active participation evident in Uganda and Senegal is shaped by the larger political cultures of each country. In both countries, community mobilization, political commitment, and international cooperation have been crucial.

Passive Adhesion: Côte d'Ivoire and Cameroon

From the outset of the epidemic, observers have noted that with few exceptions African political elites and citizens have been apathetic about HIV/AIDS. There is a widespread tendency among African states to exhibit two distinct and paradoxical phenomena: the adhesion to the officially sanctioned international discourse on AIDS and the lack of any active participation to address the epidemic. This is the model of passive adhesion. In Cameroon, state negotiations with international partners over access to ARVs since 2001 illustrate how the country has merely used AIDS as a way to gain needed financial resources from international partners. In its interactions with international organizations, Cameroon portrays the fight against AIDS as a 'national priority', while domestically, it remains apathetic. Similarly, in Burkina Faso Desclaux (1997) describes an 'epidemic of silence', or a situation characterized by 'the State against public health' (Desclaux 1995). In the passive adhesion model, civil society groups geared toward social change and particularly toward democratic change have been conspicuously absent in the fight against AIDS, an absence which has broadly strengthened African authorities in their passive attitudes.

Côte d'Ivoire fits this passive adhesion model. In 1997, the country hosted the 10th International Conference on AIDS and Sexually Transmitted Diseases in Africa. In the presence of the French president and the very active French health minister, Bernard Kouchner, President Konan Bedie publicly committed himself and his country to the fight against AIDS, a commitment which seemed logical given the spread of the disease in Africa in general and in Côte d'Ivoire in particular. However, a few months earlier, in the run up to the presidential elections, the word 'AIDS' did not appear once in Bedie's electoral program even though his campaign proposals stressed the need to improve the health of the country's citizens. This limited commitment to health is manifested in low public spending on health – only 1 per cent of gross domestic product in 2001, a decrease from 1.5 per cent in 1990 (UNDP 2004, 159). By 2001, Côte d'Ivoire had reached a deal with UNAIDS for low-cost access to ARVs for those with HIV/AIDS. Yet, there have been multiple problems with implementing this agreement. The inclusion of patients in the program's protocol has been slow, and the process of follow up on patients has been inefficient. Additionally, the public has received inadequate information about the project (Msellati, Vidal, and Moatti 2001). These problems attest to the shortcomings of public health institutions and largely could have been avoided if AIDS had been the priority that Bedie led international actors to believe it was. In its interactions with international donors, Côte d'Ivoire contrasts with Senegal, which made direct agreements with some pharmaceutical producers to lower the price of ARVs by 90 per cent (Desclaux et al. 2004). The difference between these two countries in the fight against AIDS lies not just in the epidemiological context – Côte d'Ivoire's infection rate in 2003 was an estimated 7 per cent while Senegal's was 0.8 per cent – but also in the political commitment and the mobilization of public health resources.

Cameroon provides yet another example of passive adhesion in addressing AIDS. State officials began the fight against AIDS in 1985, with the first meeting about the disease in the Ministry of Public Health. This meeting occurred before the first cases of AIDS appeared in the country. Despite this early discussion, there have been few positive results in limiting the spread of the disease. Government spending on public health has remained at 1 per cent of gross domestic product since the 1990s, despite the increase in HIV infection rates (UNDP 2004, 158). AIDS programs are unevenly spread throughout the country in patterns that reflect the interests of bilateral and multilateral donors, not the epidemiology of the disease. Within the country, international actors work without coordination because the state lacks autonomy in decision making. Each international partner gets involved in AIDS programs that meet its priorities, often resulting in duplicated and uncoordinated efforts (Eboko 2002). For example, several international organizations have been involved in training psycho-social counselors in Yaounde and Douala. Officially, the country has implemented directives from the WHO and UNAIDS, such as forming a national AIDS committee in 1987 and developing the Programme national de lutte contre le SIDA (National Program to Fight AIDS). Yet, even though adhering to international standards, Cameroon has never engaged in a political debate about AIDS. For the most part, AIDS has been left up to biomedical experts whose apolitical status has made them subservient to the state's silence on the disease (Eboko 1996, 2001, 2002).

The 1998 attempt to reform AIDS policies in Cameroon is a case in point. The country's AIDS programs suffered a decline at the same time that the WHO-led Global Program on AIDS (1986–1996) was being replaced by the more high-profile coordinating organization of UNAIDS. Officials in Cameroon maintained that the country lacked the means to address the disease, especially given the reduction of international resources for AIDS in the 1990s. Yet, when the government appointed a new health minister during a big cabinet reshuffle in 1997, these resource-based arguments were rejected (Eboko 1999a). The newly appointed health minister, Gottlieb Monnékosso, had been the regional director of the WHO for Africa from 1986 to 1996, and he intended to use his international experience to serve the National AIDS Committee. In 1998, he attempted to depersonalize the National AIDS Committee, decentralize AIDS policies, and mobilize important social groups such as HIV-infected people, youth, women, the media, and international partners for the fight against AIDS. This was the first time since the development of the National AIDS Committee in 1987 that a broad reform was carried out without being induced by international directives.

At roughly the same time, interest in AIDS in Africa was growing in the international community. As they did in many African countries, in 2000 the World Bank and UNAIDS imposed on Cameroon the establishment of a multisectoral plan to fight AIDS. The health minister was replaced and, in order to comply with the requirements of the World Bank and UNAIDS, the institutions of 1998 were replaced. The previous administrative experiences were neglected, and a World Bank-financed decision-making mechanism was established. (Starting in 2001, the World Bank provided 50 billion CFA over a span of five years for programs and institutions to fight AIDS.) Though decentralization and civil society participation remain fundamental concepts of the donor-supported multisectoral plan, the new structures have thwarted the proactive reforms of 1998 for the sake of a new beginning. The lack of continuity in state actions on AIDS has hampered efforts to halt the spread of HIV. The HIV infection rate grew from approximately 0.5 per cent in 1998 to nearly 8 per cent in 2003 (UNAIDS 2002, 2004).

Increasingly since 2001, political leaders have sought to distinguish their international actions on AIDS, for which they receive donor pressure, from their domestic policies on AIDS, for which they receive little internal pressure. Likewise, media coverage of state actions on AIDS exacerbates the tendency of the state to passively address international concerns. Because of the silence of African political authorities on AIDS until the 2001 African Summit on HIV/AIDS and Other Related Infectious Diseases in Abuja, Nigeria, and because of the distrust that African newspapers have for the information they receive from local health authorities, media coverage of state AIDS policies has been limited. The Western media has tended to provide much of the information on AIDS. State actions on AIDS often appear intended more for an international audience than for citizens.

The spread of HIV in Cameroon is situated within a context of profound economic and social crisis that occurred from the mid-1980s to the mid-1990s (Hugon 1996). These upheavals led to the collapse of public sectors such as education and health care. Cameroon has experienced negative economic growth since 1990 (UNDP 2004, 186), and this economic decline has contributed to the emergence of individualistic survival plans and strategies, some of which increase the risk that individuals will be exposed to HIV. The political unrest that accompanied the attempted democratic transition between 1990 and 1993 had long-term negative implications for the fight against AIDS. These economic and political transitions contributed to societal violence and they distracted political elites and intellectuals, who in a more stable and open political system might otherwise have devoted their energy to the fight against AIDS. The transition also led to a prevailing political culture of collective apathy. The ambient peace in the country hides an underlying resignation among citizens to live a precarious life, under the control of a political regime that has resisted popular pressure for radical change (Eboko 1999a). This citizen resignation has meant that the state feels no domestic pressure to proactively address AIDS. Because of the 'political transition-that-did-not-take-place' (Mehler 1997), Cameroon's fight against AIDS has been manifested primarily in biomedical professionals joining international research networks (Eboko 1999c). Though the issue of access to ARVs has created some national organizations of people living with HIV/AIDS that challenge state and international drug policies, the relative newness of these associations makes it difficult to evaluate their impact on state actions on AIDS. In the future, these groups may affect the political culture of apathy and breed a collective mobilization more inclined toward action. Yet for now, Cameroon, just like Côte d'Ivoire and most other African countries, best fits the model of passive adhesion. What Foucault (1997, 214) terms biopolitics, or 'the right to live and let die,' appropriately describes such a minimal state and societal role in the fight against HIV/AIDS.

Conclusion

For any public policy, the outcomes differ from the inputs, because of the numerous factors that shape the policy process (Kingdon 1984; Muller 2000,

191). The fight against AIDS in Africa is no exception. This chapter has shown how one of those inputs – the nature of political culture – shapes state actions on AIDS. The statements of Mbeki, as exemplified in his 2000 letter to world leaders, illustrate South Africa's desire to assert regional power and develop an African autonomy from the West. Further, they are rooted in a political culture that has experienced both the abuse of science to repress the black majority and the oppression of those who challenged the apartheid state. South Africa's active dissidence against international actors and AIDS policies must be understood in this context. Similarly, the active participation model evident in Uganda and Senegal reflects the leadership perceptions and societal networks in those two countries. Each country has built on relations with international organizations, either through aid organizations (as in Uganda) or scientific networks (as in Senegal). Both countries have mobilized civil society associations in the fight against AIDS, whether AIDS support organizations in Uganda or the Muslim brotherhoods in Senegal. Particularly in Uganda, the experiences that citizens have had with AIDS have shaped individual and institutional responses to the disease.

In many African states, the policy brokers in the fight against AIDS have been mostly biomedical professionals who have become public-health entrepreneurs. For example, in Cameroon, Côte d'Ivoire, and even Senegal, these officials were the main negotiators with the WHO, UNAIDS, and the World Bank in the implementation of public health directives (Gruénais 1999; Eboko 1999a). However, one of the first consequences of the emergence of these coalitions has been the division between the biomedical elites who work with international actors and the intended beneficiaries of AIDS policies, particularly people living with HIV/AIDS. This disconnect varies from one African state to another and it reflects the nature of weak state institutions with little autonomy, capacity, or legitimacy with civil society (Médard 1992).

Political culture shapes the ways civil society may pressure state leaders to address HIV/AIDS or the political space that the state provides for AIDS associations to participate in policy making. The nature of state-civil society relations illustrates one difference between countries reflecting the active participation model and those exhibiting the passive adhesion model. In the latter, the silent and apathetic attitudes of civil society toward public health demonstrate a lack of connection between the state and civil society. In Cameroon, Côte d'Ivoire, Congo, and Togo, the political liberalization and widespread popular movements of the 1990s led to the controversial election of leaders who often continued the undemocratic practices of their predecessors. In countries experiencing this chaotic process of democratization, how can society hold accountable leaders who do not owe their authority to the choice of the majority (Daloz and Quantin 1997; Daloz 1999)? The nature of democracy (e.g., distorted elections and an underdeveloped civil society) affects the fight against AIDS, in that the formal implementation of national AIDS programs has often taken precedence over the mobilization of the concerned populations and the content of AIDS policies. The passive adhesion model represents a double passivity: the passivity of African authorities toward international AIDS directives on the one hand, and the passivity of civil society toward political representatives who are most concerned with remaining in power, on the other.

In the larger sense, the AIDS issue raises questions about the place of Africa in the world. Africa's incomplete democratic transitions have contributed to AIDS policies that reflect the priorities of international donors, not affected populations. The lack of transparency and accountability in state actions is compounded by both the underdevelopment of state institutions that can autonomously coordinate AIDS actions and the dependence of African states on the resources of international donors. Presently, the most decisive illustration of this lack of democracy is the profound lack of access to health care for Africans with HIV/AIDS. How African states develop and sustain policies to provide health care that were agreed to at the global, not local, level will be a litmus test for African political cultures. The future of the continent is at stake. It is very likely that a new Africa will emerge, one divided between those states which make good use of available resources to address AIDS and those which do not. The latter may be temporarily or definitively marginalized in a world order whose fundamental inequalities have been dramatically highlighted by AIDS.

Notes

1 See Eboko (1999b, 2003) for an empirical examination of the diverse epidemiological, political, and social situations influencing the fight against AIDS in Africa.

2 One can refer, among others, to Badie (1983), Geertz (2003), Cefaï (2001a, 2001b), and Martin (2001). Studies pertaining to grassroots politics have contributed to an understanding of the relationship between politics and culture in Africa. See particularly Bayart, Mbembe, and Toulabor (1992).

3 For instance, Johannesburg has the highest rate of rape in the world.

4 See Fassin (2001) for an analysis of the scientific and political aspects of Mbeki's letter. Also see *Le Monde*, 16 May 2000.

5 Concerning apartheid's propaganda and 'successes' in Europe in the 1980s, see Marchand (1985).

6 For an analysis of other statements made by Mbeki, see the chapter by Furlong and Ball in this volume.

7 Ironically, the African media has hardly mentioned Souleymane Mboup, one of the discoverers of HIV-2. Beyond the glitz of international meetings on HIV/AIDS, the African media has not covered the role of African scientists in advancing knowledge about the disease.

References

Almond, Gabriel, and Sidney Verba. 1963. *The civic culture: Political attitudes and democracy in five nations*. Boston: Little Brown.

Badie, Bertrand. 1983. *Culture et politique.* Collection Politique Comparée. Paris: Economica.

Barbier, Jean-Claude. 1991. *L'Afrique du Sud après l'apartheid*. Paris: Editions Kimé.

Barnett, Tony, and Piers Blaikie. 1992. *AIDS in Africa*. New York: Guilford Press.

Bayart, Jean-Francois, A. Mbembe, and Comi Toulabor. 1992. *Le politique par le bas en Afrique Noire: contributions à une problématique de la démocratie*. Paris: Karthala.

Becker, Charles, Jean-Pierre Dozon, C. Obbo, and M. Touré, eds. 1999. *Vivre et penser le sida en Afrique*. Paris-Dakar: Codesria-Karthala-Institut de Recherche pour le Développement.

Benatar, Solomon R. 2001. South Africa's transition in a globalizing world: HIV/AIDS as a window and a mirror. *International Affairs* 77 (2): 347–75.

Boone, Catherine, and Jake Batsell. 2001. Politics and AIDS in Africa: Research agendas in political science and international relations. *Africa Today* 48 (2): 2–33.

Cefaï, Daniel, ed. 2001a. *Cultures politiques*. Paris: Presses Universitaires de France.

——. 2001b. Expérience, culture et politique. In *Cultures politiques*, ed. Daniel Cefaï, 93–116. Paris: Presses Universitaires de France.

Coulon, Christian. 1988. Senegal: The development and fragility of semidemocracy. In *Democracy in developing countries*, ed. Larry Diamond, Juan Linz, and Seymour Martin Lipset, 141–78. Boulder, CO: Lynne Rienner Publishers.

Daloz, Jean-Pascal, ed. 1999. *Le (non-)renouvellement des élites en Afrique*. Bordeaux: Centre d'Etude d'Afrique Noire.

Daloz, Jean-Pascal, and Patrick Quantin, eds. 1997. *Transitions démocratiques africaines*. Paris: Karthala.

Darbon, Dominique. 1993. *La République sud-africaine: etat des lieux*. Paris: Karthala.

——. 1999. *L'après-Mandela: enjeux sud-africains et régionaux*. Paris: Karthala-Maison des Sciences de l'Homme of Aquitaine.

Desclaux, Alice. 1995. L'Etat contre la santé publique? *Sociologie Santé* 13: 85–91.

——. 1997. L'épidémie invisible: anthropologie du d'un système médical à l'épreuve du sida chez l'enfant à Bobo Dioulasso, Burkina Faso. PhD diss., Aix-Marseille III.

Desclaux, Alice, Isabelle Laniece, Ibra Ndoye, and Bernard Taverne, eds. 2004. *The Senegalese antiretroviral drug access initiative: An economic, social, behavioural and biomedical analysis*. Paris: Agence Nationale de Recherche sur le sida, UNAIDS, and WHO.

Dicklitch, Susan. 1998. *The elusive promise of NGOs in Africa: Lessons from Uganda*. New York: St. Martin's Press.

Eboko, Fred. 1996. L'Etat camerounais et les cadets sociaux face à la pandémie du sida. *Politique Africaine* 64 (December): 135–45.

——. 1999a. Les élites politiques au Cameroun: le renouvellement sans renouveau? In *Le (non)renouvellement des élites en Afrique subsaharienne*, ed. Jean-Pascal Daloz, 99–133. Bordeaux: Centre d'Etude d'Afrique Noire.

——. 1999b. Introduction à la question du sida en Afrique: politique publique et dynamiques sociales. In *Politiques publiques du sida en Afrique*, ed. Dominque Kerouedan and Fred Eboko, 35–73. Travaux et Documents 61–62. Bordeaux: Centre d'Etude d'Afrique Noire.

——. 1999c. Logiques et contradictions internationales dans le champ du sida au Cameroun. *Autrepart, Le sida des autres*. Edition de l'Aube-Institut de Recherche pour le Développement, Paris 12 (December): 123–40.

——. 2000. Risque-sida, pouvoirs et sexualité: la puissance de l'etat en question au Cameroun. In *Le désarroi camerounais: l'épreuve de l'économie-monde*, ed. Georges Courade, 235–62. Paris: Karthala.

——. 2001. L'organisation de la lutte contre le sida au Cameroun: de la verticalité à la dispersion. In *Un système de santé en mutation: le cas du Cameroun*, ed. Marc-Eric Gruénais, 29–68. Bulletin de l'Association Euro-africaine pour l'Anthropologie du Changement Social et du Développement/Euro-African Association for the Anthropology of Social Change and Development, 21.

——. 2002. Pouvoirs, jeunesses et sida au Cameroun: politique publique, dynamiques sociales et constructions des sujets. PhD diss., Centre d'Etude d'Afrique Noire-Institut d'Etudes Politiques de Bordeaux, Bordeaux IV.

——. 2003. Le sida en Afrique: la perspective globale d'un drame local. In *Les pratiques de santé dans un monde globalisé*, ed. Isabelle Gobatto, 47–80. Paris, Karthala- Maison des Sciences de l'Homme of Aquitaine.

Fabing, D. 1998. Le sida en Ouganda: peut-on vaincre une épidémie sans traitements? Mémoire de Diplôme d'Etudes Supérieures Spécialisées: Développement et Coopération. Université Paris I – Panthéon-Sorbonne.

Fassin, Didier. 2000. Une crise épidémiologique dans les sociétés post-apartheid: Le sida en Afrique du Sud et en Namibie. *Afrique contemporaine* supplement: 105–35.

——. 2001. A global controversy. Paper presented at the Maison des Sciences de l'Homme of Aquitaine, Bordeaux.

——. 2002. Le sida comme cause politique: une controverse sud-africaine sur la scène global. Unpublished mimeograph.

Foucault, Michel. 1997. *Il faut défendre la société: cours au Collège de France, 1975–1976.* Collection Hautes Etudes. Paris: Gallimard/Seuil.

Galvan, Dennis. 2001. Political turnover and social change in Senegal. *Journal of Democracy* 12 (3): 51–62.

Geertz, C. 2003. L'idéologie comme système culturel. In *Cultures politiques*, ed. Daniel Cefaï, 39–91. Paris: Presses Universitaires de France.

Gruénais, Marc-Éric, ed. 1999. *L'organisation de la lutte contre le sida en Afrique: une problématique etat/société civile.* Report for the Agence Nationale de Recherche sur le sida/Institut de Recherche pour le Développement, Paris.

Hermet, Guy. 1993. *Les désenchantements de la liberté: la sortie des dictatures des années 1990.* Paris: Fayard.

Hugon, Philippe. 1996. Sortir de la récession et préparer l'après-pétrole: le préalable politique. *Politique Africaine* 62: 35–44.

Irwin, Alexander, Joyce Millen, and Dorothy Fallows. 2003. *Global AIDS: Myths and facts.* Cambridge, MA: South End Press.

Joint United Nations Program on HIV/AIDS (UNAIDS). 1999. Acting early to prevent AIDS: The case of Senegal. *UNAIDS best practice collection.* www.unaids.org/bestpractice/collection/country/senegal/senegal.html.

——. 2000a. *Le sida en Afrique pays par pays.* Geneva: UNAIDS.

——. 2000b. *Report on the global HIV/AIDS epidemic.* Geneva: UNAIDS.

——. 2001. *Le point sur l'épidémie de sida.* Geneva: UNAIDS.

——. 2002. *Le point sur l'épidémie de sida.* Geneva: UNAIDS.

——. 2004. *Report on the global AIDS epidemic.* http: //www.unaids.org/bangkok2004.html.

Kerouedan, Dominque, and Fred Eboko. 1999. *Politiques publiques du sida en Afrique.* Collection Travaux et Documents 61–62. Bordeaux: Centre d'Etude d'Afrique Noire.

Kingdon, John. 1984. *Agendas, alternatives and public policies*. Boston: Little Brown.

Low-Beer, Daniel, and Rand Stoneburner. 2004. Uganda and the challenge of HIV/AIDS. In *The political economy of AIDS in Africa*, ed. Nana Poku and Alan Whiteside, 165–90, Aldershot: Ashgate Publishers.

Marchand, Jacques. 1985. *La propagande de l'apartheid: quand l'Afrique du Sud se crée une image de marque*. Paris: Karthala.

Martin, D. C. 2001. Pratiques culturelles et organisations symboliques du politique. In *Cultures politiques*, ed. Daniel Cefaï, 117–36. Paris: Presses Universitaires de France.

Mbeki, Thabo. 2000. Untitled letter to world leaders. *New African* 397: 18–20.

Médard, J. F., ed. 1992. *Etats d'Afrique noir: formation, mécanismes et crises*. Paris: Karthala.

Mehler, A. 1997. Une transition qui n'a pas eu lieu. In *Transitions démocratiques africaines*, ed. Jean-Pascal Daloz and Patrick Quantin, 95–138. Paris: Karthala.

Moreux, C. 1982. Weber et la question de l'idéologie. *Sociologie et Sociétés* 14 (2): 9–31.

Msellati, Philippe, Laurent Vidal, and Jean-Paul Moatti, eds. 2001. *L'accès aux traitements du VIH/sida en Côte d'Iviore*. Evaluation de l'Initiative Onusiad/ Ministère Ivoirien de la Santé Publique: aspects économiques, sociaux et comportementaux. Paris: Agence Nationale de Recherche sur le Sida.

Muller, P. 2000. L'analyse cognitive des politiques publiques: vers une sociologie politique de l'action publique. *Revue Française de Science Politique* 50 (2): 189–207.

Otayek, René. 1997. Démocratie, culture politique, sociétés plurales: une approche comparative à partir de situations africaines. *Revue Française de Science Politique* 47 (6): 798–822.

Perrot, S. 1999. Les élites politiques ougandaises et le 'Mouvement': la génération Museveni. In *Le (non)renouvellement des élites en Afrique subsaharienne*, ed. Jean-Pascal Daloz, 77–98. Bordeaux: Centre d'Etude d'Afrique Noire.

Prunier, G., and B. Calas, eds. 1994. *L'Ouganda contemporain*. Paris: Karthala-Institut Français d'Afrique.

Raynaut, C., and F. Muhongayire. 1993. Chronique d'une mort annoncée: problèmes d'éthique et de méthode posés par la démarche anthropologique au suivi des familles touchées par le sida (autour du cas rwandais). In *Les sciences sociales face au sida – cas africains autour de l'exemple ivoirien*, ed. Jean-Pierre Dozon and Laurent Vidal, 299–324. Paris: GIDIS, ORSTOM.

Schoepf, Brooke Grundfest. 2001. International AIDS research in anthropology: Taking a critical perspective on a crisis. *Annual Review of Anthropology* 30 (October): 335–61.

Seytre, Bernard, and Willy Rozenbaum. 1993. *Sida: les secrets d'une polémique*. Paris: Presses Universitaires de France.

Sindjoun, L., and M. Vennesson. 2000. Unipolarité et integration régionale: l'Afrique du Sud et la 'renaissance africaine.' *Revue Française de Science Politique* 50 (5): 915–40.

The AIDS Support Organization (TASO). 2004. Background on organization. http://www.tasouganda.org.

United Nations Development Program (UNDP). 2004. *Human development report*. New York: Oxford Univ. Press.

Verboud, Mathieu. 1994. Ouganda: le sida dans sa seconde décennie. In *L'Ouganda contemporain*, ed. G. Prunier and B. Calas, 275–97. Paris: Karthala-Institut Français d'Afrique.

Chapter 4

AIDS, Politics, and NGOs in Zimbabwe

Jake Batsell

Academics, public policy makers, journalists, and activists who closely follow the impact of HIV/AIDS on sub-Saharan Africa often stress the critical role of nongovernmental organizations (NGOs) in confronting the pandemic.[1] The shrinking of state health services across the continent – a consequence of the 'hollowing of the state' caused by increased privatization and structural adjustment programs throughout the 1980s and 1990s – has placed much of the burden on NGOs to fill the gap (Mameli 1998; Turshen 1999; van de Walle 2001).[2] Since NGOs play a major role in the health sector already, it might seem that African governments would be eager to tap them for their skills and assistance in confronting AIDS. But for a variety of reasons, including political competition and a lack of resources, governments and AIDS-focused NGOs have been slow to form alliances in many African nations. In fact, relations between the two entities often have been contentious.

Such has been the case in Zimbabwe, where AIDS NGOs and the government have repeatedly clashed over territorial and financial matters and only recently have begun to work together to develop policies and programs in response to AIDS. The Zimbabwe case is a cautionary tale of how a political regime primarily concerned with preserving its own power can undermine the capacity of NGOs to respond to a public health crisis, either by overtly intimidating the NGO sector or by simply choosing not to fully engage NGOs in the fight against AIDS. While Uganda's success in reducing HIV infections demonstrates the importance of an early, multisectoral approach spearheaded by government at the highest levels (Barnett and Whiteside 2002, 319–23), Zimbabwe illustrates that the absence of such cooperation can allow a disease to spiral out of control. The first AIDS case in Zimbabwe was reported in 1985, yet for most of the 1990s, as HIV spread to over one-fifth of Zimbabwe's adult population, the government remained in denial about AIDS and failed to enlist the expertise and resources of its NGO community.

This chapter will provide an overview of the political efforts of AIDS-focused NGOs in Zimbabwe, based largely on a dozen interviews I conducted in Zimbabwe in 2000 with NGO representatives, public health officials, and political analysts. The NGO community in Zimbabwe consists of a wide spectrum of groups with varying resources, objectives, and domestic and international ties. In this chapter, I will focus mainly on indigenous organizations whose primary objective is responding to HIV/AIDS. These AIDS NGOs 'tend to be small, localized, and dispersed. Many rely on funding from Western governments or NGOs. This may force them to compete amongst themselves for the donors' largesse and to hamstring them politically by tying them to the funders' agendas' (Boone and Batsell 2001, 16).

Collectively, these AIDS NGOs form a community that has made only modest gains in the political arena. Not only have they faced obstacles imposed by an increasingly heavy-handed state, but they also have lacked political coordination. AIDS NGOs have been further limited in their impact because conservative social mores in Zimbabwe have discouraged open talk about AIDS. In recent years, the creation of a government AIDS tax has spurred AIDS NGOs to become more politically aggressive in lobbying the state. While those efforts have produced some policy victories, this chapter will show that AIDS NGOs continue to operate against a backdrop of state intimidation and a legacy of denial, which combine to curb their political clout.

By highlighting how politics has impacted responses to AIDS in Zimbabwe, I hope to make evident that the relationship between AIDS-focused NGOs and governments in Africa is a topic ripe for greater scrutiny by political science, and to encourage future work on the subject. As Mameli (1998, 2) writes:

> It is essential that researchers begin to analyze which background conditions, administrative techniques and organizational forms have worked most effectively at the national and international levels of political response as we continue to address this health crisis. Understanding the roots of success and failure in HIV/AIDS management thus far is key to plotting an effective policy path into the future.

Given the important role NGOs play in responding to Africans' medical needs, scholars and policy makers need to take a closer look at how NGOs can be incorporated into effective HIV/AIDS management strategies in Africa.

Political Dynamics between AIDS-focused NGOs and African Governments

Writing at the outset of the AIDS pandemic, Waite (1988, 156) predicted that NGO activity in Africa would play an important part in the campaign against AIDS. But she also warned that NGOs were likely to encounter resistance from the state 'as these organizations attempt to push their own mandates, and to do so in tandem with the changing policies of central governments.' This prediction proved to be the case in Kenya, where NGOs and the government clashed over NGO representation on the National AIDS Committee. Several

Kenyan NGO representatives initially were invited to sit on a subcommittee in charge of developing an AIDS prevention campaign, but they were eventually dropped because the government viewed them as 'a potential threat to what politicians perceived as the government's right to control of the agenda' (Lanegran and Hyden 1993, 251). In the early stages of the pandemic, authoritarian regimes such as the government of Daniel arap Moi in Kenya seemed to fear that if NGOs were given too prominent a role in developing AIDS policy and programs, they might commandeer the process altogether.

Discord also has characterized the relations between government and AIDS-related NGOs in South Africa. Friedman (*Mail and Guardian* [Johannesburg], 15 June 2000) has described the government-NGO relationship as 'in a word, hostile.' Among the most vocal groups has been the Treatment Action Campaign, which has gone so far as to file manslaughter charges against government ministers for presiding over thousands of AIDS-related deaths in South Africa (Associated Press, 20 March 2003). The passionate tactics of AIDS sufferers and activists are often an uncomfortable fit for traditional political protocol. 'NGOs may feel less concerned about the need to consider what is appropriate from a political point of view to say about the disease in public. Hence, government officials want to be the sole spokespersons on the subject' (Lanegran and Hyden 1993, 252). Over the past decade, relations between African governments and AIDS-related NGOs frequently have been acrimonious.

A notable exception to these tensions is Uganda, where President Yoweri Museveni created a nationwide plan in 1990 that enlisted government agencies, local and international NGOs, and international development and relief agencies in crafting and delivering public education and health services programs (Barnett and Whiteside 2002, 323). In Uganda, NGOs have been crucial contributors to outreach programs that deliver AIDS education to the country's predominantly rural population. The Joint United Nations Program on HIV/AIDS (UNAIDS) credits Uganda's inclusive prevention campaign with helping to substantially lower the country's HIV infection rate, which was estimated to be near 30 per cent in 1991 and is now around 4 per cent (UNAIDS 2002, 2; UNAIDS 2004). 'Despite practical limitations, the Ugandan government has been steadfast in opening opportunities for non-state entities to become involved with treating the ill of this pandemic' (Mameli 1998, 124). Do relations between AIDS NGOs and the government in Zimbabwe follow the participatory model of Uganda or the more contentious pattern of Kenya and South Africa?

Politics and HIV/AIDS in Zimbabwe

Zimbabwe is one of the world's most severely AIDS-stricken countries. The HIV infection rate had reached 24.6 per cent by the end of 2003 (UNAIDS 2004). The United Nations Development Program reports that a child born today in Zimbabwe is expected to live to be 33 years old, down sharply from a life expectancy of 67.5 years prior to the arrival of AIDS (*Financial Gazette* [Harare], 24 July 2003). Infant mortality is now 72 per cent higher than it would have been without AIDS (Republic of Zimbabwe 2002, 3). The back pages of daily newspapers in Harare and Bulawayo are replete with death notices, many accompanied by haunting photographs of young people cut off in their prime.

During the 1980s and 1990s, as structural adjustment programs decimated public health services, Zimbabweans came to rely more on the private sector for health care (Turshen 1999, 32–36). State spending on health dropped from 2.6 per cent of gross domestic product in 1980 to 2.2 per cent in 1997 (Republic of Zimbabwe 2002, 5). By 2001, this percentage had somewhat increased, to 2.8 per cent (UNDP 2004, 158). Structural adjustment policies were accompanied by the proliferation of health-related NGOs, many with connections to parent agencies from Western countries. Turshen (1999, 35–36) cites a 1991 study by the World Health Organization that found that NGOs provided 94 per cent of health-related services for the elderly in Zimbabwe, and church missions supplied 35 per cent of all institutional beds, including nearly 70 per cent of beds in rural areas. In 2001, the private sector accounted for 54.7 per cent of total spending on health care in Zimbabwe, with government spending accounting for the remaining 45.3 per cent (WHO 2003). Outside the formal health-care sector, there has been a formidable effort by NGOs at the grassroots level to educate and care for local populations afflicted by AIDS.[3]

Public health services, meanwhile, have been hampered not only by severely limited government funding, but also by plummeting manpower as a direct result of the disease. 'Our staff are dying', said Christina Nkomo, assistant director for the city of Bulawayo's Health Services Department (interview with author, 13 July 2000). 'They are experienced, educated staff, but they are like the rest of the population – 25 per cent is infected. We have very, very good people who are dying. We send people for training that aren't completing it, because they get sick.' In July 2000, about 100 of 400 staff positions at the Bulawayo Health Services Department were unfilled, primarily because of AIDS.

Despite the severity of the catastrophe, AIDS received little attention in Zimbabwean politics throughout the 1990s, and the government did not engage NGOs in the fight against the disease as infection rates soared. In the latter part of the decade, NGOs began to lobby the state more aggressively, and actually did register some modest victories, including mandatory AIDS education in elementary schools and a law prohibiting employers from firing a worker for being HIV positive. Still, NGOs were unable to persuade the ruling political party, President Robert Mugabe's Zimbabwe African National Union-Patriotic Front (ZANU-PF), to increase overall government spending on AIDS amid increasing inflation and economic chaos in Zimbabwe. The director of the government's National AIDS Program admitted in 1999 that state spending on AIDS prevention had, in real terms, 'certainly not increased and probably declined' since 1995 (Schoofs 1999). To tackle the unrelenting onslaught of AIDS in the twenty-first century, Zimbabwe would have to find alternative sources of funding.

The AIDS Levy

In January 2000, the government began collecting a tax of 3 per cent from workers and corporations to raise funds for AIDS care and prevention, partly because of NGO pressure that was manifested through petitions, public marches, and advocacy campaigns. Groups of people living with HIV/AIDS were the most vocal and demonstrative, while other NGOs took a quieter route and lobbied government officials behind the scenes.

The tax, known as the 'AIDS levy' throughout Zimbabwe, was welcomed by many NGOs and AIDS activists. But controversy swiftly erupted, when it was reported in April 2000 that the fund's bank account was empty, despite assurances from the government that funds would be transferred to the account immediately after being collected. After a boisterous public outcry, the government deposited nearly $4.5 million into the fund's coffers (*Financial Gazette* [Harare], 27 April 2000).[4]

By July 2000, the tax had raised more than $13 million for the newly created national AIDS fund, to be overseen by the National AIDS Council (NAC) (*Herald* [Harare], 4 July 2000). Once the money was available, the question of who would decide how to divide the funds quickly became a hotly contested issue. President Mugabe appointed a dozen members to the council's board of trustees. Board members were chosen from a variety of sectors, including public health, farmers' unions, the legal fraternity, civic organizations, traditional healers, business, the media, schools, youth, and people living with HIV/AIDS. However, only three of the 12 appointees had connections to NGOs, and only one representative was from an organization primarily focused on HIV/AIDS. The remaining two NGO appointments went to a traditional healers association and the commercial farmers' union. In March 2001, the government briefly disbanded the original NAC board (*New York Times*, 19 August 2001), although the board later resumed control of the fund and continues to distribute money for AIDS-related projects. Meanwhile, NGO representatives were appointed to three of the 17 slots on Zimbabwe's Country Coordinating Mechanism, which distributes proceeds granted by the Global Fund to Fight AIDS, Tuberculosis and Malaria (Republic of Zimbabwe 2002, 9–10).

The original appointments to the NAC board revealed the tensions between the government and NGOs in Zimbabwe. The AIDS-focused NGO community was livid at the board's composition and circulated a petition demanding that the government add more seats for NGO representatives. An NGO administrator said, 'We are the people actually doing the job, and our opinions are not being really listened to ... these exclusions from the AIDS council board are a clear indication that government doesn't feel like it wants to work with the NGOs.' This administrator said board members from fields such as business and the legal profession lack expertise on AIDS and may not channel funds to the right places. 'We feel that as NGOs who are working in the AIDS field, we know where this money is needed' (interview with author, 13 July 2000).[5] NGOs argued that because they bring specific knowledge, information, and experience to the fight against AIDS, they should be given a leading role in distributing funds; they should not be put on equal footing with individuals in fields that have had little direct contact with the disease. However, giving AIDS NGOs a larger say in HIV/AIDS policy and funding represents a political threat to the state, limiting its ability to control the agenda. And from the state's perspective, giving equal billing to other organizations with little AIDS expertise effectively dilutes the power that AIDS NGOs can wield.

In July 2000, an official from Zimbabwe's national AIDS program – which has since been folded into the NAC – disputed the notion that the government intentionally shunned NGOs in appointing members to the board, saying that NGOs were 'very well-represented. They signed a petition, and we just ignored it … I don't know if they wanted the whole board to be NGOs. We wanted that board to be multisectoral.' The central problem, the official said, was that NGO representatives wanted to dominate the process and collect most of the funds from the AIDS levy, while the government preferred to give the funds to district AIDS action committees. 'Our thinking is that the funding should go directly to the communities, because then the money will go directly to the beneficiaries. With NGOs, most money goes toward salaries, cars, or petrol' (government official, interview with author, 28 July 2000). This argument would surface again two years later, when Frenk Guni, a prominent AIDS NGO leader and NAC board member, was accused by the government of misappropriating AIDS levy funds granted to his organization.

The issue of whether NGOs allocate their resources effectively is indeed a legitimate question, as they are susceptible to excessive overhead expenses, mismanagement, and even corruption. Van de Walle (2001, 165) observes that some donor-funded NGOs in Africa have fallen victim to a degree of corruption 'that certainly rivals corruption within the state'. But in Zimbabwe, channeling the AIDS levy funds through district AIDS committees – the approach ultimately adopted by the government – also has not been efficient, and has added layers of bureaucracy that have slowed the disbursement of funds. In August 2003, the NAC announced that nearly $10 million of AIDS levy funds were lying idle because the 80 district AIDS committees, run largely by village residents, had not yet completed the proper accounting procedures for previous allotments (*Herald* [Harare], 15 August 2003). Activists also have complained that district committee members with ties to the ruling party have been the most frequent beneficiaries of the AIDS levy. 'The funds are benefiting ZANU-PF members and not those people who need them,' said Dominica Banure, a district representative for the Zimbabwe National Network of People Living with HIV/AIDS (ZNNP+) (*Financial*

Gazette [Harare], 4 July 2002). In late 2002, the country's leading opposition party, the Movement for Democratic Change (MDC), publicly demanded an independent audit of the fund, citing lapses in its transparency and accountability (Chebundo 2002). A year later, AIDS NGOs were still pressing for an audit (*Daily News* [Harare], 16 May 2003).

The levy is still actively collected in Zimbabwe, and the NAC has made a number of large payouts from the fund, including more than $18 million for antiretroviral drugs for Zimbabweans suffering from AIDS and millions more to district committees for food, home-based care kits, and school uniforms for children orphaned by AIDS (*Financial Gazette* [Harare], 4 April 2002, 29 August 2002). In 2002, each of the 80 district committees was given more than $375,000 from the fund (Republic of Zimbabwe 2002, 5). The NAC also provided approximately $37,000 to the army for HIV/AIDS military training in 2003 (*Herald* [Harare], 4 July 2003).

However, NGOs and other government watchdogs charge that the government has selectively distributed funds from the AIDS levy for political advantage. Before the March 2002 presidential elections, the government suspended disbursements to the district AIDS committees, citing the committees' inability to properly handle the funds. Proceeds from the AIDS levy were instead diverted to district councils dominated by ZANU-PF party structures – a move that critics said allowed government officials to use the AIDS levy as a form of political patronage as the election approached (*Financial Gazette* [Harare], 15 November 2001). In addition, the $18 million disbursement for antiretroviral drugs in 2002 came a month after Mugabe was reelected and was seen by local journalists as a step toward delivery of a ZANU-PF campaign promise to make such drugs available to individuals with AIDS (*Financial Gazette* [Harare], 4 April 2002). At times, Mugabe and ZANU-PF have used the AIDS levy as a political weapon, much to the chagrin of the NGOs who pressed for the levy in the first place.

The government's prudence in spending state funds also can be viewed with skepticism when considering that from 1998 to 2002, as AIDS infections were escalating and the country grappled with a financial crisis, Mugabe spent billions of Zimbabwe dollars – well over $550 million, by one journalist's measure – to send thousands of Zimbabwean soldiers to support the government of the Democratic Republic of Congo in its civil war (*Business Day* [South Africa], 30 August 2002). Most of the Zimbabwean forces were withdrawn in late 2002. Even aside from the Congo war expenditures, the state has spent lavishly on perks for government officials, including $3.7 million for a fleet of new Mercedes Benz cars for Mugabe's ministers (*Zimbabwe Independent,* 28 July 2000).

A New Emphasis on NGO Advocacy and Reactions by the State

The creation of the AIDS levy in 1999 spurred AIDS NGOs to increase their political lobbying efforts, building on their earlier policy victories in the arenas of education and labor. The Zimbabwe AIDS Network created an Advocacy Task Force in May 2000, and organized a workshop to train NGO representatives to lobby the government and media more effectively. At the workshop, organizers distributed advocacy handbooks and held sessions covering topics such as how to develop and deliver policy messages and how to write effective letters to decision makers.

Such workshops have continued, and there is reason to believe they have helped NGOs become more politically savvy. In 2001, Zimbabwe's Parliament passed the Sexual Offenses Act, which criminalized the deliberate transmission of HIV and marital rape (Agence France Presse, 24 August 2001). This was a landmark policy victory for the AIDS NGO community in a patriarchal society where women often contract HIV from their husbands. NGOs also collaborated with the government to produce a draft National Plan of Action for Orphans and Vulnerable Children, which seeks to establish a safety net for AIDS orphans (United Nations Relief and Recovery Unit 2003). A number of AIDS NGOs have become more outspoken and have challenged the government when quoted in the local media.

While these advocacy efforts have produced some successes, critics argue that AIDS NGOs have often been too timid in their dealings with government. As University of Zimbabwe population studies professor Marvellous Mhloyi said, 'There hasn't been an NGO which has really endeavored to put HIV/AIDS on the political agenda as an area of debate, to really push on it continuously and persistently. We need somebody who has a passion for it to speak about it ... we need action – somebody who will just get out and do it' (interview with author, 5 July 2000). In the same year, a US embassy official observed that 'there's no ACT UP in Zimbabwe. Nobody's out there making a big fuss about it. It's all very quiet' (interview with author, 29 June 2000).[6]

The ACT UP comparison is an interesting analogy. The United States has a longstanding tradition of voluntary organizations in civil society; in the health arena, campaigns to bring awareness to diseases such as cancer and polio are prime examples. African postcolonial societies, meanwhile, 'have seen few enduring mobilizations around health issues' and lack a strong legacy of civic activism (Misztal and Moss 1989, 240). That is not to say that public protests regarding health policy do not occur in Africa, but such protests have been slow to gain widespread legitimacy in African societies. And a host of African leaders like Mugabe, preoccupied with maintaining a veneer of national unity, have shown a penchant for clamping down hard on dissidents of any sort.

Mugabe's government has increasingly sought to stifle NGOs since 1995, when it passed the Private Voluntary Organizations (PVO) Act. The act requires NGOs to register with the government and gives ministers the power to 'suspend' NGO officials from their administrative duties whenever 'it is necessary to do so in the public interest' (Raftopolous 2000, 36). The government took things a step further in 2002 with the Public Order and Security Act, which requires NGOs to receive advance clearance from the government for meetings and workshops (*Zimbabwe Standard*, 22 June

2003). Leading opposition and civil society figures have fled Zimbabwe in recent years after reportedly receiving death threats from state security agents. Civic activists taking part in street protests to call for constitutional reforms have been arrested and taken away in vans by baton-wielding riot police (Voice of America News, 22 October 2003). In late 2004, the parliament was poised to pass legislation that would restrict NGOs – including AIDS NGOs – from receiving direct funding from organizations with any employees who are not citizens of Zimbabwe (*Christian Science Monitor*, 27 August 2004). Thus, while AIDS NGOs have become more active and better trained in their advocacy efforts, they continue to operate against a backdrop of political cooptation and repression aimed at civil society as a whole.

When told about the US embassy official's remark that 'there's no ACT UP in Zimbabwe', an NGO administrator responded:

> Remember that we are being threatened indirectly through the PVO act and all those other things … In the end, we might be compelled by the people to join them and be more ACT UP. But right now, ACT UP? No. We wouldn't want to try and get on anybody's wrong side right now. At the end of the day, you have to [ask], 'Will me standing up and jumping on tables, will it really help the man in the street?' My main concern is helping the clients – they are the main thing. Jumping in front of the president's car, I don't know if it will really help in the long, long run (interview with author, 13 July 2000).

As the political climate in Zimbabwe grew increasingly precarious for NGOs in 2002, Edith Masunda, chairperson of the Zimbabwe AIDS Network (ZAN), advised fellow AIDS NGOs against adversarial relations with the government. 'The political situation in the country has made it necessary to follow a cautious path in advocacy', Masunda told delegates at the network's annual meeting. 'We believe it is more conducive at present to network and build alliances with other stakeholders, than to confront the government head-on as this could backfire on ZAN' (*Daily News* [Harare], 25 October 2002). Being too outspoken could trigger harassment from the government, risking the very survival of organizations whose primary mission is to serve those suffering from AIDS in local communities.

In addition, the dearth of health services in Zimbabwe leaves public and private health organizations with such a Herculean task in responding to AIDS, there is often little time to worry about lobbying the state. 'At work, I don't think we even think of [politics],' said Annah Mpatsi, sister-in-charge of the Zimbabwe Family Planning Council's Matabeleland North community division. 'You are just thinking of giving quality care to the clients – that's all you really think about, how you can improve in giving quality care' (interview with author, 13 July 2000).

Zimbabwean NGOs, particularly those composed of individuals with AIDS, occasionally have deployed radical tactics. Frenk Guni, the former national coordinator for ZNNP+, is a rare example of a Zimbabwean activist who dared to cross the line between polite, respectful dissent and confrontational, disruptive behavior. Guni described how he and dozens of ZNNP+ members stood in the path of Mugabe and his entourage in December 1999, preventing the president from leaving a downtown Harare hotel after he had presided over a ceremony launching the long-awaited national HIV/AIDS policy. 'We blocked him from leaving the place until he had an audience with us. That's when he saw that we were very serious. The secret forces were there, but we told them to shoot us' (interview with author, 27 July 2000).

The combative approach apparently worked. Mugabe eventually agreed to meet with ZNNP+ and Guni was later named as the sole representative from an AIDS-focused NGO to the NAC board. Guni, who like all ZNNP+ members is HIV positive, said 'sometimes we had to go to the extreme to get to where we are. But at least now we are in a position where we can dialogue with the government. They now recognize us. They know us, they accept us, they know we are there. They know we are not just a force to be pushed aside' (interview with author, 27 July 2000). Guni, however, is no longer a leading voice in the Zimbabwean community of AIDS NGOs. In March 2002, several months after leaving Zimbabwe to seek medical treatment in the United States, Guni was accused in the state-run newspaper of misappropriating more than $750,000 of his organization's funds, some of which he allegedly used to buy houses for himself (*Herald* [Harare], 7 March 2002). ZNNP+ was the largest single recipient of funds from the AIDS levy in 2001, receiving approximately $1.8 million. The charges, true or not, tarnished the credibility of ZNNP+, and Guni is now living under political asylum in the United States (*Boston Globe*, 31 May 2003). The episode evoked the government's oft-used criticism that NGO leaders use their organizations as a means to gain access to external resources.

The flamboyant tactics exercised by Guni and other ZNNP+ members are redolent of the confrontational protest methods used by ACT UP in the United States in the 1980s, and lend credence to the belief that activists who personally suffer from a disease are more likely to break conventional norms in their political activities. Jennings and Anderson (1996, 330) argue that while suffering has always been a central source of motivation for disruptive behavior in most social movements, 'the pain and threat associated with bodily harm and death appears to carry a special potency', emboldening activists to push the envelope. Such extreme tactics have sometimes been necessary for activists to get their point across in Zimbabwe, where the government has restricted civil society through laws such as the Public Order and Security Act, has used police to break up marches and protests, and has taken measures to curtail Zimbabwe's judiciary.

Eliot Magunje, another outspoken activist with AIDS in Zimbabwe, conveyed his passion for involving NGOs in the fight against AIDS during an interview in 2000, when he was a counselor and information officer for a Harare-based AIDS hospice organization called The Center. 'We are still going to take it up seriously with the government that NGOs get a meaningful role, not sort of a "get down there and listen". We want a meaningful role where members will be in a position to be involved in policy formulation and implementation' (interview with author, 27 July 2000). Magunje died in 2003.

Another outspoken organization, the Zimbabwe Activists on HIV and AIDS (ZAHA), was formed in 2003 to advocate for the universal treatment of individuals with HIV/AIDS in Zimbabwe. ZAHA was vocal during US President George W. Bush's trip to Africa in July 2003, issuing a press release urging Bush to set politics aside and 'put Zimbabwe on his map on HIV/AIDS intervention' (ZAHA 2003). ZAHA has taken on the Mugabe administration as well. After the Ministry of Health announced that the country's adult HIV infection rate had decreased to 24.9 per cent (Agence France Presse, 21 August 2003), ZAHA challenged the credibility of the data, saying the government's survey was plagued by 'hazy' methodology and sharply differed with projections from the Joint United Nations Program on HIV/AIDS (*Zimbabwe Standard*, 5 October 2003).[7] ZAHA has publicly called for the government to make antiretroviral treatment more accessible and affordable for people with AIDS (*Zimbabwe Standard*, 4 August 2003). In its first year of existence, ZAHA proved to be a bold voice in the arena of AIDS policy, challenging government at both the domestic and international level.

A Legacy of Denial and Inaction

As HIV infections skyrocketed in Zimbabwe in the 1990s, the government largely swept AIDS under the carpet, making it more difficult for AIDS NGOs to make headway against the conservative mores of Zimbabwean society. Mugabe kept silent on AIDS until April 1999, when he publicly acknowledged for the first time that the virus was a national epidemic, with more than 1,200 Zimbabweans dying each week from the disease (*Los Angeles Times*, 19 April 1999). A US embassy official said, 'President Mugabe, although he will occasionally wear an AIDS ribbon, has never taken the sort of leadership stance that President Museveni in Uganda has, talking openly about the problem. The minister of health has, at times, spoken bluntly and honestly about the problem in productive ways. But his tack here seems to be to downplay it, to try to persuade people that no, it's not as the West says it is.' The US official observed that, 15 years after HIV arrived in Zimbabwe, AIDS NGOs in Zimbabwe were still:

> struggling to get the government to sort of step up and acknowledge the magnitude of the problem. But perhaps more importantly, the AIDS NGOs are struggling to get this very conservative society to deal with the problem. ... Just read the newspapers for a couple of weeks – so and so died after a long illness, so and so died after a short illness. In the background, people are whispering, 'It was the virus.'

> But that will not be publicly acknowledged. There's still a stigma attached to HIV/AIDS which is deeply uncomfortable for the vast majority of Zimbabweans (US embassy official, interview with author, 29 June 2000).

Not only foreign observers have reached this assessment. University of Zimbabwe Professor Mhloyi said, 'We have persistent denial in Zimbabwe, which is anchored in high-level puritanical views about society – views which are so puritanical that they are unachievable in real life' (interview with author, 5 July 2000). Consider the sentiment voiced by the state-run *Herald*, the nation's largest newspaper, in a 4 July 2000 editorial on AIDS. 'This is one area where a Government can do very little. It cannot stop people living dangerous lifestyles ... young men and women die in vast numbers because they have been indulging in risky sexual experimentation and lifestyles in their later teens and twenties.' This one-dimensional argument disregards, among other things, how Zimbabwean customs have created the perception among many married men that they are entitled to have affairs, resulting in a considerable number of HIV infections transmitted to unknowing wives, or from infected mothers to infants. But these deeply ingrained cultural roots may be exactly why the government ignored AIDS for so long. As Fredland (1998, 562) observes, government reticence on AIDS in Africa stems in part from pragmatism, since no sensible political leader would want to spend his or her time scolding people through public education campaigns about a disease 'that can only be prevented by wholesale behavioral changes' which are 'unlikely to reach fruition during any given leader's tenure in office'.

Because AIDS NGOs are generally small and fragmented, they cannot be expected to spur widespread behavioral change by themselves. Only the government has the capacity to mount a nationwide response effort, and to harness the expertise of NGOs as part of that effort. 'Governments, after all, possess the capacity to mobilize and allocate resources, to coordinate national education programs, to appeal for international funding, to supply materials such as condoms and self-destruct syringes to reduce the spread of the disease, and to supply or subsidize the cost of drug therapies' (Boone and Batsell 2001, 8). A report compiled by UNAIDS (2000, 25) observes that nearly two decades of worldwide experience in responding to HIV/AIDS has taught us 'that when governments commit their political prestige and financial resources, involve civil society fully, emphasize prevention and care, and support activities in a range of sectors, they are able to limit the spread of the epidemic and mitigate the impact.'

Since 2000, Mugabe and his administration have gradually begun to speak more openly of HIV/AIDS. In his opening address at Zimbabwe's Parliament in July 2003, Mugabe identified the disease as the country's foremost challenge (United Nations Relief and Recovery Unit 2003). A year earlier, at a UNAIDS forum in Geneva, his wife Grace Mugabe called HIV/AIDS 'the greatest threat to Zimbabwe's social and economic development since independence' (*Herald* [Harare], 18 July 2002). Health

Minister David Parirenyatwa, who took office in 2002, constantly stresses the government's commitment to fighting AIDS in speeches and when quoted in local media.

Still, many observers view the government's recent change in candor as a textbook case of too little, too late. Despite the devastating consequences AIDS has wrought in Zimbabwe, the disease remains on the periphery of the political landscape. HIV/AIDS was not a major focus for either party during the parliamentary elections of 2000 or the presidential campaign in 2002, when the prominent issues were land reform, the plummeting economy, and transparent governance. Professor Mhloyi (interview with author, 5 July 2000) was aghast that neither ZANU-PF nor the opposition MDC made AIDS a central issue in its platform. 'If I were to stand up and campaign today, my number one priority would be HIV/AIDS before I get to anything else. You can't have development without people. To me, that's the core or the center of any developmental debate.'

Obstacles to the Political Efficacy of AIDS NGOs

An additional obstacle for NGOs seeking to engage the Zimbabwean state on AIDS policies is the nature of civil society itself. Civil society in Africa is notoriously weak, hampered by the legacy of colonial rule and by post-independence governments' repression or cooptation of civic groups (van de Walle 2001, 47–48). Across Africa, when it comes to AIDS, 'NGO political capacity may be very low in general. Political science may be over-generalizing when it identifies these groups as agents of political reform or democratization' (Boone and Batsell 2001, 16–17). Many, if not most, NGOs in Africa lack resources and coordination, and these weaknesses are only further exacerbated by government intimidation. The specter of state repression is by far the largest obstacle facing AIDS NGOs in Zimbabwe. But a number of other dynamics bedevil the country's AIDS NGOs.

Lack of Cohesion among AIDS NGOs

In interviews, many NGO representatives emphasized the need to establish common ground and then engage the government as a united front. As one NGO administrator said, 'We end up competing against each other, duplicating what each other is doing, scared that you will steal my idea, personalities clashing' (interview with author, 13 July 2000). More cooperation among AIDS NGOs ultimately could lead toward better cooperation with the government in fighting HIV/AIDS. Aulora Stally, formerly of the Southern Africa Aids Information Dissemination Service (SAfAIDS), commented, 'Government in itself needs to certainly get its act together and put HIV/AIDS on the public agenda, and we definitely need more political commitment. But I think as AIDS NGOs, we also have to really galvanize our efforts and come together as one body, rather than several different individual bodies' (interview with author, 26 July 2000).

Such efforts to come together must be spearheaded by NGOs themselves, since the government would prefer to keep them splintered. ZAN has made some progress in this regard, emerging as a strong umbrella organization for AIDS NGOs in recent years. To a lesser extent, the National Association of Non-Governmental Organizations (NANGO) also has sought to coordinate the efforts of AIDS NGOs. NANGO has been working to update the national HIV/AIDS policy with segments on antiretroviral drugs and medications that reduce mother-to-child HIV transmission.

Duplication of Efforts among AIDS NGOs

Some 200 AIDS NGOs currently operate in Zimbabwe, and many of them are performing similar tasks. Some suggest that AIDS NGOs should consult with each other to come up with the best possible division of labor. 'Rather than duplicating efforts and channeling money to five NGOs that are doing the same work, why don't those NGOs come together and say, this is what we want the money for, and it gets channeled to them and then divided? There's a lot of duplication, and that may cause problems. Because if my organization is going to advocate for prevention and care, and the organization down the road is doing the same thing, I don't think government will take you seriously' (Aulora Stally, interview with author, 26 July 2000).

In recent years, organizations from the broader NGO community have launched their own HIV/AIDS efforts. For instance, in 2003 the Zimbabwe National Mental Health Association established its first AIDS program. While these are worthwhile endeavors, they also heighten the potential for duplication of HIV/AIDS programs among NGOs, and underscore the need for careful coordination to guard against redundancies.

Overreliance on Foreign Aid by AIDS NGOs

During my interviews, a consensus emerged that while NGOs should continue to tap into international resources, they should simultaneously seek ways to become more self-sustainable. On the one hand, no African country can afford to shun the international community when it comes to fighting AIDS, and there is little question that Zimbabwe simply cannot handle the epidemic by itself. Frenk Guni (interview with author, 27 July 2000) said, 'We need that support, whether we like it or not, whether it comes with political strings, whatever.' Where money for fighting AIDS comes from 'is irrelevant to us. Because we are saying, "we are dying." We need political commitment and external support.' Pointing out the recent establishment of the Global Fund, Guni said it was up to NGOs to lobby the state to claim Zimbabwe's fair share of that money. 'It's for us now to push our government, to say, "Please, take this opportunity".' In 2002, Zimbabwe was awarded

$22.9 million from the Global Fund, to be released in installments over two years to the NAC (Panafrican News Agency, 27 April 2002). In Zimbabwe's proposal to the Global Fund, money was earmarked for government ministries, church-related hospitals, and an unspecified number of NGOs to develop youth behavior-change programs, to establish voluntary counseling and testing centers, to expand programs for prevention of mother-to-child transmission, and to increase the availability of antiretroviral therapies (Republic of Zimbabwe 2002). The proposal did not specify how much money would be channeled to NGOs, but said 'perhaps 25 per cent' would go to NGOs and other organs of civil society, all of which would be required to undergo 'full financial accounting backed by a recognized accounting firm, plus external audits' (Republic of Zimbabwe 2002, 17).

AIDS NGOs cannot rely solely on donors if these NGOs hope to remain sustainable in the long run. They also must find innovative ways to generate funds for themselves. The recent exodus of international donors because of Zimbabwe's worsening political and economic crisis has highlighted the fact that AIDS NGOs must become less reliant on external sources. For example, Zimbabwe was notably excluded from President Bush's proposed $15 billion package for AIDS relief in 12 African countries (Associated Press, 30 January 2003), most likely because the United States has been at odds with Mugabe's government over human-rights abuses, alleged election fraud, and the seizure of commercial farms owned by white Zimbabweans. In another example, on 12 August 2004, the *New York Times* reported that donors, including the Global Fund, have refused to provide resources for AIDS to the country because of their distrust of Mugabe. With foreign governments and private-sector donors shunning Zimbabwe, sources of NGO funding have dwindled, a fact which has pitted NGOs against each other and against the government for resources.

There are several promising examples of income-generating projects among NGOs in Zimbabwe. SAfAIDS, funded by a variety of international donors, now provides consulting services and strategic planning for other organizations, develops company AIDS policies, and produces outside publications. Income-generating activities are targeted to make up 11 per cent of the organization's annual budget – a modest share for the time being, but an encouraging sign for the future. In addition, the Matabeleland AIDS Council in Bulawayo now offers HIV/AIDS training programs for small businesses. Members of this organization view this venture as both a fund-raising opportunity and a way to further the council's educational mission.

Indigenous NGOs in Zimbabwe also are wary of what they perceive to be a 'one-size-fits-all' mindset among foreign donors. While the experiences of Uganda, Senegal, and Thailand are praiseworthy, carbon copies of those countries' programs are not sufficient to curb the AIDS epidemic in Zimbabwe. To be sure, Zimbabwe can learn from successes achieved elsewhere, but ultimately government and NGOs must work together at the grassroots level to design the best possible AIDS programs for their own country.

'USAID, they want to make a model that you can take from Uganda and replicate it here in Zimbabwe. … We keep on telling them, "Look, this is not Uganda. Here, we don't do things like that". In Zimbabwe, the situation is different. People are more hidden about the epidemic; they're not so open' (NGO administrator, interview with author, 13 July 2000). Guni agreed, explaining that 'the practices of women in Thailand are not the same as here in Zimbabwe. So we have to develop our own innovations, based on our environment and the system around us. It's good to borrow ideas, but tailor-make them to suit our environment' (interview with author, 27 July 2000).

The impulse against foreign meddling has taken on new meaning in Zimbabwe since 2000. The political climate has been dominated by an anti-Western discourse stemming from US and British disapproval of Mugabe's decision to expel hundreds of white farmers, as well as by diplomatic flare-ups over alleged fraud during the 2002 presidential elections. In light of these developments, there is more resistance than ever in Zimbabwe to the idea of foreign solutions for local problems.

Recognizing developing countries' concerns about international domination, UNAIDS formed an International Partnership against AIDS in Africa emphasizing indigenous 'ownership and leadership' at all levels. The partnership, created in May 2000 as a precursor to the United Nations General Assembly Special Session (UNGASS) on HIV/AIDS, listed eight bedrock principles, the first of which was to allow 'country and community priorities to drive the action … implementation plans will be based on local priorities and contexts' (UNAIDS 2000, 26). A year later, UNGASS delegates crafted the Declaration of Commitment prescribing, among other things, 'a wide range of prevention programmes which take account of local circumstances, ethics and cultural values' (UNGASS 2001). Whether the rhetoric ultimately meets reality remains to be seen, but UNAIDS at least appears to intellectually recognize the pitfalls of imposing 'one-size-fits-all' remedies that neglect the nuances of individual cultures.

Conclusion

The three obstacles mentioned above – lack of cohesion, duplication of efforts, and overreliance on foreign aid – present substantial challenges to Zimbabwe's AIDS NGOs. These obstacles have prodded NGOs to come up with innovative ways to become more effective. But none of these NGO initiatives are likely to have a broad impact on society without the cooperation of a receptive government. A government like Mugabe's, which passes laws to intimidate NGOs and allegedly has used funds from the AIDS levy as a form of political patronage, can severely compound the internal problems that the NGO community already faces. And because AIDS-focused NGOs tend to be small and localized, they do not possess the political power wielded by other NGOs such as labor unions and professional associations, which 'operate in economically strategic sectors and have institutional infrastructures of national scope' (Boone and Batsell 2001, 17). AIDS NGOs are unlikely to sway the government through any sort of political clout – their advocacy efforts are based mainly on moral and humanitarian grounds, and their collective capacity relies largely on how much room the government gives them to operate.

In contrast to Uganda, where the government enthusiastically sought the help of NGOs in responding to AIDS, Zimbabwe illustrates that years of denial and a reluctance to collaborate can lead to disastrous consequences. As one prominent Zimbabwean NGO wrote in a recent policy analysis, 'Where our collective responses [to HIV/AIDS] needed to be guided by a robust, large scale, multi-sector strategy that incorporated the diverse needs and concerns of the most marginalized and deprived groups of women and men; denial, stigma, blame, fear, and selfishness have largely been the order of the day' (Tichagwa 2003, 4). Mugabe is now discussing AIDS more openly, but his government's slow-footed and denial-ridden response to AIDS in the 1990s caused the loss of incalculable lives. Aside from the economic catastrophe and political violence that Mugabe's government has foisted on its citizens in recent years, this legacy of inaction will haunt generations of Zimbabweans for years to come.

In a snapshot that illustrates the maddening inefficiency of AIDS prevention efforts in Zimbabwe, consider the fate of a multisectoral committee called the National Behavior Change Communication Strategy, headed by the Ministry of Information. Designed to create programs to work with the media on AIDS education campaigns, the committee formed in 1998. But years later, the committee was shelved after never having held a single meeting.

If Zimbabwe is to overcome the HIV/AIDS epidemic, the state will have to overcome its fear of losing control of the agenda and fully engage AIDS-focused NGOs in the fight against the disease, combining the unparalleled reach and resources of the government with the NGOs' invaluable on-the-ground expertise. As United Nations Secretary General Kofi Annan observed, Zimbabwe's predicament with AIDS 'is caused partly by the forces of nature and partly by mismanagement. We could debate endlessly which of them made the greater contribution, but the challenge now is for all Zimbabweans to work together, with each other and with the international community, to find solutions before it is too late' (Agence France Presse, 14 January 2003).

Notes

1 This chapter is an updated version of a paper first presented at the African Studies Association Conference in Nashville, Tennessee, on 16 November 2000. The paper was later incorporated into an article co-written with Catherine Boone. See Boone and Batsell (2001). The author's field work in June and July of 2000 was funded in part by generous grants from the Institute for International Education and the University Co-Operative Society in Austin, Texas.

2 For an overview of the 'hollow state' theory as it applies to the HIV/AIDS issue, see Mameli (1998). In addition, Turshen (1999) describes how structural adjustment programs shifted much of the delivery of health services from governments to NGOs in Zimbabwe, Zambia, Mozambique, and Malawi. Van de Walle (2001, 165) provides a broad overview of how NGOs came 'to undertake activities that used to be a state responsibility.'

3 One example is the Insiza Godlwayo AIDS Council, which operates in a rural pocket of southern Zimbabwe. In 1999, this organization had 500 active volunteers, as well as another 500 individuals who assist as needed. For a comparative perspective, Schoofs (1999) reported that the largest AIDS organization in New York City, the Gay Men's Health Crisis, had 500 home-care volunteers in 1994, the year before new drugs began to lower the AIDS death rate in the United States.

4 Hyperinflation has rapidly and drastically reduced the value of Zimbabwe's currency in recent years. In April 2000, the official exchange rate was roughly 38 Zimbabwe dollars to one US dollar; by September 2004, the rate was more than 5,600 to one. In this chapter I have converted Zimbabwe dollar amounts into US dollars according to official exchange rates published on the date of the news report cited, although the official rates may differ drastically from parallel market rates. Currency conversions were made at http://www.oanda.com/convert/classic.

5 To eliminate any fears of recrimination, I have not disclosed the identity of interviewees in cases where they made politically sensitive comments. This does not apply, however, if an interviewee has publicly criticized government AIDS policy.

6 ACT UP, the acronym for the AIDS Coalition to Unleash Power, is a grassroots AIDS organization that formed in 1987 in the US to challenge government policies on HIV/AIDS. It has utilized nonviolent civil disobedience.

7 UNAIDS later said it was skeptical of any *decline* in Zimbabwe's infection rate, explaining that the government's latest figures were not based on new data, but on revised numbers from 2001. UNAIDS further asserted that while HIV prevalence rates appear to have leveled off in Zimbabwe since the late 1990s, there was 'no basis' to believe the country had turned the epidemic around (UNAIDS 2003). The prevalence rates reported by UNAIDS in 2004 did, however, mirror those the government announced in 2003 (UNAIDS 2004).

References

Barnett, Tony, and Alan Whiteside. 2002. *AIDS in the twenty-first century: Disease and globalization*. Basingstoke: Palgrave Macmillan.

Boone, Catherine, and Jake Batsell. 2001. Politics and AIDS in Africa: Research agendas in political science and international relations. *Africa Today* 48(2): 2–33.

Chebundo, Blessing. 2002. MDC calls for an independent audit of the AIDS fund. Press release, 4 October. http://www.mdczimbabwe.com/archivemat/statements/socwelfare/.

Fredland, Richard A. 1998. AIDS and development: An inverse correlation? *Journal of Modern African Studies* 36 (4): 547–68.

Jennings, M. Kent, and Ellen Ann Andersen. 1996. Support for confrontational tactics among AIDS activists: A study of intra-movement divisions. *American Journal of Political Science* 40: 311–34.

Joint United Nations Program on HIV/AIDS (UNAIDS). 2000. Briefing pack. Panel to discuss HIV/AIDS: A new priority for international security, 5 June. Council on Foreign Relations, New York.

——. 2002. *Uganda: Epidemiological fact sheet on HIV/AIDS and sexually transmitted infections.* http://www.unaids.org/hivaidsinfo/statistics/fact_sheets/index_en.htm.

——. 2003. *AIDS epidemic update: December 2003.* http://www.unaids.org/wad/2003/Epiupdate2003_en/Epi03_04_.htm.

——. 2004. *Report on the global AIDS epidemic.* http://www.unaids.org/bangkok2004.html.

Lanegran, Kim, and Goran Hyden. 1993. Mapping the politics of AIDS: Illustrations from East Africa. *Population and Environment* 14 (3): 245–63.

Mameli, Peter Angelo. 1998. Sparks and embers: The HIV/AIDS pandemic, public administration, and international relations in the twenty-first century. PhD diss., Syracuse Univ.

Misztal, Barbara, and David Moss. 1989. *Action on AIDS: National policies in comparative perspective* New York: Greenwood Press.

Raftopolous, Brian. 2000. The state, NGOs and democratisation. In *NGOs, the state and politics in Zimbabwe*, ed. Sam Moyo, John Makumbe, and Brian Raftopolous, 21–46. Harare: SAPES Books.

Republic of Zimbabwe. 2002. Proposal to strengthen and scale up disease prevention and care for HIV/AIDS, TB and malaria in Zimbabwe. Submitted to the Global Fund to Fight AIDS, Tuberculosis and Malaria Interim Secretariat, Geneva.

Schoofs, Mark. 1999. Africa responds. Part 3 of AIDS – The Agony of Africa. *The Village Voice*, 17 November. http://www.villagevoice.com/specials/africa.

Tichagwa, Wilfred. 2003. *Gender and HIV/AIDS: An analysis of Zimbabwe's national policies and programs on HIV/AIDS/STIs.* Report for Zimbabwe Women's Resource Center and Network, Harare.

Turshen, Meredeth. 1999. *Privatizing health services in Africa.* New Brunswick: Rutgers Univ. Press.

United Nations Development Program (UNDP). 2004. *Human development report 2004.* New York: Oxford Univ. Press.

United Nations General Assembly Special Session on HIV/AIDS (UNGASS). 2001. *Declaration of commitment on HIV/AIDS: Global crisis – global action.* http://www.un.org/ga/aids/coverage/FinalDeclarationHIVAIDS.html.

United Nations Relief and Recovery Unit. 2003. *Zimbabwe humanitarian situation report.* http: //www.reliefweb.int.

van de Walle, Nicolas. 2001. *African economies and the politics of permanent crisis, 1979–1999.* Cambridge: Cambridge Univ. Press.

Waite, Gloria. 1988. The politics of disease: The AIDS virus and Africa. In *AIDS and Africa: The social and policy impact*, ed. Norman Miller and Richard C. Rockwell, 145–64. Lewiston: Edwin Mellen.

World Health Organization (WHO). 2003. *Zimbabwe: Core health indicators.* http://www3.who.int/whosis/country/indicators.cfm?country=zwe&language=en#economic.

Zimbabwe Activists on HIV and AIDS (ZAHA). 2003. Zimbabweans deserve help too, despite Mugabe: Statement of Zimbabwe activists on HIV & AIDS on President Bush's visit to South Africa. http://us.oneworld.net/article/view/63329/1/1879.

Chapter 5

AIDS, Democracy and International Donors in Ghana

Amy S. Patterson and Bernard Haven

Scholars have given little attention to the politics of AIDS in Ghana. Yet, Ghana provides an interesting case study of how a newly democratic country with a low HIV prevalence rate can proactively fight AIDS. The Joint United Nations Program on HIV/AIDS (UNAIDS) reported in 2004 that Ghana's HIV prevalence rate among 15 to 49 year olds was 3.1 per cent (UNAIDS 2004). Ghana's highest prevalence rates are in the two eastern regions of Volta (4.6 per cent) and Eastern (5.3 per cent), where migration and cross-border trade are prevalent and commercial sex workers to serve these migrants are numerous. HIV prevalence rates in the cities of Accra (3.6 per cent) and Kumasi (2.7 per cent) are not among the highest, though they have seen an increase in recent years. The lowest rates are in the rural northern region (1.4 per cent). Two-thirds of those infected in Ghana are women (GAC 2003; UNAIDS 2002; Oppong and Agyei-Mensah 2004). This chapter argues that while Ghana's democratic transition has provided a more open arena for discussion of AIDS, the disease has yet to become a crucial political topic. International donors play a key role in AIDS policy making, but civil society organizations have limited influence. Because few Ghanaians have been affected by AIDS, political commitment and public interest have been slow to develop. The chapter is based on media reports, government documents, and data from interviews conducted in 2003 with representatives from 20 nongovernmental organizations (NGOs), government agencies, and international donors.

Democratic Transitions and the Fight against AIDS in Africa

There are two perspectives on the impact of democratization on public health. Democracy may have a positive, long-term impact because in democratic systems, there is pressure on government to increase health spending (Ghobarah, Huth, and Russett 2003). Zweifel and Navia (2000) maintain that infant mortality rates are lower in democracies than dictatorships because democratic societies allow NGOs to address health concerns, permit the media to publicize health issues, and empower the free market to develop health products and services. Sen (2001) asserts that democracies protect the well being of their citizens, and that no democracy has ever suffered a famine. On the other hand, countries undergoing democratic transitions may face extraordinary pressure from labor unions and business groups to create jobs, bring down inflation, or promote trade. The immediate needs of the population may mean government cannot or will not invest in public health spending (Przeworski and Limongi 1993). This fact may be especially true for investments in AIDS prevention, since the impact of the disease is not seen in society until several years after citizens are infected with HIV (Barnett and Whiteside 2002).

Both of these perspectives on democracy assume that civil society associations will lobby for government policies, either to the benefit or the detriment of public health. In the United States, for example, interest groups such as the AIDS Coalition to Unleash Power or the National Hemophilia Foundation played an important role in shaping AIDS policies (Siplon 2002). Proponents of civil society in Africa argue that these organizations were crucial for the democratic transitions of the 1990s (Chazan 1993; Gyimah-Boadi 2004). However, while African civil society may reflect interests, it is often not organized to lobby the state (van de Walle 2001, 26–27). Civil society may be divided along class, gender, ethnic, and religious lines (Patterson 1998; Fatton 1995; Chabal and Daloz 1999). Associations in civil society often lack resources such as leadership, institutional capacity, and finances; the state or international donors may co-opt these organizations (Ndegwa 1996). In countries with a history of state repression and little experience with civil disobedience, there may not be a political culture of challenging government. The formation of AIDS organizations is made more problematic by the fact that people with AIDS may face social ostracism. Because potential members and leaders of AIDS groups may not want their sero-status to become public, they may not form associations (AF-AIDS eForum 2003, af-aids@healthdev.net, 1 August 2003).

Even if civil society organizations do lobby for increased public health spending, the underdevelopment of state institutions in Africa often constrains the state's ability to meet such demands. In the 1990s, public investment in Africa declined to an average of less than 6 per cent of gross domestic product (GDP). Almost all capital investment in health infrastructure throughout Africa now comes from international donors. Permanent, large state deficits have led to a dearth of highly qualified state personnel, few opportunities to audit state agencies, inefficiency in state services, and plummeting civil service salaries; the best state employees move from the public to the private sector (van de Walle 2001, 86–94). These inefficient institutions do not enhance the legitimacy of the state with its citizens. The result is a neopatrimonial state, in which political elites use patronage to reward key supporters and maintain power. Lacking revenue, state officials turn to international donors and NGOs for patronage resources. These donors also relieve political pressure on the government, since they supply many of the social welfare programs the state no longer can or will provide. However, reliance on donors means that African state leaders must put on a façade of following donor-supported policies, including those to address AIDS (Chabal and Daloz 1999). Another characteristic of the neopatrimonial state is the centralization of power and the development of high-level but relatively weak government institutions to reward key supporters (van de Walle 2001, 2003).

The Ghana Case

Under the control of Flight Lieutenant Jerry Rawlings, the military ruled Ghana from1981 until 1992.[1] Repression of potential opponents and the regime's control of key civil society associations characterized the military period (Gyimah-Boadi 1994). In 1992, President Rawlings and his National Democratic Congress (NDC) wrote a new constitution and held a multiparty election, though international observers criticized the election and the opposition boycotted it (Sandbrook and Oelbaum 1997). The 1996 multiparty elections were believed to be free and fair, despite the fact that Rawlings was reelected and the NDC maintained a majority of seats in the legislature. Barred from running for a third term in 2000, Rawlings stepped aside and his hand-picked successor John Evans Atta Mills campaigned as the NDC presidential candidate. Mills lost by a margin of 57 per cent to 43 per cent to John Kufour of the National Patriotic Party (NPP) in a run-off election; the NPP also won 100 of the 200 legislative seats (Gyimah-Boadi 2001).[2] In six 2003 by-elections, the NPP gained more legislative seats (*AllAfrica.com*, 28 April 2003). In addition to the 2000 historic victory, Ghanaian society has become more open, with an independent media challenging the regime and active opposition parties criticizing NPP policies (Freedom House 2004).

In addition to the democratic transition, Ghana has undergone economic liberalization. In reaction to declining cocoa exports, an 80 per cent decline in real wages between 1970 and 1982, a government deficit that was 15 per cent of GDP, and droughts that adversely affected agriculture, Ghana launched the Economic Recovery Program in 1983. Sponsored by the World Bank and International Monetary Fund, this program has included trade liberalization, currency devaluation, food subsidy withdrawal, labor retrenchment, and the introduction of user fees for public services. Positively, these neoliberal policies have led to increased cocoa production, growth in exports, infrastructure development, and improvements in balance of payments. Negatively, these policies have increased unemployment, made health and education less affordable, and contributed to inflation and high interest rates. In 2002, Ghana's debt was 126 per cent of its GDP and its inflation rate was 20 per cent. Poverty is widespread, with 36 per cent of urban Ghanaians living below the national poverty line (World Bank 2002, 2003a).[3] In 2003, 40 per cent of

Ghanaians reported going without food and 54 per cent reported going without medical care (Gyimah-Boadi and Mensah 2003). Despite these negative outcomes, both the NDC and the NPP are committed to a neoliberal economy (Boafa-Arthur 1999; Nugent 2001).

Ghana's AIDS Policies

It is important to note that Ghana's government policies are not the major reason that Ghana's HIV prevalence rate is relatively low in comparison to many other sub-Saharan African countries. Rather, even though the first AIDS cases were discovered in the mid-1980s, HIV has not spread as quickly as in southern Africa because of underdeveloped transportation links and limited rural-urban migration. However, predictions are that the prevalence rate will continue to rise, from 3.1 per cent in 2004, to 8.2 per cent in 2009, to 9.5 per cent in 2014 (Oppong and Agyei-Mensah 2004, 76). The country appears to be in the early stages of the epidemic; policy decisions and individual behavior choices will determine if the country reaches infection rates of 20 per cent to 30 per cent.

Before the 2000 election, President Rawlings established the Ghana AIDS Commission (GAC), though it did not meet until 2001. Prior to the formation of the GAC, the government had viewed AIDS solely as a health concern and had situated policy making in the Ministry of Health. The National AIDS Control Program developed a draft policy statement in 2000 that focused on education programs, though the draft was not formally adopted. Few state resources were channeled to the disease and high-level political leaders rarely spoke about the issue (Ghana National AIDS/STDs Control Program 2000; Ghana Ministry of Health 2001). In February 2000, First Lady Nana Konadu Agyeman Rawlings launched the 'Love Life, Stop AIDS' media campaign, but President Rawlings made no public statements on AIDS until late 2000 (*Xinhua News Service*, 4 February 2000).

In contrast, the relatively new GAC is an extension of the president's office; it is intended to set policy directives for national ministries, regional AIDS committees, and district AIDS committees (GAC 2003). This high-level body focuses on a multisectoral approach to fighting the disease. In addition to setting policy directives, the GAC distributes money from the Ghana AIDS Response Fund (GARFUND) to NGOs, community-based organizations (CBOs), and ministries, departments, and agencies (MDAs), whose prevention, care, and support projects complement the Ministry of Health's HIV/AIDS programs and the Strategic Framework for HIV/AIDS in Ghana (World Bank 2000). NGOs and MDAs apply directly to the GAC for project funding. CBOs apply to district assemblies, which in turn apply to the GAC for regional funding. The GARFUND has supported more than 2,600 projects in all regions of the country (Abedi Boafo, GAC Director of Administration, interview with author, 11 November 2003). Additionally, the government set up the Country Coordinating Mechanism (CCM), which applies to the Global Fund to Fight HIV/AIDS, Tuberculosis, and Malaria and oversees any grant money from this fund.

The Kufour government has sought to raise AIDS awareness. The president discussed AIDS in his first state of the union address, urging Ghanaians to speak frankly about sex in order to prevent the spread of the disease (*AllAfrica.com*, 16 February 2001). Both the president and first lady have worked with traditional rulers such as the Okyehene and the Queen Mothers Association to develop prevention messages for the media (*Ghanaian Chronicle*, 5 December 2001; *Ghanaian Chronicle*, 31 March 2003).[4] Ghana has sought to educate the population through media campaigns, most designed by Johns Hopkins University, and it has stressed prevention messages such as abstinence, healthy living, and faithfulness (*Accra Mail*, 10 June 2003). On all of these efforts, the president and high-level officials have urged compassion for people with the disease.

In the area of treatment, the government has publicly promised to acquire or produce antiretroviral (ARV) drugs, but it has tended to rely on international donors to fund and design such programs. In 2001, the minister of health outlined a $45 million plan to fight AIDS which included $30 million for ARVs (*BBC News*, 26 June 2001). The government announced in 2002 that it would start production of three off-patent ARVs in 2003, though the government then dropped production efforts and has worked with international donors to obtain cheap drugs (*PanAfrican News Agency*, 30 September 2002; *AllAfrica.com*, 6 July 2003). As of late 2003, the only ARVs available in Ghana were provided through Family Health International in a project funded by the US Agency for International Development (USAID). The program provides drugs at reduced costs to fewer than 200 individuals in the Eastern region, Accra, and Kumasi (Dr. Phyllis Antwi, Project Manager of Family Health International, interview with author, 6 October 2003).

Political Explanations for AIDS Policies in Ghana

Several variables have shaped Ghana's policies on AIDS. In this section, we examine how the 2000 election provided political space in which to address AIDS. Yet, we note that AIDS has not become an important political issue. Next, we illustrate the minimal role of indigenous NGOs in AIDS policy making. We maintain that limits in NGO resources, the policy-making structures advocated by international donors, and the low level of public concern about AIDS have contributed to the weakness of AIDS NGOs. We then demonstrate how neopatrimonialism has shaped the formation and implementation of AIDS policies. Finally, we examine the influence of international donors on Ghana's AIDS policies.

The 2000 Election and AIDS Policies

When the NPP was elected in 2000 it had a unique opportunity to increase state efforts against AIDS. The NPP campaigned with the slogan of 'Positive Change,' which signaled to voters that not only was the NPP a change from the NDC, but also that the party would address new issues. The excitement surrounding the democratic election gave the government initial legitimacy (Gyimah-Boadi 2001). According to a 1999 survey, 55 per cent of Ghanaians expressed satisfaction with the country's democratic process (Bratton, Lewis, and Gyimah-Boadi 2001). By 2003, that number had risen to 72 per cent. Ghanaians in 2003 also reported relatively high levels of public confidence in political leaders, with 74 per cent ranking the president's job performance as satisfactory (Gyimah-Boadi and Mensah 2003). The government benefited from this goodwill, and could use this opportunity to lead on the AIDS issue. Partially in response to this democratic opening, the government committed to the GAC structure.

However, it is important to acknowledge that AIDS was not a central issue of the 2000 presidential or legislative campaign for any political party. Rather, we maintain that once the NPP was in power, the party's urban and youth base of support did not *prevent* Kufuor from developing policies on the disease or making public statements to increase AIDS awareness. In 2000, the NPP made a calculated decision to win the youth vote, since Rawlings and the NDC were perceived to be the old establishment (Nugent 2001; Gyimah-Boadi 2001). As AIDS disproportionately impacts young people, it would be relatively unlikely that NPP actions on AIDS would anger this block of supporters. Likewise, areas with highest support for the NPP – Accra, Kumasi, and the Central regions – also face growing HIV prevalence rates. In comparison, the NDC-dominated Northern and Upper East regions have HIV rates of 1.4 per cent and 1.3 per cent, respectively. Even in the exceptional case of the Volta region (a NDC stronghold where HIV prevalence rates are 4.6 per cent), the NPP gained some voter support over its 1996 showing (GAC 2003; Nugent 2001).

As the 2000 election illustrates, however, AIDS has yet to become a top political issue. Political parties and candidates do not stake out positions on AIDS policies as they would other issues. Voters do not participate based on government actions on AIDS. The relative unimportance of AIDS as a political issue continued in the 2004 presidential election campaign. As of September 2004, neither President Kufour nor his repeat challenger Mills had mentioned AIDS in a major campaign speech. The fact that political leaders have given limited attention to the disease is one reason that international donors want high-level government officials to sit on AIDS policy-making boards like the GAC. It is also a reason why MDAs must compete for resources from the GARFUND. One official from the UK Department for International Development (DFID) commented:

> I would rather have people like members of cabinet sitting on the commission because for four years ... you know that you have people with clout who can move things forward. Rather than have people who, because they are politically acceptable to both sides, may not have the necessary clout ... because we are all trying to get the president to champion this. To get him you need people who he is closely in tune with (Dr. Victor Bampoe, HIV/AIDS advisor for DFID, interview with author, 8 December 2003).

Though the 2000 election provided opportunities for more political attention to AIDS, it is not clear that the government has fully taken advantage of these openings to make AIDS a top priority.

Weak AIDS NGOs and AIDS Policies

Despite Ghana's political liberalization, few NGOs are involved in AIDS policy making. There are three reasons for this situation. First, most of these NGOs are small and localized and they lack the funds, personnel, or training to become involved in politics. Students Against HIV/AIDS (STAIDS) illustrates these points. Formed in 1998 by eight university students, STAIDS has no office space and only sporadically holds meetings. Because its members are unable to do full-time work for STAIDS, the group has a limited ability to write proposals to the GAC to solicit funds (Theodora Obeng-Asamoa, STAIDS coordinator, interview with author, 22 September 2003).

The Ghana HIV/AIDS Network (GHANET) provides another example. An umbrella organization intended to represent AIDS NGOs in policy making and to encourage NGO capacity building, the group has suffered from internal dissent, poor communication, and limited resources. Although GHANET has taken steps to open regional offices throughout the country, it lacks funding for this plan. In late 2003, the group was housed in a small church office in Accra with an outdated phone number on its sign. The organization has a difficult time maintaining communication with its members, most of whom lack telephones and cannot easily access email (Sam Anyimadu-Amaning, GHANET chair, interview with author, 14 November 2003; GHANET meeting, author observation, 28 November 2003).

The second reason for the absence of AIDS NGOs in policy making relates to the structures of AIDS decision-making bodies. Few NGO representatives sit on the GAC or the CCM. Of the GAC's 40 members, 16 are from government and 12 represent international donors; only one is a person living with HIV/AIDS (PLWHA), four represent domestic and international NGOs or CBOs, five are from the private sector, one is from a religious group, and one is from the education sector. GHANET and the Wisdom Association, a group that represents PLWHAs, are the only two indigenous NGOs (Ghana Country Coordinating Mechanism 2002).

The lack of NGO representation, and particularly representation of PLWHAs, may harm Ghana's overall AIDS policies. Mobilizing PLWHAs can address the stigma that accompanies AIDS and that prevents individuals from being tested for HIV. Additionally, incorporation of PLWHAs into decision making exposes the organization to the unique perspectives of individuals with the disease; PLWHAs often provide needed emotional and practical support to those engaged in prevention and education activities (UNAIDS 1999). The largest of these organizations in Ghana, and the only group representing PLWHAs on these official institutions, is the Wisdom Association. Centered in Accra, this group of volunteers provides care and support through nutrition programs and counseling for 1,500 PLWHAs. Wisdom receives most of its funding from the GARFUND, with additional support from the UN Development Program (Harruna Sanusi, Administrative Manager of Wisdom Association, interview with author, 8 December 2003).

The GAC is quick to display its cooperation with Wisdom as a means to gain legitimacy for incorporating PLWHAs into decision making. GHANET and Wisdom are considered to be representatives of the NGO and PLWHA communities respectively, a practice that then precludes the involvement of other organizations in decision making. Yet GHANET represents only about 150 of the country's 1,500 AIDS NGOs, and even fewer groups are involved in its leadership. Few members attend meetings or benefit from the workshops it holds (Sam Anyimadu-Amaning, GHANET chair, interview with author, 14 November 2003; GHANET meeting, author observation, 28 November 2003). Furthermore, since these two groups benefit from the all-but-guaranteed support of donors, they have little motivation to challenge donor policies or to upset the status quo.

At the same time, groups critical of current AIDS policies and programs face exclusion from decision-making bodies. The most vocal of these groups is the Ghana AIDS Treatment Access Group (GATAG), which advocates for affordable access to ARVs on behalf of Ghana's PLWHAs. Headquartered in a small office near Accra, this group receives no money from the GARFUND or international donors and must rely on the contributions of its members to continue operations. GATAG does not sit on any national bodies and is ignored by the GAC, UNAIDS, and the CCM though it has tried to establish partnerships with these organizations. Its president has been unable to receive visas to attend international conferences, a result, he claims, of being blacklisted by the GAC, which is routinely contacted in the visa-application process:

> Most of these embassies from Europe and America want GAC to recommend you before they give you the visa. And of course GAC will not recommend us, because we are the only advocacy group that is telling them that … the prevention efforts are good but are worthless if you don't add treatment (Israel Asamoah, GATAG president, interview with author, 19 November 2003).

Because of its focus on the importance of treatment to control HIV/AIDS, something the government has yet to provide, GATAG has been excluded from the select group of voices the GAC chooses to hear. Instead, the government has partnered with Wisdom, which advocates for care and support but not treatment.

Ghana's larger political and social environment is a third variable that influences the ability of AIDS NGOs to shape government actions. Even though Freedom House (2004) ranks Ghana as 'free', civil society remains underdeveloped.[5] Most participation in civil society is concentrated in religious groups. While 53 per cent of survey respondents in 2003 described themselves as active members of a religious association, only between 15 per cent and 24 per cent reported membership in professional or business associations, trade unions or farmers' groups, and community development or self-help (voluntary) organizations (Gyimah-Boadi and Mensah 2003).[6] Discomfort with expressing political views after many years of authoritarian rule and concern about meeting immediate material needs may contribute to these low levels of participation. While some associations have created social capital that bonds members with similar social characteristics together, few organizations have bridged across religious, regional, ethnic, or class lines to address broad challenges to society such as AIDS (Bratton, Lewis, and Gyimah-Boadi 2001).[7] In a country with an underdeveloped civil society, the formation of AIDS NGOs is problematic.

AIDS NGOs are further marginalized by the fact that relatively few Ghanaians have a personal stake in AIDS policies. In 2004, only 18 per cent of Ghanaians reported having a relative or friend who had died of the disease, and only 5 per cent said they had spent more than five hours a day caring for someone with AIDS or orphaned children. (In contrast, 43 per cent of Malawians reported spending more than five hours a day on such care.) Further, just 3 per cent of citizens named AIDS as one of the top three problems the government should address (Afrobarometer 2004). Low public support for AIDS programs 'betrays evidence of a growing discomfort, among sections of the Ghanaian population, with the culturally inappropriate character of the public commentary on AIDS' (Gyimah-Boadi and Mensah 2003, 13). In addition, of the roughly 400,000 HIV-positive Ghanaians (USAID 2003), it is estimated that only about 10 per cent of them know they are HIV positive. Without such knowledge, individuals cannot begin to form organizations to combat AIDS.

Comments from the president of the GATAG reflect this social environment. He said of the organization: 'We are advocates; we didn't want to use the word "activist" because in Ghana we are, by our nature, we are not an aggressive people' (Israel Asamoah, GATAG president, interview with author, 19 November 2003). Although the group has hundreds of PLWHAs as members, it does not engage in political activism. In 2002, GATAG lobbied Coca-Cola to provide access to treatment for its Ghanaian bottling workers. After GATAG threatened to launch a protest march, one of its executives was detained by the police until pressure from treatment activists around the world secured his release. Instead of pushing ahead with its protest against

Coca-Cola, GATAG then called off its march (Israel Asamoah, GATAG president, interview with author, 19 November 2003). Even this group that is excluded from government forums and funding did not display radical opposition to harmful policies and obeyed government orders to end its protest.

The Neopatrimonial State and AIDS Policies

While AIDS in Ghana has not become politicized, in that it is not a top concern in political debates, it does have the potential to become a tool of the neopatrimonial state. Nugent (1995) argues that 'big men' have historically dominated Ghanaian politics; they provide resources to citizens in return for political support. The use of patronage, the hallmark of neopatrimonialism, has been evident in recent elections. For example, Ghana's capital budget rose in 1995 and 1996 to finance road construction in rural areas, the bastion of NDC support (Sandbrook and Oelbaum 1997). In the 2000 election, the NDC distributed patronage through district assemblies, which are allegedly nonpartisan entities. Though the opposition NPP lacked access to state resources in 2000, it too used patronage when it could tap into independent finances (Nugent 2001).

Neopatrimonialism contributes to limited state capacity in Ghana. Nearly 50 per cent of Ghanaians report difficulty in obtaining some government services (Gyimah-Boadi and Mensah 2003). The World Bank (2003b) maintains that the state's lack of transparency and accountability is a liability in fighting poverty, and it calls for reforming procurement laws and strengthening internal and external auditing procedures. Minimal transparency contributes to perceptions of corruption both inside and outside the country. In 2003, 62 per cent of citizens believed that at least some government officials are corrupt; 23 per cent said that most or all officials are corrupt; and 13 per cent reported paying a bribe in the last year (Gyimah-Boadi and Mensah 2003).[8] Transparency International (2003), an organization that surveys international business leaders about their perceptions of corruption, gives Ghana a ranking of 3.3 out of 10, with 10 being the least corrupt.

While it is difficult to prove that neopatrimonialism shapes the government's AIDS policies, aspects of the aforementioned structures seem to provide opportunities for neopatrimonial behavior. The structure of the GAC lacks efficiency; its hierarchy provides many levels at which patronage potentially could be dispersed to supporters. As mentioned above, the GAC works through regional AIDS committees, which oversee district AIDS committees; CBOs apply for funding from district AIDS committees. NGOs may apply directly to the GAC, though they must be able to contribute 10 per cent of the cost of their proposed budget. (Thus, the number of applicants from rural districts for GAC funds has been low.) In a 2001 assessment, the World Bank suggested that the roles and responsibilities of all involved parties at all levels of the hierarchy needed to be clearly defined (GAC 2003). One representative of an international donor agency recently echoed this concern, stating that the GAC structure and its funding decisions are very political (Anonymous international donor, interview with author, 8 October 2003).

Inefficiency and delays in funding to NGOs from the GAC are common. The lack of capacity in Ghana's banking sector exacerbates this situation, since funds must be transferred from the GAC to the Ministry of Finance for approval. Money then is transferred to the head office of the NGO's bank, then to the local branch of the bank, and finally to the NGO's account. The GAC gives applicants little information on the progress of grants or the reasons for the delays, prompting legitimate concerns on the part of applicants and harming the legitimacy of the process. Speaking about this delay, one NGO leader stated:

> You look at it from our side, we don't really know what is going on there … And even though the fault may not come from you, but I may feel that … you may want to take a bribe or something from me … that's why you are delaying the process (Rev. Fiifi Khan Agtarkwah, Executive Director of Multiple Motivation Foundation, interview with author, 1 December 2003).

This interviewee raises a point about the GAC structure: the potential for abuse of power. Although it is not an official requirement, all NGOs must produce a letter of endorsement from their district assembly before their GAC application will be considered. 'If they're not endorsed, you don't bring it here. Before you bring an NGO proposal here, you should have obtained the endorsement of the district assembly' (Abedi Boafo, GAC Director of Administration, interview with author, 11 November 2003). Designed to prevent duplication of projects and to encourage accountability, there is some evidence that this requirement has fostered corruption at the local level. The president of Media Response, a small NGO that publishes a monthly newspaper that chronicles projects and organizations working on HIV/AIDS, explained that the endorsement is essential and usually not given without something in return: 'It wasn't difficult. But the thing is, you have to … give something, give some tip … to whoever [is] going to give you that endorsement … without that your proposal will not be considered. It would be incomplete' (Samuel Dodoo, President of Media Response, interview with author, 12 December 2003).

The potential for political favoritism in the GAC has not been lost on government opponents. Many AIDS education programs have been organized in Accra, Kumasi, and other NPP strongholds. While these urban areas have some of the highest HIV rates, the fact that money has been channeled to these NPP bastions has raised questions about how GARFUND money is allocated. For example, the NPP's National Youth Wing received a sizeable grant from the GARFUND to conduct AIDS education programs (*Ghanaian Chronicle*, 2 December 2002; *Accra Mail*, 30 January 2003). In May 2003, CBOs in Ahafo Ano North (a traditional

NDC stronghold) accused some district committee chiefs of politicizing AIDS funds. The *Ghanaian Chronicle* (26 May 2003) reported that one district committee had warned 'the officer in charge of the AIDS programme not to accept their group's budget proposals on the grounds that the chairman is an NDC activist'.

In the most extreme case, the lack of GAC institutional capacity and the many layers of its hierarchy also may provide opportunities for blatant corruption. In 2003, the monitoring and evaluating chairman of the GAC reported that some CBOs and NGOs that took state money had not used the money for AIDS activities (*Accra Mail*, 8 May 2003). The government announced in June 2003 that officials from 11 NGOs were charged with embezzling money that the GAC gave to their organizations (*Ghanaian Chronicle*, 24 June 2003). Though it is impossible to know the level of corruption of the groups, these examples illustrate the potential for misuse of funds within Ghana's AIDS policy-making and implementing structures.

Dependence on Donors and AIDS Policies

Ghana's actions on AIDS reflect the country's high level of dependence on donors, especially in key sectors such as health and education. In 2002, 10.6 per cent of Ghana's GDP came from foreign aid (approximately $32 per capita); this amounts to approximately $650 million annually (UNDP 2004). Government spending on health as a percentage of the total government budget was 8 per cent in 2001, a decline from 9 per cent in 1998. Government spending comprised roughly 59 per cent of all health spending in 2001; the remainder came from international donors and the private sector (WHO 2002; Ghana Ministry of Finance 2002).

Ghana relies heavily on multilateral and bilateral donors to fund AIDS programs. The World Bank loaned the GAC $25 million for AIDS programs (*Accra Mail*, 3 December 2002). In 2002, USAID allocated $20 million for AIDS (out of a total of $58 million for the country) and DFID provided £20 million to the GAC (USAID 2003). In 2002, the Global Fund to Fight HIV/AIDS, Tuberculosis, and Malaria granted the country $38 million for its AIDS, tuberculosis, and malaria projects. (Roughly half of this money will go for AIDS programs.) While these donor resources will allow government and NGOs to develop and implement AIDS policies, they also can contribute to the continuation of the neopatrimonial state (van de Walle 2001). Not only do donor resources provide an opportunity to build health infrastructure, but they also finance the formation of new administrative bodies such as the GAC, the CCM, and district AIDS committees. For example, 1 per cent of Ghana's Global Fund money (roughly $378,000) will go to the CCM for administrative costs. Of the AIDS component of the Global Fund grant, most of the money is intended for government ministries and district assemblies, not NGOs, religious groups, or organizations of PLWHAs (Ghana Country Coordinating Mechanism 2002).

Donors also have played a key role in shaping structures and policies that relate to AIDS. The impetus to develop the GAC came from the UNAIDS-orchestrated International Partnership on AIDS in Africa, a program to focus international attention on AIDS and to develop political commitment among African leaders (Baylies 1999). Through the partnership, a UNAIDS-led team reviewed Ghana's AIDS policy structures and suggested the formation of a supra-ministerial, multisectoral organization to advise and coordinate AIDS policies. Other donors such as the UN Development Program and the World Bank urged the formation of such a structure (GAC 2003). The initial money for the GAC and its GARFUND came from the World Bank's $25 million loan. As the chapter by Patterson and Cieminis illustrates, the formation of Ghana's CCM reflects donor requirements for accessing the Global Fund. Additionally, Ghana's focus on healthy living and faithfulness in its media messages may partially be a response to American foreign policy demands that have stressed these aspects of HIV prevention (*US Newswire*, 3 June 2003). Even President Kufuor's public leadership on AIDS must be situated in the larger context of the country's dependence on donors. While the president's actions on AIDS no doubt reflect genuine concern for the well-being of Ghanaians, they also are a reaction to international donors who have called for more political commitment to the disease from African politicians. AIDS became a more important issue for Ghanaian politicians at roughly the same time as the UN General Assembly Special Session on HIV/AIDS in June 2001, when developed countries took a greater interest in AIDS and pledged to devote more resources to the disease.

One unintended consequence of the close involvement of donors in AIDS policy making is that the structures and programs that they fund may actually limit the creativity and independence of AIDS NGOs. Not only do donors and the GAC make AIDS policies, but they also allocate money to groups to implement those policies. It then becomes difficult for NGOs receiving funding to criticize these policies and programs. This is especially true of the GAC, since NGOs apply directly to it for money. In the ensuing environment of submission, an association like Wisdom that does not challenge the government's lack of treatment programs is not threatening to the GAC, but GATAG is. Media Response provides another example. Because it receives most of its funding from the GAC, it is hesitant to oppose government policies in its monthly newspaper. The president explained: 'Well, at most, I really tread cautiously; I still go ahead and publish, but I make sure that it is quite balanced, not necessarily against the GAC' (Samuel Dodoo, President of Media Response, interview with author, 12 December 2003).

Conclusion

The Ghana case raises questions about the relationships between democratic transitions, international donors, and AIDS policy making. Though Ghana's political environment has become more open, with free media, opportunities for civil society activism, and competitive elections, state officials have done little more than what is required by international donors to address AIDS. In comparison to countries like South Africa or Uganda, citizen activism and NGO incorporation into the AIDS fight have been limited. The lack of state capacity and the country's dependence on donors have meant that Ghana's struggle against AIDS is at times haphazard. While leaders do not deny the disease, they also do not talk about it daily, as the president of Botswana does. Furthermore, some AIDS NGOs and media officials perceive that AIDS resources have become merely another source of patronage, a fact which challenges the legitimacy and efficiency of the country's AIDS efforts.

Given Ghana's high level of debt and its dependence on foreign aid, it is likely that donors will continue to play a large role in AIDS policy making and implementation. To address some of the problems outlined in this chapter, donors should work to incorporate more NGOs into the policy-making process, including those such as GATAG that challenge the status quo. Efforts should be made to streamline the process for grant applications to the GAC, while still insisting on government accountability and transparency. Donors should encourage the media to cover AIDS stories, not only to increase AIDS awareness, but also to make the policy process more transparent and salient to citizens. Donors also should urge political leaders to debate various proposals on AIDS, and more broadly public health, during elections.

The Ghana case raises an additional question: Must AIDS reach epidemic proportions before citizens and state officials pay attention to it? Part of the *political* difficulty in addressing AIDS in Ghana is that the public sees little urgency in the disease. Oppong and Agyei-Mensah (2004, 78) write: 'While high levels of HIV/AIDS awareness (over 90 per cent) prevail throughout the country, over 70 per cent did not consider themselves or their families to be at risk of HIV infection. People seemed to perceive AIDS as a problem that affected "other people".' Yet, the case of Senegal provides a counterexample. In that country, officials publicly discussed the disease and mobilized key sectors in society before HIV rates reached 2 per cent. Though there were other societal reasons for Senegal's success such as strong social cohesion and the country's limited migration, Senegal illustrates that it is possible for a government to lead, not follow, public opinion and proactively develop AIDS policies.

Placing HIV/AIDS high on the political agenda may be Ghana's best chance to successfully contain the disease. As the chapter by Furlong and Ball in this volume illustrates, when AIDS becomes a political issue that mobilizes citizens, government is more likely to act. As the DFID official said:

> Politics and HIV/AIDS are not necessarily a bad thing. I mean, Uganda's success has been primarily because Museveni politicized HIV/AIDS. And we are actually looking for more politicization of HIV/AIDS so that it becomes one of the big

> things that every political organization talks about in their bid to win power in Ghana (Dr. Victor Bampoe, HIV/AIDS Advisor for DFID, interview with author, 8 December 2003).

For the sake of the millions of Ghanaians at risk of HIV infection, and the thousands who are already HIV positive, one can hope that AIDS becomes central to the country's politics.

Notes

1 Ghana experienced previous periods of military rule from 1966 to 1969 and from 1972 to 1978.
2 The first round of the presidential election was much closer, with Mills winning 45 per cent of the vote and Kufour, 48 per cent. Smith (2002) argues that the NPP legislative victory may actually have been inflated because of malapportionment and bloated voter registration rolls.
3 These statistics on urban poverty in Ghana do not provide a complete picture since most Ghanaians live in rural areas, where poverty is more widespread. As another indicator, the US Department of State (2002) reports that 80 per cent of the work force is employed in the informal sector.
4 The Okyehene (the king of the Akyem people, who traditionally inhabit the Eastern region) broke traditions when he ran in a marathon to draw attention to the campaign against HIV/AIDS. After the race, he publicly had an HIV test, in order to encourage others to be tested.
5 Using Freedom House's scale of 1 to 7, with 1 being the 'most free', Ghana received a rating of 2 for political rights and 2 for civil liberties in 2003. Political rights include the right to form political parties that represent a range of voter choices and that have leaders who freely compete for office. Civil liberties include religious, ethnic, economic, linguistic, and gender rights; freedom of the press; and freedom of association.
6 The percentage varied with the type of group.
7 Warren (2001) argues that bridging social capital, not bonding social capital, is essential for addressing large social problems, such as poverty, economic inequality, and discrimination.
8 The survey's authors speculate that the percentage of citizens paying a bribe is much higher.

References

Afrobarometer. 2004. Public opinion and HIV/AIDS: Facing up to the future. Briefing paper no. 12. http://www.afrobarometer.org.

Barnett, Tony, and Alan Whiteside. 2002. *AIDS in the twenty-first century: Disease and globalisation.* Basingstoke: Palgrave Macmillan.

Baylies, Carolyn. 1999. International partnership in the fight against AIDS: Addressing need and redressing injustice? *Review of African Political Economy* 81: 387–414.

Boafo-Arthur, Kwame. 1999. Structural adjustment, democratization, and the politics of continuity in Ghana. *African Studies Review* 42 (2): 41–72.

Bratton, Michael, Peter Lewis, and E. Gyimah-Boadi. 2001. Constituencies for reform in Ghana. *Journal of Modern African Studies* 39 (2): 231–59.

Chabal, Patrick, and Jean-Pascal Daloz. 1999. *Africa works: Disorder as political instrument.* Bloomington: Indiana Univ. Press.

Chazan, Naomi. 1993. Africa's democratic challenge. *World Policy Journal* 9 (2): 280–311.

Fatton, Robert. 1995. Africa in the age of democratization: The civic limitations of civil society. *African Studies Review* 38 (2): 67–110.

Freedom House. 2004. Ghana. http://www.freedomhouse.org/research/freeworld/2004/countryratings/ghana.htm.

Ghana AIDS Commission (GAC). 2003. *Annual report.* http://www.ghanaids.gov/gh/about/annualreport.asp?subnav=annualreport.

Ghana Country Coordinating Mechanism. 2002. Proposal to the Global Fund to Fight HIV/AIDS, Tuberculosis, and Malaria. http://www.globalfundatm.org.

Ghana Ministry of Finance. 2002. *Annual budget.* http://www.finance.gov.gh/Budget-2002.pdf.

Ghana Ministry of Health. 2001. *HIV/AIDS in Ghana: Background, projections, impacts, interventions, and policy.* Accra: Government of Ghana.

Ghana National AIDS/STDs Control Program. 2000. *Draft for national HIV/AIDS and STI policy.* Accra: Government of Ghana.

Ghobarah, Hazem, Paul Huth, and Bruce Russett. 2003. Civil wars kill and maim people – Long after the shooting stops. *American Political Science Review* 97 (2): 189–202.

Gyimah-Boadi, E. 1994. Associational life, civil society, and democratization in Ghana. In *Civil society and the state in Africa*, ed. John Harbeson, Donald Rothchild, and Naomi Chazan, 125–48. Boulder, CO: Lynne Rienner.

——. 2001. A peaceful turnover in Ghana. *Journal of Democracy* 12 (2): 103–17.

——. 2004. Civil society and democratic development. In *Democratic reform in Africa: The quality of progress*, ed. E. Gyimah-Boadi, 99–119. Boulder, CO: Lynne Rienner.

Gyimah-Boadi, E., and Kwabena Amoah Awuah Mensah. 2003. The growth of democracy in Ghana despite economic dissatisfaction: A power alternation bonus? Afrobarometer paper no. 28. http://www.afrobarometer.org.

Joint United Nations Program on HIV/AIDS (UNAIDS). 1999. *From principle to practice: Greater involvement of people living with or affected by HIV/AIDS.* http://www.unaids.org/publications/documents/persons/una9943e.pdf.

——. 2002. Ghana: Epidemiological fact sheet. http://www.unaids.org.

——. 2004. *Report on the global AIDS epidemic.* http://www.unaids.org/bangkok2004.html.

Ndegwa, Stephen. 1996. *The two faces of civil society: NGOs and politics in Africa.* West Hartford, CT: Kumarian Press.

Nugent, Paul. 1995. *Big men, small boys and politics in Ghana: Power, ideology, and the burden of history, 1982–1994.* New York: Francis Pinter.

——. 2001. Winners, losers and also rans: Money, moral authority and voting patterns in the Ghana 2000 election. *African Affairs* 100: 405–28.

Oppong, Joseph, and Samuel Agyei-Mensah. 2004. HIV/AIDS in West Africa: The case of Senegal, Ghana, and Nigeria. In *HIV & AIDS in Africa: Beyond epidemi-*

ology, ed. Ezekiel Kalipeni, Susan Craddock, Joseph Oppong, and Jayati Ghosh, 70–82. Malden, MA: Blackwell Publishing.

Patterson, Amy. 1998. A reappraisal of democracy in civil society: Evidence from rural Senegal. *The Journal of Modern African Studies* 36 (3): 423–41.

Przeworski, Adam, and Fernando Limongi. 1993. Political regimes and economic growth. *Journal of Economic Perspectives* 7: 51–69.

Sandbrook, Richard, and Jay Oelbaum.1997. Reforming dysfunctional institutions through democratization? Reflections on Ghana. *The Journal of Modern African Studies* 35 (4): 603–46.

Sen, Amartya. 2001. Democracy as a universal value. In *The global divergence of democracies*, ed. Larry Diamond and Marc Plattner, 3–17. Baltimore: Johns Hopkins Univ. Press.

Siplon, Patricia. 2002. *AIDS and the policy struggle in the United States*. Washington, DC: Georgetown Univ. Press.

Smith, Daniel. 2002. Consolidating democracy? The structural underpinnings of Ghana's 2000 elections. *Journal of Modern African Studies* 40 (2): 621–50.

Transparency International. 2003. Corruption perceptions index. http://www.transparency.org.

United Nations Development Program (UNDP). 2004. *Human development report.* New York: Oxford University Press.

US Agency for International Development (USAID). 2003. Ghana budget justification. http://www.usaid.gov/policy/budget/dbj2004/sub-saharan_africa/Ghana.pdf.

US Department of State. 2002. *Country reports on human rights practices.* http://www.state.gov/g/drl/rls/hrrpt/2002/18206.htm.

van de Walle, Nicolas. 2001. *African economies and the politics of permanent crisis, 1979–1999*. New York: Cambridge Univ. Press.

——. 2003. Presidentialism and clientelism in Africa's emerging party systems. *Journal of Modern African Studies* 41 (2): 297–321.

Warren, Mark. 2001. *Dry bones rattling*. Princeton: Princeton Univ. Press.

World Bank. 2000. *Project appraisal document on a proposed credit in the amount of SDR 19.6 million to the Republic of Ghana for AIDS response project (GARFUND)*. Unpublished report. Accra: World Bank.

——. 2002. Ghana at a glance. http://www.worldbank.org.

——. 2003a. Ghana data profile. http://www.worldbank.org.

——. 2003b. Joint staff assessment of the poverty reduction strategy. Paper prepared for World Bank. http://poverty.worldbank.org/prsp/index/php?view=ctry&id=66.

World Health Organization (WHO). 2002. Ghana health indicators. http://www3.who.int/whosis/country/indicators.cfm?country=gha&language=en.

Zweifel, Thomas, and Patricio Navia. 2000. Democracy, dictatorship and infant mortality. *Journal of Democracy* 11(2): 99–114.

Chapter 6

The Economic, Social, and Political Drivers of the AIDS Epidemic in Swaziland: A Case Study

Alan Whiteside

Several features distinguish Swaziland from other African countries. It is the second smallest country on the continent. Its system of government is baffling to most outsiders. It managed reasonable economic growth until recently, and has not experienced any major political, social, or economic upheavals. But Swaziland also has a uniquely severe AIDS epidemic. HIV prevalence among antenatal clinic (ANC) attendees is 38.8 per cent, the highest rate in the world in 2004 (UNAIDS 2004). The chapter looks at the AIDS epidemic and what is driving it in this small African country. It suggests that the state is crucial, both in fueling the epidemic and in addressing it, and also considers why the epidemic is so serious and what features of Swazi society have made it so.

The original research for this chapter came from a report prepared for the National Emergency Response Committee on HIV/AIDS (NERCHA) in Swaziland (Whiteside et al. 2003).[1] The report sought to address the three different questions: (1) Why is HIV prevalence in Swaziland so high? (2) What can be done about it? (3) What are the innovative responses to the AIDS epidemic? The report was compiled in several stages. A draft was prepared using material collected by the Joint United Nations Program on HIV/AIDS (UNAIDS) and NERCHA, documents at the University of Natal's Health Economics and HIV/AIDS Division, and information from online data bases. This draft was circulated to all stakeholders and presented at a workshop in Swaziland, where participants commented on it. The final draft was presented a month later at a meeting of NERCHA staff, who made final comments and agreed on the text for publication.

The HIV/AIDS Epidemic in Swaziland

The first HIV infection in Swaziland was identified in 1986. The government responded rapidly by establishing the National AIDS Prevention and Control Program (NAPCP) – later renamed the Swaziland National AIDS/Sexually Transmitted Infections (STI) Program – with support from the World Health

Organization's Global Program on AIDS. By the end of the 1990s, a standard package of interventions had been established. These included mandatory screening of all donated blood; information, education, and communication programs; condom promotion and distribution; and the establishment of AIDS Information and Support Centers.

The response to the epidemic was in accordance with internationally accepted standard practices at that time, and in many cases, went beyond them. For example, leadership and political commitment have been identified as crucial for fighting HIV/AIDS. As early as 1993, the NAPCP conducted a one-day retreat for the cabinet, during which a commitment was made to fight the disease. Swaziland was one of the first African countries to make mention of HIV in its national development plan and to commission a study on the socioeconomic impact of HIV/AIDS (Whiteside and Wood 1994). A senior government diplomat was open about his HIV-positive status and the need for behavioral change as early as the mid-1990s.

But the response went beyond government, with small programs initiated by the private sector, nongovernmental organizations (NGOs), religious groups, and communities. These happened with the tacit support of the government, although the transfer of resources to these groups was limited. The donor agencies, particularly the European Union and the US Agency for International Development, were concerned about the epidemic and made funds and technical assistance available to support interventions. Despite these activities, HIV prevalence rose inexorably.

In December 2001 the government created the NERCHA and mandated it to coordinate and mobilize resources for an expanded and coordinated response to AIDS. NERCHA is a statutory council, with the task of putting into action the National Strategic Plan for HIV/AIDS produced by the HIV/AIDS Crisis Management and Technical Committee. The National Director of NERCHA reports directly to the prime minister (NERCHA 2003).

The Data

The research for the original NERCHA report first sought to examine if the available data reflect the true scale of HIV infection in Swaziland. Is the epidemic as serious as the data suggest? We looked at data collection and analysis for the *Report on the 8th sentinel survey* (Government of Swaziland 2002), and concluded that the antenatal survey in Swaziland was conducted using global best standards in epidemiological sampling and statistical principles.[2] It was estimated that 2,157 samples would be needed in order to give a confidence interval of 95 per cent. In this survey, 2,787 samples were collected. The World Health Organization requires only one enzyme-linked immunosorbent assay (ELISA) test for surveys. But in Swaziland, when a sample was positive, an additional test was carried out to confirm the result.

The survey provides sound information on HIV prevalence among pregnant women in Swaziland, and it outlines clear trends in HIV prevalence since 1992. To what extent can these ANC data be a proxy for the general population? As the 2002 survey notes:

> The use of pregnant mothers attending antenatal clinics raises issues on the representativeness of this sentinel population to the general population or even women in general. Sentinel surveillance in ANC clinics has an inherent selection bias against women using modern contraceptives. Women who have adopted safer sexual behaviours such as consistent condom use are unlikely to become pregnant and therefore not attend antenatal care. Women with infertility are not likely to be captured in the ANC clinics. Infertility caused by STIs would tend to result in an underestimation of HIV prevalence rates especially in the older age groups where infertility is most common. However, infertility due to STIs and HIV are unlikely to affect the HIV prevalence rates in the young age groups 15–19 years. Fortunately enough the ANC based data has been found to closely reflect the HIV prevalence in the reproductive age group (Government of Swaziland 2002, 21).

Certainly in the rest of southern Africa, these data are accepted as providing a good measure of HIV prevalence in the general adult population. Indeed, a concern is that ANC data may underestimate HIV prevalence in more mature epidemics because of falling fertility among HIV-positive women. A 2002 study of 4,183, mainly male, workers at the Royal Swazi Sugar Corporation found HIV prevalence to be 37.5 per cent. This survey used saliva tests and had a 60 per cent compliance rate (employee of Royal Swazi Sugar Corporation, correspondence with author, February 2003). These results suggest that the ANC data are representative of infection rates in the adult Swazi population.

Is Swaziland's epidemic trajectory unique for the region? Figure 6.1 shows national data for Botswana, Namibia, and South Africa through 2002. The data illustrate the high prevalence rate among ANC attendees in Swaziland. Comparative data from the border areas of southern Mozambique, and Mpumalanga and KwaZulu-Natal provinces in South Africa, show that the HIV prevalence rate in KwaZulu-Natal was 36.5 per cent in 2002, while in Mpumalanga it remained around 29 per cent. The only location with a significantly lower prevalence was Mozambique's Maputo province, which adjoins Swaziland and where the prevalence rate was 13 per cent in 2002 (UNAIDS 2002b). By 2003, adult HIV prevalence rates in Zimbabwe and Lesotho were 24.6 per cent and 28.9 per cent, respectively (UNAIDS 2004).

The AIDS epidemic in Swaziland is distinctive in how uniformly severe it is. There is little difference between rural and urban areas in terms of HIV prevalence rates. This is indicative of population mobility and close links between rural and urban areas in Swaziland, a pattern also found in Botswana. In 2002, there was also minimal difference in HIV prevalence between districts: Hhohho had the lowest HIV prevalence rate, 36.6 per cent and

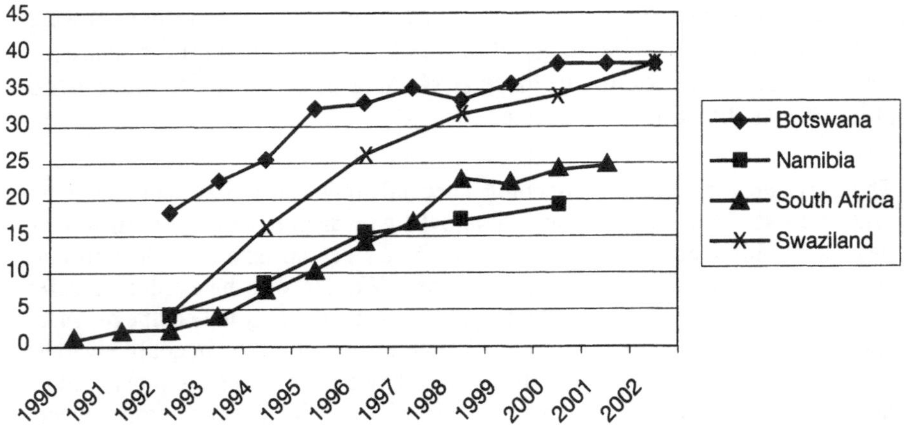

Source: Compiled by author from antenatal surveys from the Health Economics and HIV/AIDS Division, University of Natal, Durban.

Figure 6.1 National trends in HIV prevalence (%)

Manzini the highest, 41.2 per cent. Hhohho and Manzini are the country's richer and more urbanized districts, while the poorer and more rural districts of Lubombo and Shiselweni had HIV prevalence rates of 38.5 per cent and 37.9 per cent, respectively. These rates have remain relatively constant since 2002.

The original report questioned how high prevalence rates might go, noting that HIV prevalence has consistently risen higher than expected. In 2002, UNAIDS reported:

> The worst of the epidemic clearly has not yet passed, even in southern Africa where rampant epidemics are under way. In four southern African countries, national adult HIV prevalence has risen higher than thought possible, exceeding 30 per cent: Botswana (38.8 per cent), Lesotho (31 per cent), Swaziland (33.4 per cent) and Zimbabwe (33.7 per cent) (UNAIDS 2002a, 16).

Though it revised prevalence rates downward for Lesotho and Zimbabwe between 2002 and 2004, UNAIDS wrote in 2004 that 'prevalence is still rising in some countries such as Madagascar and Swaziland' (UNAIDS 2004, 6).

As of 2004, there were no instances where national prevalence rates exceeded 40 per cent. Where HIV prevalence has reached about 40 per cent of pregnant women, the epidemic seems to plateau. There are 'hotspots' where HIV prevalence among ANC attendees has reached more than 60 per cent. (In 2000, HIV the prevalence in Chiredzi, a sugar plantation area in Zimbabwe, was 70.7 per cent. See *AIDS Analysis Africa* 2002.) The present data do not show any such hotspots in Swaziland, but they also do not show prevalence leveling out. Figure 6.2 illustrates the national trend in HIV prevalence, while Table 6.1 breaks down the data by region.

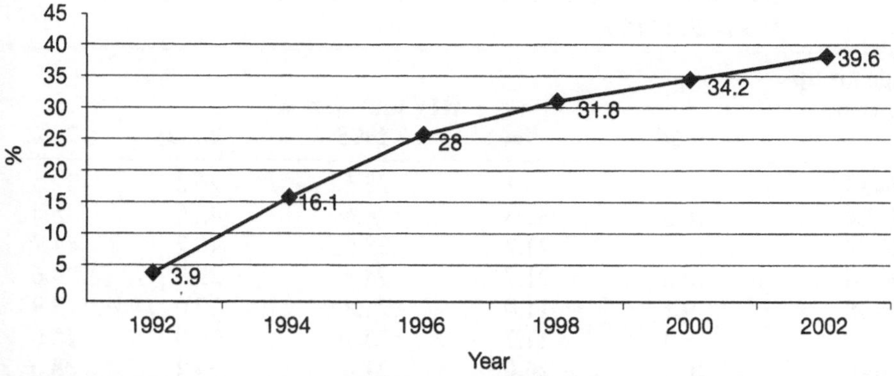

Source: Government of Swaziland. 2002. *Report on the 8th sentinel survey*. Mbabane: Government of Swaziland.

Figure 6.2 HIV prevalence among ANC respondents in Swaziland, 1999–2002 (%)

Table 6.1 HIV infection trends among ANC respondents by Swazi region, 1994–2002 (%)

Region	HIV prevalence				
	1994	1996	1998	2000	2002
Hhohho	15.5	26.3	30.3	32.3	36.6
Lubombo	16.8	26.5	31.5	34.5	38.5
Manzini	15.6	27.7	34.8	41.0	41.2
Shiselweni	16.8	23.9	29.6	27.0	37.9

Source: Government of Swaziland. 2002. *Report on the 8th sentinel survey*. Mbabane: Government of Swaziland.

There is little good news in the data. An early indication of HIV being brought under control through successful prevention programs would be a decline in prevalence among young women. Table 6.2 illustrates HIV prevalence in various age groups. The increase in prevalence in the 15 to 19 and 20 to 24 age groups shows that Swaziland still has a long way to go in halting the spread of HIV. The country, however, may be beginning to see changes in prevalence rates in some of these age groups. A study by UNICEF in 2004 found that only 6 per cent of girls 15 to 18 years old tested HIV positive. However, some researchers cautioned that the study was preliminary (Reuters, 27 August 2004). If prevalence remains high among young people, and if there is not a massive delivery of antiretroviral drugs, there will be a rise in illness and death for at least another six to eight years, because of the time it takes for an infected person to develop the illness.

Table 6.2 HIV prevalence among ANC respondents by age group, 1994–2002 (%)

Age group in years	HIV prevalence				
	1994	1996	1998	2000	2002
15–19	17.8	24.1	25.6	26.3	32.5
20–24	18.8	32.3	38.4	42.5	45.4
25–29	14.3	27.2	38.0	40.7	47.7
30–34	10.8	21.7	24.8	29.7	29.6
35–39	9.1	11.0	21.8	17.0	23.9
40+	18.3	11.7	25.7	26.9	25.0
Total	**16.1**	**26.0**	**31.6**	**34.2**	**38.6**

Source: Government of Swaziland. 2002. *Report on the 8th sentinel survey*. Mbabane: Government of Swaziland.

The Drivers of the Epidemic

Why is the heterosexual epidemic so bad in Swaziland? Table 6.3 shows the proximate and distal causes of the epidemic (Barnett and Whiteside 2002). Multiple factors contributing to the spread of HIV include biological and behavioral variables, the age structure of a population, access to knowledge about HIV and prevention practices, cultural beliefs, economic upheavals, and political and economic transitions.

Biological and Behavioral Factors Shaping the Epidemic

In order for people to be infected, they need to be exposed to the virus. Even then, exposure does not necessarily lead to infection. Sufficient viral particles must penetrate the body's defenses and enter the blood for infection to occur. Several biological factors determine how likely that is to occur: At the early and later stages of the infection, an infected HIV-positive person has a higher viral load, which increases the risk of exposure for partners. Women are more likely to be infected than men, because semen enters their bodies and remains there; and younger women are more prone to infection as the vaginal tissues are less mature and more prone to tearing. Linked to this, violence increases the chance of HIV infection, especially for women. For men, there is a growing body of evidence that circumcised men are less likely to be infected and thus, infect their partners. (Circumcision is only protective if it is carried out prior to sexual debut.)[3] Additionally, the presence of other STIs greatly increases the chance of HIV infection, because the open ulcers associated with STIs ease the spread of HIV. In women, STIs concentrate the specific type of cells that HIV targets (T cells) in the cervix, where the virus enters the body. Finally, poor nutrition and bad general health mean the body's immune system is less able to fight an infection (Stillwagon 2000).

Table 6.3 Proximal and distal causes of sexual transmission of HIV/AIDS

Determinants	Distal determinants		Proximal determinants	
	Macro environment	**Microenvironment**	**Behavior**	**Biology**
	Wealth or poverty	Mobility	Rate of partner change	Age
	Income distribution	Urbanization	Prevalence of concurrent partners	Stage of infection and virus sub-types
		Education		
		Access to health care	Sexual mixing patterns	
	Culture	Levels of violence	Sexual practices and condom use	Presence of other STIs
	Religion	Women's rights and status	Age of sexual debut	Gender
	Governance		Levels of sexual and physical abuse	Circumcision
Interventions	Social policy – redistribution	Social policy	Behavior change	STI treatment
		Economic policy	Condom use	Condom promotion
	Legal reform – human rights	Legal reform	Delay sexual debut	Antiretroviral therapy during pregnancy
		Employment	Fewer partners	
	Taxation	Legislation	Communication	Blood safety
	Debt relief		Address abuse and violence	Post-exposure prophylaxis
	Terms of trade			

Source: Barnett, Tony, and Alan Whiteside. 2002. *AIDS in the twenty-first century: Disease and globalisation.* Basingstoke: Palgrave Macmillian.

In order for these factors to matter, individuals have to have sex with a partner who is infected. If someone does not have sex, or has sex with only one uninfected partner who is also faithful, then the individual will not have sexual exposure to HIV.[4] Thus, there are a number of behavioral factors that affect the likelihood of infection. First, the more sexual partners that individuals have, the more likely they are to come into contact with someone with HIV. Second, the rate of concurrent partnering increases the risk of exposure to HIV. If a person has more than one partner at the same time, and if any of these individuals are infected, HIV is more likely to be transmitted. Third, patterns of sexual mixing affect the spread of HIV. For example, a person who works in Mbabane, has a rural home in Nhlangano, travels regularly to Durban, and has partners in each location could spread any STI very rapidly and widely. Some sexual practices also are conducive to the spread of HIV. These include sex with young partners and 'dry sex', a practice in which women use traditional herbs, or a range of other substances from toothpaste to detergent, to dry out the vagina before sexual intercourse, increasing the risk of tearing, bleeding, and exposure to infection. Other practices, such as consistent and correct use of condoms and late sexual debut, help prevent the spread of HIV.

The level of STIs in Swaziland provides insight into the increased risk of the spread of HIV in the country. In 1992, HIV prevalence was 3.9 per cent among ANC attendees in Swaziland and 11.1 per cent among people with STIs. The Government of Swaziland (2002) found that of those who tested positive for syphilis, 53 per cent were HIV positive. Among those who tested negative for syphilis, 37.9 per cent were HIV positive. However, there has been a decline in syphilis prevalence. Since 1994 syphilis prevalence among ANC attendees has fallen from 11.6 per cent to 4.2 per cent. Of greater concern for the AIDS epidemic are ulcerative STIs, since they facilitate the transmission of HIV. Table 6.4 illustrates STI incidence in 2003 among occupational groups based on various sexual behaviors. The data demonstrate the clear linkage between behavior, particular occupations, and STI transmission. There are very high levels of STIs among female factory workers, female sex workers, seasonal workers, the military, and the police.

The *Annual statistical bulletin* shows a small decline in outpatient visits for genital disorders over the period 1997 to 1999. However, the drop from 118,293 to 106,515 must be seen in the context of a decline in total outpatient visits from 1,485,685 in 1997 to 1,270,020 in 1999 (Government of Swaziland 1999a). Participants in discussions about the preliminary NERCHA report identified STIs as one of the drivers of the AIDS epidemic, and there is little evidence STIs are under control. The pressures on the health system and the general economic situation will only exacerbate the difficulty of combating the spread of STIs.

Another variable that influences the likelihood of the transmission of HIV is the age structure of the population. If a given population has a relatively large number of young people, there is a greater potential for the spread of

Table 6.4 STI incidence and behaviors, by occupation

	Military	Police	Seasonal workers	Watch men	Kombi drivers and assistants*	Long-distance drivers	Female factory workers	Female sex workers
Reported STIs episode in last 12 months	12.1%	6.5%	10.0%	4.8%	4.3%	5.7%	14.7%	16.1%
Sex with nonregular partner in last 12 months	54.8%	38.4%	30.7%	49.1%	57.7%	28.5%	32.5%	N/A
Condom use at last sex with nonregular partner	59.4%	73.2%	29.9%	59.8%	59.8%	57.1%	48%	60%

Source: Government of Swaziland. Ministry of Health and Social Welfare, and Family Life Association of Swaziland. 2003. *National behavioural surveillance survey.* Mbabane: Government of Swaziland.

*A kombi is a mini-bus taxi, which holds 12 or 16 passengers.

HIV, since young people often are the most sexually active individuals in a society. The most recent census carried out in 1997 puts the Swazi population at just under a million inhabitants, with an annual population growth rate of 2.9 per cent. Though the annual growth rate of urban areas is 3 per cent, most Swazis (77 per cent) still live in rural areas, predominantly on homesteads (Government of Swaziland n.d.). The major urban areas are the commercial and industrial conurbation of Manzini and Mataspha and the administrative capital Mbabane. The Swaziland age pyramid and population data (Figure 6.3) show a youthful population. According to the 1991 Demographic and Housing Survey, 43.5 per cent of the population is below 15 years old (Government of Swaziland 1992). This is a serious concern because it means that without behavior change, the potential for a sustained epidemic remains. We know that young people become sexually active and as they do, they are more likely to have several partners and less likely, in the absence of AIDS interventions, to use protection.

The *National behavioural surveillance survey* found that the majority of youth in Swaziland were not sexually active (Government of Swaziland 2003). Table 6.5 illustrates that more than 70 per cent of young people in school have never had sex, while almost 70 per cent of out-of-school youth

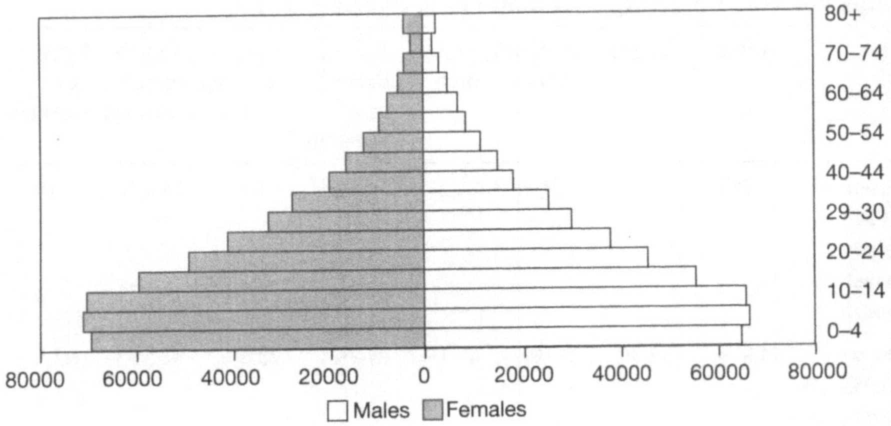

Source: Government of Swaziland Central Statistics Office, n.d. *Report on the 1997 Swaziland population and housing census*, Vol 4 of *Analytical report*, Mbabane: Government of Swaziland.

Figure 6.3 Swaziland population structure, 1997

have had sex.[5] It is clear that once youth leave school, they become sexually active. Why is this? Part of the reason may be that sexual intercourse is viewed as part of the normal rite of passage to adulthood. Once people leave school, they have more freedom. But there are other factors at work. Because of Swaziland's poor economy, the majority of youth will not find formal employment. They will be forced into poverty and dependence on others and they will be unoccupied for much of the time.

The information in Table 6.5 on age at sexual debut is somewhat limited and counterintuitive, since the data illustrate that in-school youth have a younger

Table 6.5 Sexual behavior of in- and out-of-school youth

	Ever had sexual intercourse (%)	Age at first sexual intercourse (in years)	Mean age of sexual partner (in years)
In-school youth			
Male	28.3	16.3	15.1
Female	28.3	16.1	20
Out-of-school youth			
Male	69.3	19.8	22.4
Female	69.3	18.3	28.7

Source: Government of Swaziland. Ministry of Health and Social Welfare, and Family Life Association of Swaziland. 2003. *National behavioural surveillance survey*. Mbabane: Government of Swaziland.

age of sexual debut. Although out-of-school youth's sexual debut may be at an older age, it is striking that their sexual partners uniformly have been older than the partners of in-school youth. This fact may indicate that out-of-school youth are involved in exploitative relationships. The relationship between older men and younger women has been identified as crucial for the transmission of HIV elsewhere in southern Africa (UNDP 2000).

To better interpret these data, it is important to know the proportion of Swazi youth who are enrolled in school. Enrollment ratios in the primary school years are above 100 per cent, indicating high numbers of students who repeat years. However, enrollment rates drop precipitously for secondary school years, with only 60 per cent of youth enrolled in school, including those repeating years (UNESCO 2002). There are a number of reasons for this decline, including the costs of school fees, uniforms, and books. Children who fail the standard five examination after the final year of primary education are not admitted to secondary school. Finally, some children feel that because of the low prospects for employment, there is little value in attending school.

Sexually active youth also are at risk of contracting STIs. Table 6.6 shows STI incidence and patterns of sexual behavior for in- and out-of-school youth. As mentioned above, STIs further increase the risk of HIV infection for an individual. Among youth in school, STI rates are negligible, while STI rates are significant for out-of-school youth.

As Table 6.3 demonstrates, condom use and access to information about the spread of HIV are two AIDS interventions. There is good evidence that condom use is increasing in Swaziland. In 1991, 86 per cent of all respondents surveyed knew about condoms, but only 18 per cent of these individuals had ever used condoms (Project Hope and FLAS 1991). By 1999, 62.3 per cent of youth surveyed said they used condoms when they last had sex (FLAS and UNICEF 1999). Table 6.4 illustrates that in all occupational groups – except seasonal workers (29.9 per cent) and female factory workers (48 per cent) – most individuals reported using a condom during their last sexual encounter with a nonregular partner. (In the case of the police, the figure was 73.2 per cent.) Table 6.6 shows that among in-school youth, condom use during first sexual encounter ranged by region from 59.5 per cent to 89.5 per cent, and from 83.3 per cent to 96.1 per cent during sex with a noncommercial partner. For out-of-school youth, rates of condom use were lower, from 33.3 per cent to 41.2 per cent during first sexual experience and from 41.6 per cent to 57 per cent during sex with a noncommercial partner. However, participants involved in writing the NERCHA report expressed concern over the messages used in the social marketing of condoms. Social events often promote a lifestyle that many individuals, particularly out-of-school youth, cannot afford, and the promotional events often take place in settings that do not encourage safe sexual behavior. While this type of social marketing may successfully target employed, urban young people who are wealthier than most Swazi youth, this marketing also may provide different messages to the majority of young people, who are rural, unemployed, and poor.

Table 6.6 Behavior of in- and out-of-school youth by region (%)

	Hhohho region	Lubombo region	Manzini region	National average
Male and female in-school youth				
Ever had sexual intercourse	26.8% (86/321)	31.1% (37/119)	28.6% (151/525)	28.3% (274/967)
Condom use at first sexual intercourse	89.5% (77/86)*	59.5% (22/37)*	69.5% (105/151)	74.5% (204/274)
Reported episode of STI in the last 12 months	0% (0/321)	0.8% (1/119)	0.8% (4/528)	0.5% (5/968)
Sex with noncommercial sexual partners in the last 12 months	13.7% (44/321)	20.2% (24/119)	15.9% (84/528)	15.7% (152/968)
Condom use with last noncommercial partner	96.1% (44/321)	83.3% (20/24)	83.3% (71/84)	84.8% (129/152)
Male and female out-of-school youth				
Ever had sexual intercourse	73.3% (328/448)	71% (489/689)	64.6% (413/639)	69.3% (1230/1776)
Condom use at first sexual intercourse	38.6% (126/328)	33.3% (163/489)	41.2% (170/413)	37.3% (459/1230)
Reported episode of STI in the last 12 months	4.7% (21/448)	7.4% (51/689)	4.9% (31/639)	5.8% (103/1776)
Sex with noncommercial partner in the last 12 months	52.7% (236/448)	47.8% (329/689)	48.4% (309/639)	49.2% (874/1776)
Condom use at last noncommercial sex	52.1% (123/236)	41.6% (137/329)	57% (176/309)	49.9% (436/874)

Source: Government of Swaziland. Ministry of Health and Social Welfare, and Family Life Association of Swaziland. 2003. *National behavioural surveillance survey.* Mbabane: Government of Swaziland.

* The sample size is too small to make a meaningful inference.

The data on knowledge around HIV in Swaziland are encouraging (Project Hope and FLAS 1991; Government of Swaziland 2003; Schools Health and Population Education 2003). People understand what HIV is and how it is spread. The *National behavioural surveillance survey* concludes, 'The Swazi people are highly knowledgeable about HIV/AIDS/STIs, though this knowledge has not translated into desirable behavioural change' (Government of Swaziland 2003). However, these reports also show that while people may be knowledgeable about how HIV is transmitted and how to protect themselves from the virus, they are confused about many other aspects of the disease, such as its progression and manifestations. A Ministry of Education report echoes this ambiguity. Based on interviews with teachers, parents, and students, the authors concluded that a central theme about AIDS in Swazi society is 'We are confused' (Government of Swaziland 1999b).

Social and Cultural Factors Shaping the Epidemic

In addition to biological and behavioral factors, social and cultural variables affect the spread of HIV. As the chapter by Siplon in this volume illustrates, the poor status of women can contribute to the AIDS epidemic. Swaziland is a society where polygamy is practiced; indeed, the Swazi king has nine wives and traditionally chooses a new one each year. Polygamy does not in itself lead to greater risk of contracting HIV. As one of the early AIDS prevention posters in Swaziland instructed, 'Be faithful in your polygamous family.' If partners are faithful to one another, and if all partners are HIV negative, then HIV is not a threat. However if one partner is unfaithful, then it is more likely that an infection will spread throughout the household. In addition, the level of trust among all members of a polygamous relationship must be greater than the level of trust in a monogamous relationship, since the number of partners is higher.

In traditional Swazi society, polygamous unions were no more likely to lead to nonregular partnering than monogamous ones. However, in traditional Swazi society, sex outside marriage was also not culturally acceptable. Boys and girls were permitted to experiment through practices such as thigh sex, but they were expected to stop before engaging in penetrative intercourse. Virginity was greatly valued. For example, a 2003 study found that 10.8 per cent of pupils reported having thigh sex (Schools Health and Population Education 2003). Because of economic and social disruptions that have strained traditional institutions, beliefs about premarital and extramarital sex are changing in Swazi society.

In Swaziland, men have more political power and legal rights than women. Politically, women serve in many senior positions in the civil service, but hold only 3 per cent of the seats in parliament. Almost all chiefs and traditional leaders are men. Legally, women are considered minors and cannot open bank accounts or own property without the approval of their husbands. The employment of women also has decreased, a fact that exacerbates women's lack of power in society. Between 1990 and 2001, the female share of nonagricultural wage labor fell from 35 per cent to 30 per cent (UNDP 2003). The upbringing of boys and girls also contributes to a situation in which boys are expected to seek sex and girls are expected to be more compliant. Boys are pressured at an early age to experience sex and prove their masculinity. The pressure to have sex and many partners is a socially expected competition among boys; for girls, there is a cultural belief that they are not women until they give birth. These beliefs increase the risk of the spread of HIV in Swaziland.

The issue of women's status in Swaziland is controversial. As of 2003, only one source in the literature examined the relationship between gender and the HIV/AIDS epidemic. This study (UNDP 2002, 1) reports:

> women's vulnerability to HIV/AIDS infection is increased by economic, social and cultural factors and by different forms of violence, (particularly sexual), that

place them at a disadvantage within relationships, the family, the economy and society at large. Women's economic dependence on men, their high poverty levels and lack of access to opportunities and resources, contribute to their vulnerability to HIV/AIDS infection. Because of the economic dependence on men, women are unable to take control of their lives and protect themselves against HIV infection. This is because the men can withdraw the economic support if women refuse to do as they want. Most cultural expectations and practices were found to contribute to women's vulnerability to HIV/AIDS. The Swazi society expects women to be subordinate and submissive; allows men to have multiple sexual partners; and polygamy, which exposes women to HIV infection, is legal in the country.

Additionally, the UNDP (2002) states that women's limited power means that, although basic information on HIV/AIDS is available to women, this knowledge does not assist them in making decisions to avoid risky sexual behavior. Table 6.7 illustrates this point. More specifically, women's inability to use knowledge about HIV/AIDS to protect themselves is evident among students in teritiary institutions. Though female students have marginally better knowledge about HIV/AIDS than male students, only 55.4 per cent of female students used condoms with nonregular partners, while 86.9 per cent of males did. These female students also are more likely to report STIs than male students. (The rates are 6.6 per cent for females and 3.7 per cent for males.) (Government of Swaziland 2003)

The 2002 UNDP study was based on interviews with only 32 women and 26 men. Nonetheless, the small-scale study echoes the concerns of participants in the NERCHA discussion, who noted that some cultural practices contribute to the spread of HIV. These include polygamy, arranged marriages, widow inheritance, and *umhlanga*, a traditional dance when young women bring reeds to repair the royal kraal and the king chooses a wife from among them. In contrast, other practices were thought to prevent the spread of HIV. These include virginity tests for young women and men and sexual abstinence until young people are mature enough to make meaningful decisions

Table 6.7 Can women use information/knowledge on HIV/AIDS to negotiate safer sex? (%)

Region	Yes	No	Don't Know
Hhohho	17	83	–
Manzini	50	25	25
Shiselweni	33	50	17
Lubombo	33	67	–

Source: UNDP. 2002. *Gender focused responses to HIV/AIDS in Swaziland: The needs of women infected and affected by HIV/AIDS*. Mbabane: UNDP.

Note: The anomalous response from Manzini may be because it is the only region where there were more men than women participating in the survey.

about their bodies and sexual relationships. NERCHA participants viewed *umcwasho*, the wearing of woollen tassles by young girls to indicate virginity, to be a positive traditional practice in the fight against HIV/AIDS. Likewise, the practice of *lusekwane,* the assignment of all Swazi males to an age regiment which comes together for various traditional activities, can contribute to HIV prevention.

Social norms and expectations about relationships also differ greatly between young men and women in Swaziland. Data from the Family Life Association of Swaziland (1995) illustrate the confusion evident in these relationships. When asked what they expect from boys, 36.2 per cent of female participants said money, 30.4 per cent said sex, 16.9 per cent reported fidelity, 5.8 per cent said gifts and entertainment, and 1.8 per cent did not know what they expected. When males were asked what they believed females expect from their boyfriends, 38.8 per cent said women expect money, 18.1 per cent reported that women expect sex, 14.3 per cent said females expect love, hugs, kisses, and to be cared for, and 8.9 per cent said women expect love, sex, and money. What is particularly interesting about this study is that it asked boys what they thought girls wanted, and it asked girls what they wanted. However, it never asked boys what they actually wanted or girls what they thought boys wanted.

The survey also reported that 69.8 per cent of males said their current girlfriend was not their first sexual partner. More males (65 per cent) than females (47.5 per cent) admitted to being sexually active. Among the females, 87 per cent believed that their boyfriend was the one who 'pressured' them into having sexual intercourse. In contrast, only 7.8 per cent of females believed sexual intercourse was no one's fault and had happened spontaneously; 2.6 per cent of women admitted to having insisted on having sexual relations, and 1.9 per cent of females believed sex occurred through mutual consent. On the issue of multiple sexual partners, 29.6 per cent of female respondents reported having sex with more than one person in their lifetime, and 29.9 per cent indicated that the primary cause of promiscuity was that 'girls want more money from their boyfriends'. However, 69.6 per cent of the female respondents felt that it was not a good idea to engage in sex before completing one's formal education, and 18.4 per cent thought engaging in sex was unwise because it could lead to dropping out of school because of pregnancy (FLAS 1995).

Economic Factors Shaping the Epidemic

The economic situation of a country shapes the context in which HIV may spread. Table 6.8 illustrates that until 2002 Swaziland's economic growth was fairly steady and gross domestic product (GDP) per capita was rising. According to the African Development Bank (2003), real GDP grew 2.6 per cent between 1998 and 2001, though only 1.6 per cent between 2001 and 2002. The gross national income per capita in 2001 was $1,300, compared to South Africa's $2,900, Mozambique's $210, and Lesotho's $550.[6] GDP per capita increased only 0.1 per cent between 1990 and 2002 (UNDP 2004, 186).

Table 6.8 Macroeconomic indicators

	1995/1996	1996/1997	1997/1998	1998/1999	1999/2000	2000/2001
Total GDP in millions of emalangeni (E)	1,251	1,304	1,355	1,405	1,483	1,504
% change in total GDP	3.7	4.2	3.9	3.7	5.6	1.5
GDP per capita (E)	1,399	1,430	1,457	1,485	1,518	1,540
% change GDP per capita	1	2.2	1.9	1.9	2.2	1.4

Source: Economist Intelligence Unit. 2002. *Swaziland country profile 2002*. London: Economist.

The continued food crisis in southern Africa is of great concern for the overall economy of Swaziland. Food production in the country has steadily declined. Maize production was 113,000 metric tons in 1999 but has decreased every year since then; in 2002, production was 70,000 metric tons (de Waal and Whiteside 2003). It is unclear the extent to which poor rainfall is responsible, but state policies have not helped to prevent the crisis. Crop failure may result in rural-to-urban migration and may increase poverty. Stillwagon (2000) has shown 'that HIV prevalence is highly correlated with falling calorie consumption, falling protein consumption, unequal distribution of income and other variables conventionally associated with susceptibility to infectious disease, however transmitted.' Malnutrition and parasite infestation depress both specific and nonspecific immune responses by weakening epithelial integrity and the effectiveness of cells in the immune system. Protein-energy malnutrition, iron-deficiency anemia, and vitamin-A deficiency – all poverty related conditions – decrease resistance to diseases including HIV. Reciprocally, the AIDS epidemic in southern Africa makes recovery from the food crisis more difficult. The African Development Bank (2003, 125) reports, 'Lesotho, Malawi, Swaziland and Zambia will be strongly affected by food security issues, growth recovery largely hinging on a return to normal weather conditions in time for the next harvests in April–June. The high incidence of HIV/AIDS on some of these countries' productive capacity make an economic rebound unlikely in the medium term.'

Swaziland's uncertain economic situation has discouraged foreign investment flows, which are crucial for job creation. The failure of the 2003 World Trade Organization talks in Cancun, which were intended to open the markets of developed countries to goods from the developing world, has harmed the economic prospects for Swaziland. Swaziland also may face some specific problems accessing US markets through the African Growth and Opportunities Act (AGOA) and the Generalized System of Preferences.

As of 2003, the AGOA allows duty-free entrance of Swazi products into the American market. However, in 2003 the US Department of Treasury accepted a petition from the American Federation of Labor-Congress of Industrial Organizations (AFL-CIO) to investigate Swaziland's labor practices. Participation in the AGOA is linked to a country's commitment to good governance, political reform, and the protection of human rights. Though the Swazi government passed the Industrial Relations Act in 2000, which gives workers the right to organize and bargain collectively, there have been widespread allegations that manufacturers, especially in the garment industry, have not complied with these labor laws. Likewise, the government has not actively enforced this legislation (US Department of State 2003). In response to possible loss of access to the US market, Taiwanese companies in the garment industry have warned the Swazi government that they will leave the country if preferential status for exports under the AGOA is lost (*AllAfrica*, 15 September 2003).

In order to attract foreign investment, the Swazi government and major international financial institutions have formed the Swaziland Industrial Development Company Limited. Yet, in the long run, the selling points for foreign investors may contribute to greater economic inequality and limit the rights of workers. Policies to attract foreign investment include generous tax allowances, including a five-year tax holiday; low corporate tax rates; free repatriation of dividends, interest, and profits; and a prohibition against expropriation and nationalization. The workforce in Swaziland is described to potential investors as educated, easily trainable, bilingual in English and siSwati, highly productive, and available at a competitive wage. Reading between the lines, these descriptions mean that labor is cheap, and that there are few laws to protect the rights of workers.

The structure of the economy and the type of employment available have implications for the spread of HIV in Swaziland. Table 6.9 shows that there has been a real decline in the total number of people employed in the formal sector. More people are forced to make a living in the informal sector, through subsistence agriculture or migration to South Africa. The Central Bank of Swaziland (n.d.) notes that the majority of jobs have been created in the textile sector, for low-paid female workers. As table 6.4 indicates, these workers have high levels of STIs, a significant number of nonregular sexual partners, and low levels of condom use (Government of Swaziland 2003). The environmental impact analyses for the garment industry factories, which were undertaken prior to the factories' construction, warned that HIV would be a real problem. The analyses suggested that education and communication programs and other interventions should have been put in place as soon as the factories opened (Environmental Consulting Services 2000a, 2000b). This puissant warning was ignored.

The decline in GDP, the lack of formal employment opportunities, and the uncertainty of foreign investment contribute to poverty and inequality in Swaziland. Table 6.10 provides a picture of poverty in southern Africa. The table displays the proportions of people in several countries who say they

Table 6.9 Employment in Swaziland

Year	1998	1999	2000	2001
Private sector employment	59,983	61,003	61,613	60,381
Public sector employment	31,891	32,210	32,693	33,216
Total formal employment	91,874	93,213	94,306	93,597
% change	–	1.46	1.17	–0.75

Source: Central Bank of Swaziland. n.d. *Annual reports*. Mbabane: Central Bank of Swaziland.

'sometimes' or 'often' do without particular things. Though the survey was not conducted in Swaziland, the findings can be applied to Swaziland because of the similarities among many southern African countries. These data show widespread poverty. Significant proportions of respondents say they or their families have gone without basic necessities at least occasionally, if not frequently. Southern Africans were most likely to have been short of cash income and least likely to experience homelessness. Significant proportions of people sometimes or often went without food, medical treatment, clean water, and fuel for heating or cooking.

With specific reference to Swaziland, World Vision (2003) reports:

> Poverty assessment surveys done by the World Bank and UNDP show that 66 per cent of Swazis live in absolute poverty. For rural areas, the percentage of people living in absolute poverty is even higher, in some areas it is at 80 per cent. Furthermore, the data show high inequalities in the distribution of income, with 10 per cent of the population obtaining 60 per cent of the country's income, and 90 per cent of the population receiving only 40 per cent of the income.This gap is increasing. This is one of the major causes of poverty in the country. The high rates of HIV/AIDS have further contributed to the declining standards of living.

Swaziland's Gini coefficient of 60.9 is an additional indicator of inequality in the country. (The Gini coefficient is a value on a scale from 0 to 100, where perfect equality is 0 and perfect inequality is 100.) This number compares with 59.3 in South Africa, 70.7 in Namibia and 63 in Botswana (UNDP 2003). Approximately 40 per cent of the population lives below the national poverty line (UNDP 2004).

Poverty and inequality have several effects on the AIDS epidemic in Swaziland. Poverty increases the likelihood that poor women will be forced into transactional sex as a survival strategy.[7] Orphans and vulnerable children are more likely to be exploited in situations of poverty; this exploitation may include sexual exploitation and abuse. Greater inequality in society also means that rich males may exploit poorer females, a practice which spurs the spread of HIV/AIDS.

The poor economic situation of Swaziland contributes to a high level of mobility within the country and across borders. In 1993, 54 per cent of all

Table 6.10 Shortages of basic goods and services, southern Africa, 1999–2000 (% answering 'sometimes' or 'often')

	Botswana	Zimbabwe	Zambia	Malawi	Lesotho	Namibia	South Africa	Average
Shelter	6	4	5	14	13	16	5	9
Enough fuel to heat your home or cook food	31	43	29	41	38	40	28	36
Enough clean water to drink and cook	16	46	30	47	50	41	24	36
Medicine or medical treatment that you needed	16	38	49	58	69	54	38	46
Enough food to eat	49	60	38	54	61	50	34	49
A cash income	52	77	69	69	80	71	47	66

Source: Bratton, Michael, and Robert Mattes. 2000. *Popular economic values and economic reform in southern Africa*. Afrobarometer Paper 10. Cape Town: The Institute for Democracy in South Africa.

Note: The survey asked, 'In the last twelve months, how often have you or your family gone without ____________? Was it often, sometimes, rarely or never?'

urban households maintained linkages with a rural homestead, with people from the urban areas visiting their rural homes at least once in the past month (Government of Swaziland 1993). Because Swaziland is a small country with good infrastructure, it is easy for urban dwellers to maintain contact with their rural homesteads. In addition, there is considerable cross border mobility, particularly to South Africa. Migrant miners, formally employed through the Employment Bureau of Africa, travel as single men for periods of up to a year to South Africa. There were 10,336 Swazi men employed in the mines in 1998 (TEBA 1999). Many other Swazis seek formal and informal employment in South Africa. These individuals range from unskilled workers to workers with professional qualifications and postgraduate degrees, who can earn three or four times what they would in comparable jobs in Swaziland.

Mobility provides the opportunity for and increases the likelihood of having nonregular sexual partners. When people travel, they are likely to be lonelier, to drink more alcohol, and to behave differently than they would in their home community. The long-term study of the mining community of Carletonville, South Africa, about 100 km from Johannesburg and 50 km from Soweto, provides insights into the relationship between AIDS and mobility. Many of the Swazi migrants traveling to the mines and farms of South Africa will find themselves in a social and economic situation similar to that of Carletonville, and some women from Swaziland will end up as sex workers in comparable communities. In Carletonville, the rate of HIV infection among adolescent girls is nearly 60 per cent. A large number of men in this community live in mine hostels. There are adjacent 'hot spots' in which more than 50 per cent of the women say they are commercial sex workers. The study shows that a range of factors raise individual susceptibility to infection. These variables include active or poorly treated STIs, use of alcohol, and high numbers of life-time sexual partners. For men, factors that decrease the risk of HIV infection are membership in a sports club and circumcision. (The study found that about half of the men are circumcised.) Among women, an important protective factor is membership in a burial society or church. For all, living in a squatter area raises the chance of exposure to HIV infection (Gilgen et al. 2000). All of the risk factors are associated with low levels of social cohesion, poverty among women, and economic inequality between men and women.

The Carletonville study confirms the fact that if people are in circumstances where they cannot maintain stable relationships, where they are mobile, where life is risky, and where pleasures are few and necessarily cheap, then STIs will be rampant. Furthermore, if there are inadequate medical services and limited accessible and effective treatments for STIs, HIV will spread rapidly. Some of the people in Carletonville such as the miners and sex workers had relatively high incomes. But these individuals were situated in a poor community; inequality and mobility contributed to the spread of HIV/AIDS.

Economic and Political Transitions as Factors Shaping the Epidemic

There is not a simple causal relationship between the AIDS epidemic and poverty. Part of the answer may lie in the type of economic growth or decline a country faces. Rapid economic growth brings problems such as disruption, deprivation, disease, and death. Quick economic growth disrupts traditional norms and cultures and people cannot adapt to the changes in society (Younde 2001). Szreter (2001) argues that economic growth is always accompanied by disturbances in the physical and biological environment and that growth necessitates cultural negotiation of new values. Economic growth skews income distribution and changes distribution patterns. Figure 6.4 illustrates that there is some relationship between a country's per capita income and its adult HIV prevalence rate. But, economic growth is not sufficient to fully explain the spread of the AIDS epidemic. For example, there has been little real per capita growth in South Africa since 1994. In that year, the per capita income was R18,786. In 1997, it was R14,249; but by 1999, it had fallen to R14,013. Yet the AIDS epidemic in South Africa has spread rapidly. Because exploitative sexual relationships contribute to the AIDS epidemic, a country's income distribution is probably as important as its level of economic growth for determining the spread of HIV. Income inequalities that result from uneven economic growth may fuel the AIDS epidemic.

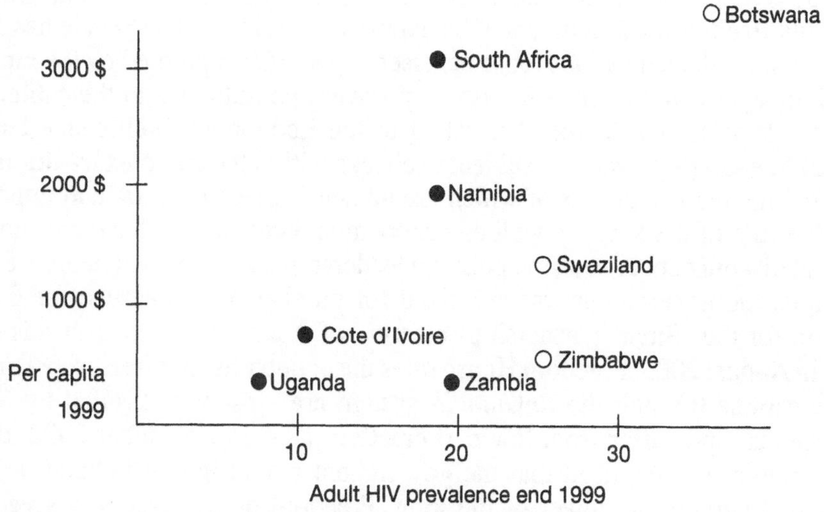

Source: Whiteside, Alan, Robert Mattes, Samantha Willan and Ryann Manning. 2002. *Examining HIV/AIDS in southern Africa through the eyes of ordinary southern Africans*. Centre for Social Research working paper 11, Cape Town: University of Cape Town.

Figure 6.4 Per capita GDP and HIV prevalence in select African countries

The relations among economic growth, income distribution, and AIDS are complicated because economic change may occur without an overall change in macroeconomic indicators. Again, South Africa illustrates this point. Though economic output has grown in real terms, this growth disguises fundamental changes in the structure of the economy. The primary sector (agriculture, forestry, and mining) and secondary sector (manufacturing, utilities, and construction) are shrinking as contributors to GDP, while the tertiary sector (banking, insurance, trade, and tourism) is growing. This new economic structure has resulted in a real decline in the number of people in formal employment. Unskilled workers have been the most affected in society. This change has occurred while the number of economically active people is growing. Swaziland presents a similar situation: formal employment is stagnant while informal employment is increasing. Swaziland's overall economic uncertainty, in terms of limited foreign investment, the ongoing drought, and the future of agriculture, creates a situation in which the continued spread of HIV is likely.

Economic transitions can lead to political conflict and societal challenges to political institutions (Szreter 2001). At best, Swaziland can be described as a dual system of rule with the monarchy of King Mswati III and a bicameral parliament. At worst, the system can be viewed as an autocracy. Fifty-five members of the House of Assembly are indirectly elected by an electoral college. Citizens in the local constituencies (*tinkhundla*) choose the electoral college by secret ballot. This traditional system was introduced by King Mswati's father after he suspended the constitution in 1973. The king appoints 10 additional members of the House of Assembly. The Senate has 30 members, 10 elected by the House of Assembly and 20 appointed by the king. The king appoints the prime minister, approves appointments to the cabinet, and can legislate by decree. According to the Economist Intelligence Unit (2002) 'the king's powers are subject to checks within the complex traditional system, the inner workings of which are unclear'. The autocratic and unpredictable rule of the king, as well as nepotism and corruption, have created a general disconnect between the political leadership and the Swazi people. For example, the government was criticized for purchasing a marquee for E13 million for the 'Smart partnership' meeting of Asian and African heads of state in August 2003. Freedom House rates the country as 'not free', reporting that elections through the *tinkhundla* system are closely controlled by the government and suffer from low participation rates. In December 2002, the prime minister announced that the government would ignore judicial decisions that curbed the power of the king. Freedom of expression is greatly restricted (Freedom House 2004). Traditional and modern institutions coexist, although this relationship is becoming more uneasy with the passage of time. The recent economic stagnation, the HIV/AIDS epidemic, and growing concerns over misuse of national resources contribute to this decline in legitimacy for the current political system. The 2003 election in Swaziland illustrates the difficulties of the political transition. In the country's first election in many years, opposition parties, which are illegal and banned by the government, called for a boycott. Instead of free and fair elections, candidates were nominated with little popular input under the *tinkhundla* system. Although there have been promises that the constitution will be revised, as of June 2004, this had yet to occur (UN Integrated Regional Information Network, 18 June 2004). The uncertainties that accompany periods of economic and political transitions create a dangerous environment for the spread of HIV. More research needs to be done to better understand the relationship between economic inequality, political change, and communicable diseases such as AIDS.

The AIDS Epidemic and the State in Swaziland

The particular nature of the Swazi state has contributed to the spread of HIV and has resulted in the country having the worst epidemic in the world in 2004. In its national development policies, the state has emphasized inward investment and has sustained an economic structure that has contributed to high levels of labor migration. In an attempt to compete in the global market, the Swazi government has promoted neoliberal policies, including low wages and limited protection of workers' rights. The worker mobility and economic inequality that have resulted from these strategies have created a climate in which HIV has spread easily. Additionally, the nature of the political system has made it difficult for the state to respond to economic and social crises, such as unemployment, inequality, and HIV/AIDS. The state lacks accountability to civil society groups such as opposition parties and trade unions. The lack of political freedom, the limited state transparency in decision making, and the relative isolation of political elites from citizens have hampered the policy-making process. The political system, with its emphasis on male-dominated power structures, polygamy in the royal family, and minimal rights for women, amplifies the gender inequality that contributes to the spread of HIV. Indeed, the most vulnerable group in Swaziland is out-of-school youth, especially young women. These women are probably the core transmitter group for the virus. However, because these women are exploited by society at large, and by older men in particular, it is inevitable that they will transmit HIV to others.

In addition, the lack of capacity of the Swazi state hampers its ability to address HIV/AIDS. Corruption and nepotism, as well as modern and traditional institutions that coexist in tension, complicate state actions on HIV/AIDS. The AIDS epidemic itself has diminished state capacity and the ability of the state to effectively serve its citizens. This pattern is becoming more apparent in the realms of health care, education, and public safety. In 1998, the Ministry of Health studied HIV prevalence rates among patients in selected hospitals. The resulting data showed that 49.5 per cent of patients were HIV positive, with 52.8 per cent being female and 45.6 per cent being male. The highest numbers of AIDS patients were between 20 and 39 years old (Government of Swaziland 1998). It is believed that since the study, HIV-positive patients occupy a greater number of hospital beds, and this burden on the public sector continues to increase. A study of bereavement notices in the *Times of Swaziland* from 1 July 1994 to 30 June 1999 revealed that the total number of deaths in Swaziland rose substantially during this period. The majority of individuals who died were between 26 and 40 years old (Whiteside et al. 2002a). A 2001 assessment of the impact of HIV/AIDS on the Ministry of Economic Planning and Development, the Ministry of Finance, and the Ministry of Public Service and Information estimated that AIDS will negatively impact personnel and ministry resources. To simply maintain current staff levels, 1.6 per cent of personnel will have to be replaced annually between 2001 and 2021. The epidemic will result in increased pension fund contributions, higher costs for sick and compassionate leave, and increased training costs. The study conservatively estimated the cost of the epidemic to the three ministries to be E10,535,994 from 2002 to 2010. This amount equates to roughly 1.5 per cent of the annual salary budget for the three ministries. Such costs mean that in the long term, the state's ability to effectively address HIV/AIDS, as well as other social development and economic concerns, will be strained (Government of Swaziland 2001).

AIDS also will affect the education sector. In 1999, it was noted that primary school enrollment will decline rapidly from 2003 to 2011, and will only begin to level off after 2012. By 2016, there will be almost 45,000 fewer Swazis of secondary school age because of the AIDS epidemic; this is a decrease of 22.7 per cent. In addition to the decline in number of students, AIDS will negatively impact teachers. Rather than training 5,093 new teachers during this period, over 13,000 will need to be trained to meet the AIDS-induced teacher shortage. Without an expansion in the number of newly trained teachers entering the education system, by 2006 the pupil-to-teacher ratio will increase to over 50: 1. It is predicted that this high ratio will remain for the foreseeable future (Government of Swaziland 1999b). Over time, the decline in the number of teachers will negatively impact the quality of education in Swaziland and will reverse educational gains that the country has achieved since independence. This situation creates a paradox: To effectively address the economic and political transition and the AIDS epidemic, Swaziland needs an educated citizenry; yet, AIDS itself is detrimental to education.

The decline in education and the rise in the number of children who have lost one or both parents to AIDS may challenge the future stability of Swazi society. Even if children have not lost parents to AIDS, they may be affected by the epidemic if they belong to a household which has absorbed AIDS orphans or which has adults that are ill. In 2003, more than 15 per cent of Swazi children below the age of 15 years old were orphaned. Estimates from 2003 indicate that there are 65,000 AIDS orphans in the country; by 2010, there will be roughly 120,000 AIDS orphans (Whiteside et al. 2003; UNAIDS 2004). Although there is little hard evidence illustrating the impact of large numbers of orphans on society, Schönteich (1999, 2001) has predicted that in South Africa, AIDS orphans will contribute to an increase in crime. Patterson (2003) has questioned the long-term impact of AIDS orphans and other vulnerable children on the democratic transitions that have occurred in many African states. AIDS challenges the ability of the Swazi state to provide for the security of its citizens, and it further complicates the economic and political transitions occurring in that country.

Given the challenges that AIDS presents to Swaziland, how might the state respond? The state could begin to address some of the key drivers of the epidemic that are outlined in this chapter: the lack of opportunities for young people; the inability of youth to stay in school; women's lack of power; the breakdown of societal norms; mobility; poverty; inequality; and the uncertain economic and political transitions. State actions might include ensuring that youth complete schooling, since being in school is a protection against HIV. The state also could provide recreational facilities for young people, to provide positive ways for them to occupy themselves. If youth are sexually active, state programs should encouraged them to be faithful and to use condoms.

The Swazi state could provide greater leadership and political commitment to the AIDS issue. In some ways, the state response has been quite path breaking. Because of the failure of early HIV/AIDS prevention programs, in 1998 the Cabinet developed and approved a new HIV/AIDS policy that focused on prevention, care, support, and impact mitigation. In February 1999, the King declared HIV/AIDS a national disaster, and the Cabinet Committee on HIV/AIDS and the Crisis Management and Technical Committee were created and launched. In 2001, the NERCHA was developed. As a coordinating body, NERCHA has become effective and efficient because of its dynamic leadership and excellent staff. Despite these positive changes, the state needs to fight AIDS through additional strategies. In the long term, job creation and economic development could address the factors such as economic inequality, poverty, and mobility that are determinants of the epidemic. Additionally, state officials should address the breakdown in social and cultural norms that has fueled the epidemic. There is a tendency for political, economic, and cultural leaders to say 'do as I say, not as I do'. Typically, older men advocate abstinence and fidelity, but their behavior contradicts this. In the context of economic stagnation, young people often are not receptive to such messages. As the Carletonville study illustrates, HIV spreads more easily in environments where there is little social cohesion. Though building such social cohesion has not been seen as a role for the state in the past, the Swazi state may need to think about how it can promote membership in grassroots efforts as a way to build ties in communities. NERCHA has begun to try to address this question, through providing small grants to a multiplicity of organizations. In 2003, Swaziland was awarded two grants from the Global Fund for AIDS, Tuberculosis and Malaria. The total amount over a five-year period is $56,736,900, but funding is only guaranteed for the first two years for a total of $30,610,400. This funding provides real possibilities to foster social cohesion for addressing the AIDS epidemic.

It is possible for Swaziland to reverse the spread of AIDS. This can be done through a variety of interventions, programs to empower people, and the construction of a stronger society. But such policies require political reform that creates strong, representative leadership. This leadership must not merely issue instructions, but also should seek to create an environment in which AIDS messages are viewed to be legitimate and are fully implemented. The Ugandan experience is instructive, because political leaders created a context in which local organizations, neighbors, and family members could openly discuss AIDS and could develop grassroots prevention, support, and care programs (Low-Beer and Stoneburner 2004). Swaziland has real opportunities to address the epidemic. Only time will tell if they are taken up.

Notes

1 Permission to use the NERCHA report is gratefully acknowledged. The report is available on the following websites http://www.nercha.org.sz/report/HEARD_report.pdf and http://www.und.ac.za/und/heard/publications/HEARD_swaziland_report_fin.pdf.
2 The survey methodology is described in Chapter 4 of the *Report on the 8th sentinel survey* (Government of Swaziland 2002).
3 There is a growing literature on circumcision, but since it is not practiced in Swaziland, this chapter does not further cover the topic.
4 Terminology is fraught with difficulty. This chapter defines 'faithful' as not having any other sexual partners.
5 The *National behavioural surveillance survey* systematically sampled and interviewed in-school youth between 15 and 19 years old from 30 schools around the country. Out-of-school youth were identified using a Probability Proportional to Size (PPS) sampling technique. Out-of-school youth between 15 and 24 years old, who were unmarried and who were not cohabiting, were selected from 90 enumeration areas, 30 youth from each of the three regions covered for in-school youth. See Government of Swaziland 2003.
6 These figures mask gross income inequality.
7 This includes commercial sex when people sell sex for money, as well as situations when a person exchanges sex for food, shelter, or protection.

References

African Development Bank. 2003. *African development report 2003: Africa in the world economy, globalization and Africa's development, economic and social statistics on Africa.* New York: Oxford Univ. Press.

AIDS Analysis Africa. 2002. Antenatal HIV prevalence survey indicates marginalized groups need greater attention in Zimbabwe. June–July: 1.

Barnett, Tony, and Alan Whiteside. 2002. *AIDS in the twenty-first century: Disease and globalisation.* Basingstoke: Palgrave Macmillan.

Bratton, Michael, and Robert Mattes. 2000. *Popular economic values and economic reform in southern Africa*. Afrobarometer paper 10. Cape Town: Institute for Democracy in South Africa.

Central Bank of Swaziland. n.d. *Annual reports*. Mbabane: Central Bank of Swaziland.

de Waal, Alex, and Alan Whiteside. 2003. New variant famine: AIDS and food crisis in southern Africa. *Lancet* 362 (October 11): 1234–37.

Economist Intelligence Unit. 2002. *Swaziland country profile 2002*. London: Economist.

Employment Bureau of Africa (TEBA). 1999. *Annual report*. Johannesburg: TEBA.

Environmental Consulting Services. 2000a. *Environmental impact assessment, garment factory, Nhlangano 2000/01*. Mbabane: Environmental Consulting Services.

——. 2000b. *Scoping report garment factory, Matspaha 2000/01*. Mbabane: Environmental Consulting Services.

Family Life Association of Swaziland. 1995. *In and out of school youth: Family health needs and sexual behaviours, attitudes and family planning practices – Manzini and Lubombo*. Mbabane: FLAS.

Family Life Association of Swaziland (FLAS), and United Nations Children's Fund (UNICEF). 1999. *Sexual and reproductive health services and HIV/AIDS peer education and counselling for youth and parents project: KAP baseline study*. Mbabane: FLAS.

Freedom House. 2004. Swaziland. http://www.freedomhouse.org/research/freeworld/2004/countryratings/swaziland.htm.

Gilgen, D., C. Campbell, B. Williams, D. Taljaard, and C. MacPhail. 2000. *The natural history of HIV/AIDS in South Africa: A biomedical and social survey in Carletonville*. Johannesburg: Council for Scientific and Industrial Research.

Government of Swaziland. Central Statistics Office. 1992. *1991 demographic and housing survey*. Mbabane: Government of Swaziland.

——. Ministry of Housing and Urban Development. 1993. *Land and housing market survey*. Mbabane: Urban Development Project.

——. Ministry of Health and Social Welfare. 1998. *Report on HIV prevalence among inpatients in selected hospitals*. Mbabane: Government of Swaziland.

——. Central Statistics Office. 1999a. *Annual statistical bulletin*. Mbabane: Government of Swaziland.

——. Ministry of Education. 1999b. *Assessment of the impact of HIV/AIDS on the education sector*. Mbabane: Government of Swaziland.

——. Ministry of Finance. 2001. *Assessment of the impact of HIV/AIDS in central ministries*. Mbabane: Government of Swaziland.

——. 2002. *Report on the 8th sentinel survey*. Mbabane: Government of Swaziland.

——. Ministry of Health and Social Welfare, and Family Life Association of Swaziland. 2003. *National behavioural surveillance survey 2003*. Mbabane: Government of Swaziland.

——. Central Statistics Office. n.d. *Report on the 1997 Swaziland population and housing census*. Vol. 4 of *Analytical report*. Mbabane: Government of Swaziland.

Joint United Nations Program on HIV/AIDS (UNAIDS). 2002a. *AIDS epidemic update*. Geneva: UNAIDS.

——. 2002b. *Report on the global HIV/AIDS epidemic*. Geneva: UNAIDS.

——. 2004. *Report on the global AIDS epidemic*. http://www.unaids.org/bangkok2004.html.

Low-Beer, Daniel, and Rand Stoneburner. 2004. Uganda and the challenge of HIV/AIDS. In *The political economy of AIDS in Africa*, ed. Nana Poku and Alan Whiteside, 165–90. Aldershot: Ashgate Publishers.

National Emergency Response Committee on HIV/AIDS (NERCHA). 2003. Background. http://www.nercha.org.sz/background.html.

Patterson, Amy. 2003. AIDS, orphans, and the future of democracy in Africa. In *The children of Africa confront AIDS*, ed. Arvind Singhal and W. Stephen Howard, 13–39. Athens: Ohio Univ. Press.

Project Hope, and Family Life Association of Swaziland. 1991. *Knowledge, attitudes, beliefs and practices on AIDS: A national survey of Swaziland.* Mbabane: Project Hope.

Schönteich, Martin. 1999. AIDS and age: South Africa's crime time bomb. *AIDS Analysis Africa* 10 (2): 1–4.

——. 2001. A generation at risk: AIDS orphans, vulnerable children and human security in Africa. Paper presented at a conference of the Nordic Africa Institute, Uppsala, Sweden.

Schools Health and Population Education. 2003. *The baseline study for the Swaziland in-school HIV and AIDS prevention programme: Draft report.* Mbabane: Schools Health and Population Education.

Stillwagon, Eileen. 2000. HIV transmission in Latin America: Comparison with Africa and policy implications. *South African Journal of Economics* 68 (5): 985–1011.

Szreter, Simon. 2001. Economic growth, disruption, deprivation, disease and death: On the importance of the politics of public health for development. In *Plagues and politics: Infectious disease and international policy*, ed. Andrew T. Price-Smith, 76–116. Basingstoke: Palgrave Macmillan.

United Nations Development Program (UNDP). 2000. *Botswana human development report 2000: Towards an AIDS-free generation.* http://www.undp.org/hiv/hdr2000/index.html.

——. 2002. *Gender focused responses to HIV/AIDS in Swaziland: The needs of women infected and affected by HIV/AIDS*. Mbabane: UNDP.

——. 2003. *Human development report 2003*. New York: Oxford Univ. Press.

——. 2004. *Human development report 2004*. New York: Oxford Univ. Press.

United Nations Educational, Scientific and Cultural Organization (UNESCO). 2002. *Education for all: Is the world on track?* Paris: UNESCO.

US Department of State. 2003. *Country reports on human rights practices: Swaziland.* http://www.state.gov/g/drl/rls/hrrpt/2002/18229.htm.

Whiteside, Alan, and Greg Wood. 1994. *Socio-economic impact of HIV/AIDS in Swaziland.* Report for the Ministry of Economic Planning and Development. Mbabane: Government of Swaziland.

Whiteside, Alan, Chris Desmond, John King, Jane Tomlinson, and Conway Sithungo. 2002a. Evidence of AIDS mortality from an alternative source: A Swaziland case study. *African Journal of AIDS Research* 1 (4): 37–40.

Whiteside, Alan, Robert Mattes, Samantha Willan, and Ryann Manning. 2002b. *Examining HIV/AIDS in southern Africa through the eyes of ordinary southern Africans.* Centre for Social Science Research working paper 11. Cape Town: Univ. of Cape Town.

Whiteside, Alan, Nkosinathi Ngcobo, Jane Tomlinson, and Alison Hickey. 2003. *What is driving the HIV/AIDS epidemic in Swaziland and what more can we do about it?* Report for the National Emergency Response Committee on HIV/AIDS (NERCHA) and United Nations Program on HIV/AIDS (UNAIDS). http://www.nercha.org.sz/report/HEARD_report.pdf.

World Vision. 2003. Swaziland background. http://www.wvi.org.za/countries/Swaziland.htm.

Youde, Jeremy. 2001. All the voters will be dead: HIV/AIDS and democratic legitimacy and stability in Africa. Paper for Charles and Kathleen Manatt Democracy Studies Program. Ames: Univ. of Iowa.

Chapter 7

The More Things Change: AIDS and the State in South Africa, 1987–2003

Patrick Furlong and Karen Ball

In 1999, the current president of South Africa, Thabo Mbeki, strongly questioned the scientific evidence that HIV is the sole cause of AIDS, an action for which he was condemned at home and abroad. His controversial stance on AIDS confuted an orthodoxy that contrasts state responses to AIDS in South Africa before and after the landmark 1994 democratic election. According to this view, the pre-1994 National Party (NP) apartheid regime, hidebound by puritanism and racism, ignored or at best paid lip service to the AIDS threat. African National Congress (ANC) rule, however, allegedly meant a dramatic improvement, as the party had condemned its predecessor's response to AIDS and was committed to helping the poor or marginalized, from whom most AIDS sufferers came. The belief was that a democratic state with broad legitimacy would focus on fighting AIDS. This chapter challenges the orthodox view through a systematic examination of AIDS policies during both periods.

Because apartheid created gross inequalities in health care (Price 1986; Packard 1989; Baldwin-Ragaven 1999; McCulloch 2002), it is logical to assume that the apartheid government would pay little attention to AIDS, a disease that disproportionately affected blacks. Zwi and Bachmayer (1990) condemn early state responses to AIDS as inadequate, inappropriate, or, as with the policy of repatriating infected migrant black miners, discriminatory. Grundlingh (1999, 2001b) argues that homophobia, racism, and puritanism thwarted a timely, effective reaction, and that the state's lack of credibility among the black majority undercut its belated response. Whiteside and Sunter (2000, 119) note how apartheid caused poverty, overcrowding, inequality, fatalism, and conflict, all of which promote the spread of HIV/AIDS. The NP regime, supported primarily by conservative Afrikaners, was notoriously prudish about issues such as sex education, and censors routinely banned 'obscene' books, films, and objects. Frank discussion of sexually transmitted infections (STIs) such as AIDS was hugely problematic in such a society.

Several scholars maintain that state attention to AIDS dramatically increased under the post-apartheid government. Phillips (2001, 23) claims that democratization 'introduced a sea-change in state policy' on AIDS. Whiteside and Van Niftrik (1990) contrast the NP regime's lack of commitment with the ANC's deep concern about the AIDS threat. Gevisser

(1994b) declared in the *Mail & Guardian Weekly*: 'Finally, the state gets serious about AIDS.' Mary Crewe (1992, 63, 71–73) compares the ineffectual response of a regime with no credibility among blacks with the ANC's commitment to making AIDS a priority.

Problems with the Orthodox View

This image of sharply contrasting state responses to AIDS is, however, too simplistic. From the late 1980s, official bodies, notably the Department of National Health (DOH) and the Medical Research Council (MRC), addressed AIDS, even while AIDS activists, public health experts, and opposition leaders decried state inaction and ineffectual strategies. Many lower-level civil servants and scientists in health-related public agencies seemed aware of the AIDS threat, although many senior government figures seemed blind to the problem. This remained true in the post-1994 period. The new government was relatively slow to address the disease, developing contradictory policies and sometimes questioning basic scientific findings about AIDS. Just as in the apartheid period, the AIDS policy-making process after 1994 could be characterized by a gap between rhetoric and reality, lack of political will, inadequate funding, slow policy development and implementation, and tensions between the state and civil society.

These similarities in state responses to AIDS before and after 1994 illustrate much about the economic, political, and social challenges to the South African state. The post-1994 government faced many problems that characterize governance throughout sub-Saharan Africa. Artificial colonial and apartheid borders and institutions weakened state legitimacy and hindered the implementation of any type of policy. The post-1994 administration found that governance proved harder than criticism; without a tradition of political pluralism or tolerance, the former rulers' centralizing, authoritarian tendencies were alluring (Southall 1998; Hawker 2000; Gouws and Gibson 2001). Just as other African states suffered from the economic legacy of colonialism, post-apartheid South Africa needed vast sums for education, housing, electricity, water, jobs, and public safety. These problems required resources even greater than those needed to defend apartheid; AIDS was only one of many problems the state faced. In the aftermath of apartheid, poverty and insecurity facilitated the spread of HIV, as they have elsewhere in Africa.

However, South Africa differs from many African states engaged in fighting AIDS in notable ways. The transition from apartheid to democracy has been time consuming and politically distracting. If negotiating a new order hampered F. W. de Klerk's government (1989–1994) from focusing on AIDS, the need to transform the state after 1994 slowed AIDS efforts. Furthermore, the end of apartheid entailed changes in government structures, such as integration of the black homelands into the previously 'white' South Africa and the devolution of some powers to nine new provinces. Apartheid-era bureaucrats, whose jobs were protected from 1994 until 1999, often clashed with new state employees. Though the struggle against AIDS has been hindered throughout Africa by an unwillingness to discuss sexual behavior, in South Africa such attitudes were compounded by many whites and blacks viewing AIDS in racial terms. Like many other African leaders, both NP and ANC politicians failed to address AIDS in a timely manner. However, unlike many of their African counterparts, some South African leaders have confused the public with their extraordinary views about the disease.

Pre-1994 AIDS Policies

During the pre-1994 period, especially before 1990, there was much denial in official circles about AIDS. The militaristic and puritanical climate under P.W. Botha (president from 1984 to 1989) made it difficult to act against AIDS, even after the disease spread into the heterosexual black majority. Once the government began to recognize the need to do more, it was distracted by other issues. Black resistance to Botha's unwillingness to end apartheid forced his successor, F. W. de Klerk, to focus on seeking a negotiated solution with black leaders. Reformists in the state bureaucracy also had to fight rearguard battles with conservatives who were suspicious of new initiatives, such as AIDS-education campaigns. Prudishness among both white and black South Africans hindered frank discussion about how AIDS is transmitted, and the government's lack of legitimacy among the black majority hampered the credibility of its most well-intentioned efforts to fight AIDS.

Early Reactions to AIDS: Denial, Discomfort, and Racism

As late as 1987, the state response to AIDS displayed little urgency. Conservative white voters saw AIDS as limited to homosexual men and 'licentious' blacks (Crewe 1992, 14–16). Some clergy, notably in the powerful Afrikaans Reformed churches, dismissed AIDS as punishment for sin (Grundlingh 2001a, 98–99). Scientists in the regime's secret chemical and biological warfare program showed interest in AIDS only insofar as HIV infection among guerrillas based in neighboring states might lead to their defeat. For example, microbiologist Mike Odendaal recounted being given a vial of blood from a dying AIDS patient to use against regime opponents (Burger and Gould 2002, 31–32, 147–48).

When DOH annual reports first discussed AIDS in 1985, they focused on how all 21 diagnosed cases were male; of these individuals, 20 were white, 16 were gay, and one was bisexual. The three heterosexual cases had 'some contact with Zaire'; one additional case was because of a blood transfusion (DOH 1986, 1). The 1986 report noted that the overwhelming majority of 13 new cases were among homosexual men (DOH 1987, 10). In 1987, the DOH reported a total AIDS caseload of 64 South African citizens plus 20 individuals 'from countries to the north'. While the report stated that 10 per cent to 20 per cent of high-risk groups (e.g., gay men) were 'definitely carriers', it claimed that HIV prevalence among the general population was low (DOH 1988, 7).

That year, Jack Metz, MRC director and chair of the government's newly appointed expert advisory group on AIDS, argued that AIDS would remain a minor disease if high-risk groups cooperated; he explained the low incidence in South Africa by the country's geographic isolation (Grundlingh 2001a, 92). In 1985, the government had taken the very modest step of setting up the advisory group, which was mandated to gather information, provide disease surveillance, liaise with counterparts abroad, inform high-risk groups of dangerous practices such as donating blood, and advise health personnel on practical preventive measures (DOH 1986, 1). However, the group's work was limited by its membership, which largely comprised economists, scientists, and clinicians. Reflecting the ultra-conservative and technocratic ethos of the Botha era, this group lacked representatives from civil society, such as gay organizations or black groups (Perlman 1988, 1989; Grundlingh 2001b, 131). Without such input, it was impossible to develop effective strategies for outreach before the epidemic began to take hold in those communities.

Even the MRC, a state-controlled but relatively autonomous body charged with researching public health threats, only paid serious attention to AIDS in 1987, when its president warned that the disease challenged the idea of 'first' versus 'third world' diseases. AIDS remained absent, however, from the report's overview of activities and research highlights (MRC 1988, 3–5, 7–8, 10–12). Furthermore, in 1987, the DOH was still negotiating over a nationwide AIDS information campaign (DOH 1988, 7). A year later a senior advisory group member complained that state guidance had been 'singularly lacking' (Perlman 1988). As late as 1988, a DOH spokesperson argued that other countries had started anti-AIDS campaigns 'too early, too heavy'; the state was still denying the potential impact of the disease on the population (Grundlingh 2001b, 126–27).

The puritanical and racist apartheid mentality also undercut the state's meager AIDS efforts during this period. For example, the first national anti-AIDS education campaign, developed in 1988, was racially segregated. It tried to scare blacks with images of a coffin and a funeral, while showing whites vague images of graffiti that suggested promiscuous relationships, but did not mention specific risky behaviors (Zwi and Bachmayer 1990, 321). Even after the de Klerk government abandoned most remaining apartheid laws such as those mandating racial classification at birth or requiring segregation of residential areas, public amenities, and political parties, it remained constrained by discomfort with sexual matters. The regime was caught between opponents of reform in the Conservative Party, which played on racist sentiment by claiming that integrated swimming pools and nursery schools would spread HIV (Van Niftrik 1990/1991), and criticism by white liberals such as Democratic Party health spokesman Mike Ellis, who attacked the government's reluctance to introduce AIDS-related sex education in schools (Ellis 1991). As late as 1993, the Publications Control Board banned two safe-sex educational videos (SAIRR 1994, 144). In the racially polarized atmosphere before the 1994 election, many blacks also viewed any safe-sex campaign as part of a 'genocidal' effort to lower their birth rate (Van der Vliet 2001, 154–55).

There are numerous political reasons why the South African state underrated the AIDS threat. In the 1980s, Botha's regime faced economic sanctions, foreign isolation, hostile neighbors, anarchy in urban black areas, and an ANC-led guerrilla campaign. In response, the government offered expensive but inadequate reforms, such as giving limited powers to new mixed race 'colored' and Indian (but not African) chambers in the previously all-white parliament. At the same time, the state became increasingly repressive and intolerant, even of whites who rejected its notions of warrior masculinity. For instance, a 1999 MRC coauthored study alleged that some gay white military conscripts suffered electrical shock or chemical treatment intended to alter their sexual orientation; there are also claims that the military performed some 900 sex-change operations on gay conscripts (Van Zyl et al. 1999; Kaplan 2001).[1] The state was so focused on preserving white rule that Botha's 'total strategy' left few resources for a disease that challenged the regime's conservative views and seemed to strike the most marginalized groups.

The Apartheid State Reacts

By the late 1980s, the state had begun to react to AIDS. Though the authoritarian Botha regime was notoriously impervious to criticism, increasing evidence of a potentially broader epidemic led to the development of new AIDS policies (Grundlingh 2001a, 102). Government preoccupation at the top with containing unrest in black areas and with allaying the growing fears of whites also provided space for lesser, but more enlightened, DOH and MRC officials to shift policy direction.

In 1987, the MRC established an AIDS research unit, which soon noted a 'disquieting increase' in heterosexual transmission, though most cases were in the black community (MRC 1989, 9, 17). That year the MRC hosted and published the proceedings of an international AIDS research symposium (MRC 1989, 7). Press reports of AIDS 'spreading among African miners and into the communities surrounding the compounds' confirmed the threat to the general population (Van Niekerk 1988). The 1988 DOH report reflected greater concern about the disease and acknowledged the difficulty of AIDS education because of 'taboo subjects, such as sex, blood and death' (DOH 1989, 17). This increased awareness that AIDS could no longer be dismissed as affecting a tiny minority was apparent in the aforementioned 1988 DOH education campaign. Despite its prudishness and the apartheid mindset in which it was framed, the campaign was progressive in one respect: it stressed high-risk practices rather than high-risk groups (DOH 1989, 17).

The 1988 DOH annual report also warned prophetically that awareness was not enough and that the state could not solve the AIDS problem alone: 'It is a community-based endeavour which involves states, private sector [*sic*] and the broader community' (DOH 1989, 17). This emphasis may reflect the regime's keenness to privatize many state activities, at a time when economic sanctions, the high costs of the total strategy, and admiration for the economic policies of the Thatcher and Reagan governments encouraged abandonment of NP state intervention. The DOH also may have recognized the limited capacity of a state with dubious legitimacy, especially among blacks. Facing enormous political and economic pressure, the Botha regime clearly needed to involve more stakeholders in the AIDS issue, but only after the pragmatic de Klerk replaced Botha in 1989 did the state begin to take more seriously the idea of a partnership with civil society to fight AIDS.

In March 1990, within weeks of legalizing the liberation movements, the de Klerk government met the ANC to discuss AIDS, leading to a joint funding request to the World Health Organization. In April the ANC took a leading role in an international AIDS conference in Maputo, Mozambique, where the participants agreed on the need for a national AIDS task force in South Africa. By this point, the government had already created DOH-funded AIDS training and information counseling centers (ATICCs) in major cities (Whiteside and Van Niftrik 1990). In January 1992, the DOH AIDS unit convened a preparatory meeting for a national conference. The DOH and the ANC appointed a steering committee that included church, union, and business representatives to organize the National AIDS Convention of South Africa. The convention incorporated education, political, insurance, health, sports, women's, and AIDS service and activist organizations, and established the National AIDS Council of South Africa (NACOSA) to coordinate a countrywide response (Fleming 1992/1993, 7). As a sign of increased state concern, the foreign affairs department provided the secretariat for the convention (Gevisser 1992c).

The ANC later claimed that it and its alliance partners had developed NACOSA (ANC 1993). Yet the state was very involved. On the other hand, while Nelson Mandela addressed the convention, neither the health minister, Rina Venter, nor any other minister attended (Fleming 1992/1993, 7). This puts in question NP leaders' (as opposed to DOH professionals') commitment to fight AIDS, although the cabinet perhaps feared alienating more white voters by prioritizing the disease. Bitter disagreements marred the convention. There were more divisions between civil society groups and the political parties (both the ANC and NP) than there were between the ANC and the apartheid regime. A major issue was the omission from the convention steering committee of the community-based National Progressive Primary Health Care Network, mandated in 1989 by the ANC to handle AIDS work (Gevisser and Stober 1992). Even the 11 ATICCs were criticized because they were located where they served almost exclusively whites; only in mid-1993 was one for Soweto approved (Fleming 1993). In hindsight, these disagreements between political authorities and civil society foreshadowed future tensions.

In theory, the government had begun to embrace a more progressive general health policy. Minister Venter announced in her 1990 budget speech a plan to 'reconstruct' health services, with less racial or ethnic fragmentation, more equity in funds, and access for all (MRC 1990, 4). The plan did not necessarily mean an improved response to AIDS, but it recognized that the apartheid approach of segregated health agencies was inefficient and unfair, and any reform that reached out to *all* South Africans might improve the state's ability to fight AIDS. Venter warned, however, that economic constraints made dramatic adjustments in her budget impossible for many years (MRC 1990, 5). The liberal *Business Day* derided her 1991 announcement of a huge AIDS education program, arguing that even doubling spending on AIDS was not enough (APRG 1991). Though the state AIDS budget quadrupled between the 1991/92 and 1992/93 fiscal years (SAIRR 1993, 285), it dropped slightly from 1992/93 to 1993/94. Much of the budget shifted from direct education to research and surveillance or the aforementioned ATICCs and nongovernmental organizations (NGOs), which were thought to be more credible than state agencies (SAIRR 1994, 139).

The state's lack of financial resources hampered its AIDS efforts. The MRC complained that funding remained inadequate for behavioral and epidemiological AIDS research (MRC 1991, 3–4). In fact, there were no reliable statistics on the number of AIDS deaths in the country. While official reports showed 26 AIDS deaths in the first nine months of 1992, 153 people had died of AIDS in just one hospital in Natal (Van Niftrik 1992/1993, 1). As was true after 1994, financial constraints also were used to justify state reluctance to offer AIDS drugs; AZT, then the one registered drug proven to slow the progression of AIDS, was provided free only to hemophiliacs infected by blood transfusions and to health-care workers infected on the job by contaminated needles (Gevisser 1992b).

Divisions in the AIDS bureaucracy complicated the state's AIDS efforts. In a period of great flux in the state apparatus, conservative, usually male Afrikaners who had dominated the senior levels of the bureaucracy increasingly diverged from de Klerk's reformist NP. English-speaking whites, somewhat more liberal than either faction, now filled key positions in the DOH AIDS unit, a possible sign of de Klerk's efforts at more inclusiveness. However, these individuals often lacked their bosses' political clout or connections. For example, bureaucratic infighting may have been behind orders by the DOH to investigate alleged irregularities in running the AIDS unit and alleged complaints about the acting unit head, Manda Holmshaw. Holmshaw countered these charges by noting that she and her deputy had complained that their advice on AIDS prevention often was ignored, and that they had opposed efforts to transfer a third of the AIDS budget to the state immunization program (SAIRR 1993, 286; Ellis 1991). Holmshaw, a clinical psychologist, was replaced by a nurse, Natalie Stockton, who seemed better able to negotiate the murky politics of a still relatively conservative civil service. One casualty of the lack of a unified, well-coordinated DOH effort was a new AIDS educational kit geared especially to schools. Its early withdrawal may have been as much because of bureaucratic infighting as because of the irrelevance of this educational material to poor black communities (SAIRR 1993, 286; SAIRR 1994, 143; Gevisser 1992a; Gevisser 1993).

Nevertheless, despite financial constraints and bureaucratic conflicts, the state gave new attention to AIDS. This concern manifested itself in several ways, some of which foreshadowed the best of post-1994 methods. The MRC, working with the DOH at the grassroots level, now emphasized relevant community health research. The MRC shifted from a narrowly biomedical AIDS focus to one involving psychologists, educators, social workers, sociologists, health economists, a social marketing expert, and social anthropologists (MRC 1992, 9). One MRC division worked on likely projections of the epidemic; another studied high-school children's sexual practices, which helped the DOH develop a national school-based educational program. In 1991 the MRC funded a survey of informal shops in African townships on the topic of offering AIDS education and selling condoms (MRC 1992, 9). That same year, the MRC used private funding to create a two-page newspaper supplement that explicitly advocated condom use to a general audience (APRG 1991). Corporate funding also helped to promote the Macmillan Boleswa AIDS awareness program, which reached children with limited English skills in a simple, non-moralizing way (MRC 1994, 31; APRG 1994). The MRC national AIDS research program helped to develop *Roxy*, a teen-oriented comic book that showed the impact of AIDS on relationships. The MRC also began assessing the use of traditional healers as AIDS educators or condom distributors (MRC 1994, 31, 39).

In summary, early denial, lack of funding, little political will, and puritanical, racist attitudes shaped AIDS policies during the Botha and de Klerk administrations. It is untrue that there was *no* movement on AIDS before 1994. State-funded research on AIDS began even in the Botha era and by the early 1990s there were some preliminary efforts at AIDS education programs, even if these suffered from inadequate input from the targeted communities. The de Klerk government did try to reach out to civil society and even involved the ANC in discussions on a plan to fight AIDS. Yet, none of these early initiatives significantly curbed the spread of HIV. Political pressure on recalcitrant officials from the president's office or the relevant minister could have given more direction and urgency to fighting AIDS. For example, presidential pressure on the state broadcasting corporation, which had often accommodated the NP, could have overridden the corporation's refusal to air unambiguous AIDS prevention messages and condom commercials (Van Niftrik 1993). Furthermore, although the state faced financial problems, innovative partnerships with the private sector and changes in spending priorities could have led to more AIDS programs. Big business was often willing to help fund AIDS education programs, and with the end of the occupation of Namibia in 1989, some defense funds could have been redirected to AIDS. By the 1990s, unwillingness to address AIDS was not because the state was unaware of the scale of the problem. On the contrary, Venter projected in 1993 that without adequate intervention one in five South Africans would be HIV positive by 2010 (SAIRR 1994, 144–45).

Post-1994 Policies

There were undoubtedly some notable changes after April 1994. AIDS awareness was one of 22 presidential priorities in the Reconstruction and Development Program (RDP), the centerpiece of the ANC's 1994 election platform (DOH 1995, 11). Grassroots organizations such as the Congress of South African Trade Unions (COSATU) had drafted much of the RDP (Terreblanche 2002, 108), which illustrates the ANC's initial support from civil society. Although the pattern of health-care expenditure by the end of the de Klerk era was progressive by African standards, after 1994 state budgets shifted significantly more money from affluent to poor communities (Nattrass and Seekings 2001, 56–57). Since poverty and soaring HIV rates are closely linked in Africa (Terreblanche 2002, 44), such changes were essential to combat AIDS. At the end of 1994, Mandela's government of national unity (composed of ministers from the ANC, NP, and the Inkatha Freedom Party) accepted a national AIDS plan. This plan included key MRC recommendations for greater control of STIs and educational programs for in- and out-of-school youth (MRC 1995, 10).

In July 1994, the health minister, Nkosazana Zuma, announced plans to double the AIDS budget by reallocating other DOH funds to AIDS (Gevisser 1994a). The 1995 AIDS budget was doubled yet again, with a quarter of it going to NGOs. The government wanted to mandate sex education for school children, run media information campaigns, improve STI treatment, develop care and support programs for infected persons, and ban discrimination against those with the disease. In the 1995/96 fiscal year, the state distributed over 97 million free condoms. Zuma promised hardnosed pragmatism: 'In the long-term perhaps we do need to change the values of this society, so that it can be more acceptable for young people not to be sexually active. But in the short term, let's face it, condoms are useful' (Phillips 2001, 23; SAIRR 1996, 199; Gevisser 1994a).

In 1997, the government formed an interministerial committee to coordinate AIDS efforts, complemented in 1998 by the Partnership Against AIDS, a program to reach out to civil society to implement an AIDS action plan. By 2000, the South African National AIDS Council (SANAC) promoted a multisectoral HIV/AIDS strategic plan. As a demonstration of high-level attention to AIDS, Deputy President Jacob Zuma chaired SANAC (Whiteside and

Sunter 2000, 124–27). By 2000 the DOH could list many further AIDS initiatives: national implementation of 'life skills and HIV/AIDS education' in high schools and parallel pilot programs in primary schools; training of key trade unionists to lobby for workplace AIDS programs; training of 270 traditional healers in HIV/AIDS counseling and care; and pilot programs of home-based care to reduce the burden on hospitals (DOH 2000, 11–13). State support for MRC research increased dramatically. From 1999 the MRC coordinated the ambitious new South African AIDS Vaccine Initiative, a collaborative state-industry-NGO-academe project (MRC 1999, 8; Tucker 2001). MRC-funded scientists also developed a system designed to reduce HIV transmission to infants by heating infected mothers' breast milk to kill HIV (MRC 2000, 35). By 2001, the state was distributing 250 million condoms per year; it had expanded sites for a rapid HIV test, established 18 research and training sites for prevention of mother-to-child transmission (PMTCT), and set up 256 outlets to distribute Diflucan, a drug for AIDS-related infections (DOH 2001a; DOH 2001b, 1).[2] And, most notably, in late 2003, the state agreed to provide antiretroviral (ARV) treatment to all South Africans needing it.

Despite these successes, the post-apartheid state has been slow to engage AIDS, often developing contradictory policies and sending confusing messages. Several overarching themes characterize state responses to AIDS during the Mandela and Mbeki presidencies. The continued lack of political will and a tendency to view AIDS solely as a health issue are reflected in the Mandela-era responses. AIDS policies in this period were further complicated by the move from a distributive economic plan to a neoliberal agenda, tensions between societal attitudes and the new liberal constitution, and a tendency to centralize policy making. Several of these themes continued in the Mbeki period, but AIDS policies became even more problematic, due to the denial of established science on HIV/AIDS, increased tension between the state and civil society, and controversy over providing treatment for those with AIDS.

The Mandela Presidency, 1994–1999

In June 1994, Clive Evian, Johannesburg AIDS chief and an architect of the NACOSA AIDS plan, hailed the appointment of Nkosazana Zuma as health minister. Zuma was an outspoken critic of the NP government's AIDS policies and a former chair of NACOSA's strategy subcommittee. Evian warned, however, that apart from Zuma there had been 'no real demonstration of political will from the heavies up there, except for Mandela, who has highlighted the issue from time to time' (Gevisser 1994a). This pattern of limited political attention to AIDS was apparent at the 1997 ANC national conference, when President Mandela, in a long final speech as ANC leader, mentioned AIDS just once.[3] In his closing comments, Mandela referred to 'the intensification of the struggle against HIV/AIDS' in a list of 12 'important issues' (ANC 1997). Similarly, an ANC-commissioned 1999 audit of the RDP only mentioned AIDS in a footnote (Bond and Khosa 1999, 101).

Like the preceding government, the Mandela administration tended to define AIDS narrowly as a health issue. The 1994 ANC election platform mentioned AIDS as part of a promise to direct 'major resources' to combat tuberculosis, AIDS and other STIs, cancer, and 'other plagues' (ANC 1994b, 11). The Kwazulu-Natal ANC, reflecting the early spread of HIV there, repeated this promise in an election flyer entitled 'A Better Life for All' (ANC 1994a, 1994c).[4] The RDP mentioned AIDS only once, in the document's health section. It advocated active and early treatment, mass education, especially in rural areas, and an end to discrimination against people with the disease (ANC 1994d, 48). Despite this brief recognition of the need to address AIDS, the DOH rather than the RDP fund paid for AIDS programs (Hambridge 1995). Major policy documents, such as those on housing, rural development, welfare, and population, minimized AIDS (Thomas and Howard 1998, 100). In the secretary general's report on the 1994 ANC national conference, apart from a claim by the youth league to have initiated a local and regional AIDS campaign, AIDS appeared only in Zuma's report on the health ministry (ANC 1994e, 71, 77, 131).

Just as the previous government was financially constrained, the post-apartheid government faced its own economic challenges that hampered the fight against AIDS. Though the RDP appeared to stress redistributive economic policies, it proved hard to implement because of massive costs and unrealistic targets. As part of the price of a political settlement, in late 1993 the ANC had accepted the fiscal priorities of expense containment, deficit reduction, and a competitive tax structure. In late 1994, a government white paper added fiscal prudence to the RDP goals, undercutting the program's redistributive thrust. At the same time, however, the government ignored the fiscal challenges of the RDP and adopted a budget for NACOSA's national AIDS plan that was unrealistically ten times the national AIDS budget for 1994 (Whiteside and Sunter 2000, 119–20).

Though the politically popular RDP remained the official policy framework of the ANC-COSATU-Communist Party alliance, President Mandela closed the RDP office in March 1996; instead, regular government departments were now to implement the RDP (Terreblanche 2002, 96–112). That year the ANC replaced the RDP with the Growth, Employment and Redistribution Strategy (GEAR), despite COSATU and Communist Party criticism. GEAR sought to marry democratic transformation with the fiscally cautious, market-oriented reforms favored by the International Monetary Fund and the World Bank (Houston and Muthien 2000, 54–55). The adoption of GEAR shows that, as before 1994, the state would not ignore the concerns of domestic or overseas investors and financiers. The move from the RDP to the GEAR hampered funding prospects for a costly AIDS campaign. GEAR did not mention HIV, but, reminiscent of the Venter era, aimed to 'limit additional state expenditure on social needs' (Thomas and Howard 1998, 100–101).

The Mandela government's shift to neoliberalism paradoxically coincided with a shift in the nature of international assistance in the fight against AIDS. Once the South African state was no longer tainted by apartheid, foreign donors increasingly switched support from NGOs to the state (Whiteside and Sunter 2000, 125). Yet, because the donors insisted on fiscal prudence, the state was less willing to fund needed AIDS programs. This shift especially hurt private initiatives that had hitherto depended on international efforts. For instance, despite longstanding political alignment with the ANC, in April 1995 lack of funding halted the National Progressive Primary Health Care Network's AIDS program, which provided nationwide community-based counseling and support (SAIRR 1996, 202; Maurice 1992). Funding constraints also hurt public sector programs; for example, overcrowding and limited staff caused Johannesburg Hospital to turn away patients with AIDS (SAIRR 1996, 203). As the DOH estimated 3.6 million HIV-positive South Africans by the end of 1998, future costs of the epidemic seemed daunting (SAIRR 2000, 207).

Just as the apartheid regime had used high costs to rationalize limited access to AIDS treatment, Zuma and the nine provincial health ministers ended a limited AZT program for PMTCT in 1998. (AZT can substantially reduce transmission of HIV from a pregnant mother to her child.) *Preventing* infection of mothers, Zuma argued, was a better use of resources (Barrell 1998). Though the government paid much more to provide free maternity care to poor mothers and free health care to all children under six years old than for the modest PMTCT program, Zuma refused to budge, even when the manufacturer of AZT heavily discounted the drug's price. In May 1999 Zuma asked for more proof that ARVs worked, although AZT had been shown to reduce HIV transmission in potentially infected health-care workers (to whom, in a somewhat contradictory policy, the state continued the NP policy of offering free AZT) (Nicodemus 1999a). When the NP-controlled Western Cape government began pilot PMTCT programs providing free AZT, the ANC complained of using AIDS as a 'political football'. Zuma accused white critics in opposition parties, the media, and AIDS NGOs of 'racism' (Van der Vliet 2001, 167–68).

Another problem bedeviling AIDS policies during the Mandela presidency was the difficulty of merging the ANC's liberal position on human rights with the societal prudishness about sexual behavior that had constrained policy reform in the de Klerk era. This tension was particularly evident in the controversy over AIDS among prisoners. After the 1994 election, the University of the Witwatersrand's AIDS Law Project began fighting the nonconsensual HIV testing of prisoners and the continued isolation of HIV-positive prisoners (Gevisser 1994b). Such discriminatory policies recalled the Botha regime's efforts to expel Malawian miners with AIDS. Moreover, given the window period between HIV infection and the appearance of HIV antibodies in blood tests, testing or isolation could not prevent newly infected convicts from spreading HIV. In July 1995, Lawyers for Human Rights also petitioned the minister of correctional services to end the segregation of HIV-positive prisoners and to distribute condoms in prisons (SAIRR 1996, 203). The ministry refused to hand out condoms on the ground that apartheid-era statutes prohibiting sexual activity between those of the same gender still existed (Davis 1996).

These prison practices contradicted the ANC position on discrimination. The ANC sought 'nondiscrimination against infected individuals' as early as 1993 (ANC 1993; ANC 1996a). The ANC had been the first major South African political party to support including sexual orientation in a bill of rights, though there had been some opposition inside the ANC to recognizing gay and lesbian rights (Croucher 2002, 319–20). A ban on discrimination on grounds of sexual orientation was included in the 1993 and 1996 Bills of Rights. Nevertheless, it was only on 17 May 1996 that the corrections minister announced the end of HIV-positive prisoner segregation and the start of condom distribution in prisons (ANC 1996b).

The prison cases illustrate not only that the government was reticent about engaging the difficult topic of sexual behavior despite the liberal constitution, but also that neither the ANC president nor the ANC-dominated legislature was willing to use its power to end discriminatory policies. As chief executive, President Mandela could have ordered changes in prison policies as early as 1994. It took the correctional services committee of the National Assembly two years to make the changes sought by the AIDS Law Project. Likewise, it took a high court ruling in 1998, rather than ANC-sponsored legislation, to overturn laws criminalizing intimate homosexual behavior (ANC 1998). One reason for the aging president's seeming lack of leadership may have been that he was turning over many day-to-day tasks to his deputy, Thabo Mbeki, who lacked his authority and charisma (Lodge 1999, 114). For example, when Mandela was scheduled to give a nationally broadcast speech on AIDS entitled 'Ten Minutes to Save the Nation', audiences discovered that he had delegated the task to Mbeki at the last minute (Van der Vliet 2001, 165).

Without strong political leadership on the AIDS issue, competing bureaucratic priorities and centralizing tendencies undercut post-1994 AIDS efforts. Old and new bureaucrats squabbled, while national, provincial, and local authorities battled over funding allocations, program design, and policy decisions (Van der Vliet 2001, 161). In June 1996, DOH AIDS project chief Quarraisha Karim complained of waiting nearly eight months for contract approval for a STI program, during which she could not hire permanent staff (Gevisser 1997). In May 1997 complaints arose that of R65 million allotted for HIV education only half had been used.[5] None of the R4.4 million intended for research on care and support had been spent and the R18 million designated for the provinces was bogged down in bureaucratic red tape. AIDS training for high school educators was only scheduled to start that same month (Day 1997).

These bureaucratic problems contributed to some AIDS schemes that embarrassed the new government. In 1996, Public Protector Selby Baqwa reported that the DOH had used R14.2 million on an AIDS educational musical, Sarafina II. Zuma claimed the funds came from the European Union (EU), but the EU denied knowledge of the production. Baqwa concluded that the contract submission process for the play was fraudulent and that the play was ineffective in fighting AIDS (SAIRR 1997, 550).[6] The tickets were certainly too expensive for the poor target audience (Mvoko 1996). Sarafina II was mounted despite massive NGO criticism (Mvoko and Pearce 1996; Maharaj 1996). Gary Lamont of Wola Nani, a Cape Town AIDS support group, claimed that 'just about every Aids agency' was losing faith in Zuma (Rossouw 1996).

Despite the new democratic, quasi-federal constitution, the pre-1994 tendency to centralize AIDS programs at the national level and to limit dialogue with civil society groups remained. Though NACOSA's AIDS plan had advocated a national manager in the president's office and regional authorities in the provincial premiers' offices, Zuma preferred to manage AIDS programs from the DOH (Gevisser 1994a). Like her predecessor, Zuma was increasingly criticized for making decisions without adequate consultation (Davis 1992; Van der Vliet 2001, 162–63). This propensity for centralization was apparent in a second disastrous state AIDS intervention. Facing growing numbers of desperate AIDS patients and the high cost of ARVs, the government appeared to back an experimental drug, virodene, developed by three Afrikaner scientists (Cowling 1997). Though American researchers had shown that virodene, which contains a toxic industrial solvent causing liver damage, actually activates HIV (SAIRR 1998, 221; Gledhill 1998a), Zuma and Mbeki arranged a meeting between the scientists and the cabinet. When the Medicines Control Council (MCC) repeatedly denied applications for human virodene trials, Zuma, Mbeki, and the ANC secretary general Kgalema Motlhanthe attacked the MCC for blocking the drug while so many faced death (Edmunds 1998; Lodge 2002, 256). In response, Zuma announced she would replace the MCC with a reformed body (SAIRR 1998, 216, 221). This decision, as well as Zuma's move to reform the HIV/AIDS and Sexually Transmitted Diseases Advisory Committee after it opposed her scheme to make AIDS a notifiable disease (Gledhill 1998b),[7] demonstrated Zuma's desire to control AIDS policies. The High Court in Pretoria later struck down Zuma's decision on the MCC and in December 1998, the MCC rejected an application for virodene clinical trials (SAIRR 2000, 236, 242). Nevertheless, the politicization of science in order to achieve central control over policy making hurt the fight against AIDS during the first years after apartheid, much as politicization of health policy had hurt AIDS efforts in the apartheid era.

The Mbeki Presidency (1999–2003)

When Mbeki became president in 1999, he replaced Zuma with Mantho Tshabalala-Msimang. The new president, who was strongly supported by his minister, became controversial for his AIDS policies. He was soon criticized for questioning the link between HIV and AIDS. In 2000, Mbeki appointed an expert commission to investigate several aspects of HIV and AIDS, such as the causes of the immunodeficiency that makes AIDS fatal, appropriate responses to these causes, and why AIDS in sub-Saharan Africa is 'heterosexually transmitted while in the western world it is said to be largely homosexually transmitted'. This framework reflected Mbeki's interest in the views of 'dissident' scientists on the panel. For example, Peter Duesberg and Roberto Giraldo denied that HIV causes AIDS, while David Rasnick claimed that AIDS would 'instantaneously disappear if all HIV testing was outlawed and the use of anti-retroviral drugs was terminated' (Presidential AIDS Panel 2001, 11–12, 15). The March 2001 panel report showed such division that orthodox and dissident panelists produced two sets of recommendations; the dissidents proposed to investigate the 'real meaning' of HIV tests and to compare whether HIV itself or anti-HIV *drugs* were more harmful (Presidential AIDS Panel 2001, 103, 106).

The MRC president Malegapuru Makgoba, himself an ardent black nationalist like Mbeki, criticized this approach in the American journal *Science*. He noted that, despite Mbeki's rejection of imposing 'Western experience on African reality,' his views on AIDS came from 'dissident' Western scientists, and that other 'politically driven decisions' on AIDS included his enthusiastic support for virodene, the refusal to give ARVs to pregnant women, and the 'politically motivated suggestion' that malnutrition and poverty caused AIDS in Africa. He concluded that South Africa could become fertile ground for the 'pseudoscience often embraced by politicians' (Makgoba 2000). In some ways, Mbeki's politicization of science and his fascination with its fringes recalled the fantastic schemes of the apartheid biological and chemical warfare program (Burger and Gould 2002, 24, 31–33).

Mbeki's ideas led to increased state-civil society tensions over AIDS policies. The opposition Democratic Alliance, the liberal media, COSATU, and AIDS NGOs such as the Treatment Action Committee (TAC) increasingly criticized the government. In the de Klerk era, NP reforms pitted Afrikaner modernizers against conservatives, but most NP hardliners had joined the Far Right. In contrast, the ANC's critics were often its political allies and supporters. For example, in 2000 COSATU blamed GEAR for the state's 'lack of a comprehensive and coherent response to the demands for access to effective treatment of HIV' and for 'inadequate social infrastructural resources' to combat AIDS. COSATU asked the government to 'end its scientific speculation' and expand its efforts 'on the basis that HIV is the medical cause of AIDS.' COSATU insisted that ARVs be given to pregnant women and rape victims (COSATU 2000). Openly gay high court judge Edwin Cameron, an appointee of the post-apartheid regime, denounced the president for creating confusion, while Nelson Mandela urged a more rapid response to AIDS (Van der Vliet 2001, 172–78; SAIRR 2001, 221). Zackie Achmat, the fiery TAC leader who insisted he was both an ANC and

Communist Party member, sued the government and advocated civil disobedience to persuade Mbeki to provide ARVs (Achmat 2002). The TAC complained that SANAC was insufficiently representative of civil society, lacked adequate staff or funding, seldom met, and was dominated or marginalized by the health minister and president's office (TAC 2002). When SANAC was launched in 2000, it included several cabinet ministers and government officials, two traditional healers, and a little known American to represent NGOs; there were no scientists, physicians, nurses, or MRC or MCC representatives on the council (Powell 2000).

The state responded to criticism from civil society in several ways. First, Mbeki claimed that the AIDS threat had been exaggerated, though he based this conclusion on 1995 data. In August 2001, he asked minister Tshabalala-Msimang to review health spending in light of the 1995 estimates. Meanwhile, the MRC reported a marked increase in AIDS mortality figures, but the government blocked release of the MRC report until the end of 2001 (Bateman 2001), and commissioned Statistics South Africa, a state agency, to develop a new report. Released in November 2002, the new report confirmed Mbeki's assessment, showing that AIDS caused only 9 per cent of deaths from 1997 to 2001, rather than the 25 per cent suggested by the MRC (Statistics South Africa 2002). The MRC's Debbie Bradshaw explained that while the new report relied on the actual listing of AIDS on death certificates, the MRC looked for HIV/AIDS as the underlying cause of death (MRC 2002). The latter method makes more sense, as HIV status is often unknown and families may pressure doctors to report other, less-stigmatized causes of death.

A second, and more recent, state response to criticism from traditional supporters was the cabinet's dramatic recommitment on 17 April 2002 to fighting AIDS. This included massively expanding the AIDS budget from R350 million in 2001/2 to R1 billion in 2002/03 (DOH 2002d). As part of this renewed interest in AIDS, the state defensively heralded recent successes. In October 2002, the cabinet claimed a 90 per cent AIDS awareness level, use of nontraditional outlets for condom distribution (such as informal shops and bars in black townships), and rapid progress toward a vaccine. The cabinet also asserted that universal rollout of PMTCT drugs and supportive programs for rape survivors were 'on track' (DOH 2002a). In the same year, the DOH claimed that HIV infection rates among teenagers had dropped for a third year, and that there was an 'insignificant' increase in overall HIV prevalence from 24.8 per cent to 26.5 per cent between 2001 and 2002 (DOH 2002f; DOH 2003). While such figures suggest some success in education, they are problematic. In 2002, the Joint United Nations Program on HIV/AIDS (UNAIDS) noted a continued rise in infection among older pregnant women (UNAIDS 2002, 16). UNAIDS (2004, 191) reported that prevalence rates had increased from 20.9 per cent in 2001 to 21.5 per cent in 2003. Further, scholars continue to question the reliability of extrapolating general prevalence patterns from state antenatal clinic data.[8]

Nowhere has the tension between the state and civil society been more apparent than over the issue of ARV treatment. From its inception, Mbeki's administration was reluctant to offer ARV therapy, even if the drugs were cheap and provided on a limited basis to rape victims and for PMTCT. As had her predecessor, Tshabala-Msimang repeatedly expressed concerns about AZT's toxicity, despite studies showing that the benefits of AZT outweigh its risks (Nicodemus 1999b). This remained true even after the cabinet appeared in April 2002 to have recommitted itself to fighting AIDS. In May Tshabala-Msimang announced that the cabinet had decided that ARVs would at least be offered to sexual-assault victims (DOH 2002c). In October, the cabinet stressed the importance of counseling rape survivors on the 'effectiveness and risks' of using as preventive drugs the very ARVs that it had made available in such cases (DOH 2002e).

To force the administration to provide the drug nevirapine (which is cheaper than AZT) for PMTCT, the TAC sued the government. In March 2002, the High Court in Pretoria ordered the government to provide nevirapine to HIV-positive pregnant women. Only when the Constitutional Court in Johannesburg upheld this decision (despite a strenuous government effort to have it overturned, ostensibly to defend the separation of powers), did the state agree to introduce universal roll-out of nevirapine. Even in accepting the court ruling in July 2002, Tshabalala-Msimang stressed that the DOH would offer the drug beyond existing sites only where a 'relevant' health authority determined 'appropriate capacity' (DOH 2002e). The cabinet warned of the challenges of 'training, budget, proper health facilities and community attitudes' (DOH 2002a). Despite the expansion of PMTCT in Kwazulu-Natal, the Western Cape, and Gauteng provinces by 2003, in the other six provinces few nevirapine programs were available beyond pilot sites. (The only ANC-controlled province with substantial PMTCT programs was Gauteng.) Insufficient staff, limited access to HIV testing or counseling, and little direction from the DOH exacerbated the situation (Thom 2003, 23).

If providing ARVs for PMTCT has proven difficult, the issue of *universal* access to ARVS for the broader HIV-positive population is even more complex. In October 2002, the cabinet announced that a joint DOH-treasury task team would investigate the costs and benefits of a free universal ARV program. At this point, the TAC agreed to delay a civil disobedience campaign, given signs of possible adoption of a national AIDS treatment plan (Thom 2002). Yet, when the report was finished in February 2003, the cabinet delayed its consideration and the health minister and president's office subsequently sent it back to its drafters. In response, the TAC leaked the report to the press (TAC 2003a). In February 2003, approximately 20,000 people marched in Cape Town to demand treatment. Speakers included the COSATU president Willie Madisha, the Anglican archbishop Njongonkulu Ndungane, and the radical opposition member of parliament Patricia de Lille (Galloway 2003).

In the face of this public outrage and TAC civil disobedience, some ANC party leaders began to view the issue of universal treatment as a political concern. Though most ANC leaders had been reluctant to differ openly with Mbeki (Lodge 2002, 262–63), concern about fallout in the 2004 election encouraged a shift in the positions of some ANC members. Education minister Kader Asmal, ex-DOH director-general Olive Shisana, ANC elections chief Manne Dipico, and party chief strategist Joel Netshitenze reportedly labored behind the scenes to support access to ARVs. Against Mbeki and Tshabala-Msimang's opposition, in August 2003 they persuaded the cabinet to endorse the report favoring universal rollout and to request the DOH to urgently develop an operational plan (Kindra 2003). On 19 November, the cabinet announced it had approved a plan to provide at least one service point with free ARVs in each DOH district within one year and one service point in every municipality in five years (TAC 2003b).

Tshabalala-Msimang showed little enthusiasm for implementing this program and even supporters of the policy were concerned about adequate health infrastructure for rapid implementation (Kindra 2003). There were concerns that such therapy would undercut prevention efforts by reducing funds for prevention or causing public complacency about the dangers of HIV infection (Sanderson 2001). In a country with so many poor, remote communities, the five-year time scale for ARV stations in every municipality also meant further delay in saving lives. In response, the TAC continued to criticize the government's hesitancy, its inefficient procurement of drugs, and its lack of communication with citizens, civil society, and provincial health centers (TAC 2004).

The MCC's objections in July 2003 about the testing of nevirapine for PMTCT further bolstered state opponents to ARVs.[9] If the MCC withdrew its approval of nevirapine, a national treatment plan would be threatened (*Economist* 2003b). Cabinet approval of a general ARV treatment program, like that for PMTCT, was predicated on using the cheaper drug nevirapine, not its more costly alternative AZT. In September, the MCC allowed the manufacturer of nevirapine more time to provide more data to allay the council's concerns and reassured the public that nevirapine could still be used for PMTCT or for broader treatment of HIV and AIDS (MCC 2003). These MCC quibbles may threaten more than PMTCT by reopening the debate about the toxicity of ARVs.

The Mbeki government has, despite its belated agreement to offer treatment to the vast majority of South African AIDS patients, seriously damaged its reputation. The administration focused on fears of toxicity and practical difficulties in implementation to block provision of ARVs even when the claim of impossible costs was rendered hollow by drug companies' offer of heavily discounted or even free drugs and by Mbeki's authorization of spending billions of rands on arms (Bond 2003, 71). Costs alone, however, do not explain Mbeki's response to providing ARVs, any more than they explain his recent assertion that he does not know anybody who has died of AIDS or his silence on World AIDS Day in 2003 (*Economist* 2003a).

The Mbeki government's seemingly baffling AIDS policies reflect much larger contradictions inside the post-apartheid regime. Despite his administration's public commitment to democracy, transparency, and accountability, behind the scenes the government has become entangled in a close if sometimes strained alliance with big business advocates of neoliberal economic policies. These links increased with the emergence of a small but growing black bourgeoisie. The shift away from idealistic redistributive policies that had begun under Mandela helps explain Mbeki's reluctance to embrace expensive programs to fight AIDS. Yet, while Mbeki has denounced international capitalists (such as drug companies) as exploiters, he also has shown little enthusiasm for importing or manufacturing cheap generic versions of ARVs. He has attacked white liberal critics of his policies as 'racists,' while he has denounced socialist critics as 'ultra-leftists' or dupes of white liberal 'enemies of transformation' (Calland and Jacobs 2003; Lodge 2002, 162–65).

Such apparently contradictory messages reflect the regime's increasing difficulty in retaining the 'broad church' tradition of the ANC, while obscuring a fiscal conservatism that reassures foreign and domestic investors. This was already a challenge under the charismatic Mandela, but it is more difficult for the cerebral and rather aloof Mbeki, who must hold together the often disparate communist, trade unionist, social democratic, neoliberal, and black nationalist elements that constitute the ANC-COSATU-Communist Party alliance. Mbeki's attraction to romantic black nationalism, a fact which partly explains his apparent suspicion of mainstream Western medical science, and his use of populist rhetoric are aimed at maintaining the support of an aspiring black bourgeoisie and the impoverished black masses. Yet, populist rhetoric has been insufficient to meet the demands of both black and white South Africans for state action against an AIDS enemy that threatens to be even more destructive than the apartheid regime.

Conclusion

Despite nearly five million HIV-positive South Africans, by 2003 state responses to AIDS continued to be characterized by a gap between rhetoric and reality. The lost opportunities, the grandiose yet ineffective initiatives, and endless delays in policy implementation remained even as official statements of determination to fight AIDS intensified and allotted funds grew geometrically. To be fair, there were some promising efforts, notably in AIDS education. Yet the post-apartheid state response to AIDS often recalled that of the pre-1994 era. The defensiveness and intolerance of the Mbeki administration in particular, like its often difficult relationship with civil society and its love-hate relationship with capitalism, are reminiscent of the previous era. Ready recourse to charges of racism has replaced the communist fear mongering of the apartheid regime, while the Mbeki administration's attacks on liberals and ultra-leftists mirror NP rhetoric under apartheid. Mbeki's defense of pseudoscience as an African right to seek autonomy from white scientific and cultural domination (although most of the leading denialist scientists are white) demonstrates an ideological and populist response to AIDS like the racist and prudish responses of the apartheid regime. The authoritarian centralism that barred giving ARVs to rape victims and that led to confrontation with groups such as the TAC mirrors the authoritarian mentality of the Botha era, when the total strategy and the apartheid mindset shaped a different kind of denial regarding AIDS. The tendency to micro-manage the war against AIDS is another parallel, and one that even the more pragmatic de Klerk and Mandela administrations could not escape. Like the apartheid regime, the Mbeki government resisted spending money on ARVs, on cost grounds, even as it authorized massive spending on arms. Finally, the state's response to AIDS has produced a close parallel to the pre-1994 mass democratic movement: the emerging alliance of COSATU, the TAC, liberal church leaders, dissatisfied ANC elements, and black civic organizations which has engaged in peaceful protest for universal rollout of ARVs.

These parallels with the apartheid era suggest that in some respects the democratization of the South African state has some way to go. Periods of transition have been difficult for all African states as they sought to negotiate the change from colonialism to independence and later from one-party states to multiparty democracies. These transitions have not been entirely successful, but South Africa has done better than most African countries, with a widely admired constitution and a Truth and Reconciliation Commission that sought a middle ground between bloody retributive justice and silence about past repression. Democratic South Africa's cautious macroeconomic policies have given it greater autonomy from international financial institutions than most African countries. However, the post-apartheid regime, in seeking to be an even bigger regional player than its predecessor, continues to spend large sums on arms while claiming that it cannot afford the redistributive policies that helped bring it to power. The post-apartheid state, like its predecessor, still finds it hard to accept criticism or advice. The AIDS crisis, however, has demonstrated one critical difference between the past and the present: this time in South Africa, many of the loudest voices of dissent come from those same oppressed masses which supported the ANC's liberation struggle. This fact has given them a credibility that eventually could not be ignored. Those masses understand that AIDS, rather than recalcitrant whites, uncaring overseas corporations, or leftwing critics, threatens most menacingly to wipe out the gains of the liberation struggle. This realization, and its manifestation in renewed citizen activism, provides some hope for the long-term fight against AIDS in South Africa's new democracy.

Notes

1 See also Letters to the editor 2001.

2 Diflucan (fluconazole) is used to treat cryptococcal meningitis and oesophageal candidiasis.

3 Mbeki succeeded Mandela as ANC leader, but became president only after the June 1999 election.

4 In 1990 there were already signs of a marked upswing in HIV rates in Natal (Pudifin and Windsor 1990, 4–5).

5 Currency conversion rates for the South African rand provide limited information, because of the currency's extreme volatility. Valued at under R1 per US dollar in the late 1970s, the currency plunged to more than R10 per US dollar at the end of the 1990s. In September 2004, the exchange rate was R6.42 per US dollar.

6 A year later, in a puzzling turnaround, Baqwa cleared Zuma of any wrongdoing (SAIRR 1998, 475).

7 In 2002, the DOH reported that AIDS would not be listed as a notifiable disease that doctors must report to the department (DOH 2002b). As of late 2004, AIDS is still not a notifiable disease. The lack of this data makes it harder to track the AIDS epidemic. Nevertheless, listing AIDS as a notifiable disease is controversial, since those who believe they may be infected with HIV or have full-blown AIDS may be reluctant to seek medical assistance if they fear that their anonymity will not be protected.

8 Antenatal clinics 'anonymously' test only consenting pregnant women, a practice that omits adult men, children, women who are not pregnant, and an unknown percentage of pregnant women who do not use the clinics or who come to the clinics but refuse to be tested. A disproportionate percentage of women who refuse to be tested may be HIV positive. The stigma attached to AIDS and blacks' mistrust of authorities may make patients suspicious of claims that their anonymity will be protected. It is impossible, however, for statisticians to build into their data assumptions about the percentage of women who decline to be tested, since the DOH does not provide any information on this subject. Skeptics of antenatal data also argue that over time, women attending antenatal clinics may become less representative of individuals with AIDS. This is because HIV-induced infertility, increased use of nonbarrier contraception methods, and abortion (legalized by the post-1994 government) may have reduced pregnancy rates, but not women's vulnerability to HIV (Shell et al. n.d., 4). The authors wish to thank Dr. Shell for sharing his research on this subject.

9 Boehringer-Ingelheim had its application to the US Federal Drug Administration for PMTCT use of nevirapine rejected, but primarily for bureaucratic reasons and not questions of safety. The World Health Organization has endorsed nevirapine for PMTCT (*Mail & Guardian* 2003, 24).

References

Achmat, Zackie. 2002. Letter to the editor. *Mail & Guardian*, 18–24 October, 14.

African National Congress (ANC). 1993. World AIDS Day. Department of Information and Publicity press release. http://www.anc.org.za/ancdocs/pr/1993/pr1201.html.

——. 1994a. A better life for all: Vote ANC! Mimeograph election flyer distributed by ANC, Durban.

——. 1994b. *A better life for all: Working together for jobs, peace and freedom.* Johannesburg: ANC.

——. 1994c. Building our future: A summary of the reconstruction and development program (RDP) for canvassers. Mimeograph flyer distributed by ANC.

——. 1994d. *The reconstruction and development programme: A policy framework.* Johannesburg: Umanyano Publications for the African National Congress.

——. 1994e. From resistance to reconstruction and nation-building. Secretary General's report for the 49th national conference, Bloemfontein, 17–21 December.
——. 1996a. HIV in prisons. Department of Information and Publicity press release. http://www.anc.org.za/ ancdocs/pr/1996/pr0312.html.
——. 1996b. The treatment of HIV-positive prisoners. Press release of ANC study group on correctional services. http://www.anc.org.za/ ancdocs/r/1996/pr0517a.html.
——. 1997. Political report of the president Nelson Mandela to the 50th national conference of the African National Congress. http://www.anc.org.za/ ancdocs/pr/1997/pr1216.html.
——. 1998. High court judgment on same sex conduct. Department of Information and Publicity press release. http://www.anc.org/anc.docs/pr/1998/pr0508.html.
AIDS Policy Research Group (APRG). 1991. South African press brings AIDS education to all. *AIDS Analysis Africa* (southern Africa edition) 2 (1): 12.
——. 1994. The Macmillan Boleswa AIDS Awareness Program. *AIDS Analysis Africa* (southern Africa edition) 5 (3): 9.
Baldwin-Ragaven, Laurel, Jeanelle de Gruchy, and Leslie London, eds. 1999. *An ambulance of the wrong colour: Health professionals, human rights and ethics in South Africa*. Rondebosch: University of Cape Town Press.
Barrell, Howard. 1998. Zuma defends AZT policy. *Mail & Guardian*, 16–22 October.
Bateman, Chris. 2001. Guarding the citadels of AIDS statistics. *South African Medical Journal* 91 (11): 932–33.
Bond, Patrick. 2003. Thabo Mbeki and NEPAD: Breaking or shining the chains of global apartheid? In *Thabo Mbeki's world: The politics and ideology of the South African president*, ed. Sean Jacobs and Richard Calland, 53–81. London: Zed Books.
Bond, Patrick, and Meshack Khosa, eds. 1999. *An RDP policy audit*. Pretoria: Human Sciences Research Council.
Burger, Marléne, and Chandré Gould. 2002. *Secrets and lies: Wouter Basson and South Africa's chemical and biological warfare programme*. Cape Town: Zebra Press.
Calland, Richard, and Sean Jacobs. 2003. Thabo Mbeki: Politics and ideology. In *Thabo Mbeki's world: The politics and ideology of the South African president*, ed. Sean Jacobs and Richard Calland, 257–74. London: Zed Books.
Congress of South African Trade Unions (COSATU). 2000. 8 resolutions on HIV/AIDS. COSATU 7th national congress resolutions. http://www.cosatu.org.za/congress/cong2000/resoce.htm#8.
Cowling, Lesley. 1997. Aids 'breakthrough' broke all the rules. *Mail & Guardian*, 24–30 January.
Crewe, Mary. 1992. *AIDS in South Africa: The myth and the reality*. Harmondsworth, England: Penguin.
Croucher, Sheila. 2002. South Africa's democratisation and the politics of gay liberation. *Journal of Southern African Studies* 28 (2): 315–30.
Davis, Gaye. 1992. This may hurt a little, says Dr. Venter. *Weekly Mail*, 21–27 February.
——. 1996. Prisoners 'should get condoms.' *Mail & Guardian*, 1–7 March.
Day, Jim. 1997. Bureaucrats dither as HIV invades. *Mail & Guardian*, 2–8 May.
Department of National Health and Population Development. 1986. *Report of the Director-General for Health and Population Development for the year 1985*. Pretoria: Government of South Africa.

——. 1987. *Report of the Director-General for Health and Population Development for 1986*. Pretoria: Government of South Africa.
——. 1988. *Report of the Director-General for Health and Population Development for 1987*. Pretoria: Government of South Africa.
——. 1989. *Report of the Director-General for Health and Population Development for the year 1988*. Pretoria: Government of South Africa.
Department of Health. 1995. *Report of the Directorate-General for the Department of Health for the year 1994*. Pretoria: Government of South Africa.
——. 2000. *Report of the Directorate-General of the Department of Health for the year 1999/2000*. Pretoria: Government of South Africa.
——. 2001a. Court case on mother-to-child transmission of HIV. Press release by Dr. Ayanda Ntsaluba, DOH Director-General. http://www.doh.gov.za/docs/pr/2001/ pr1123.html.
——. 2001b. Diflucan partnership programme. *HIV/AIDS and TB Newsletter* 15 (7 December): 1.
——. 2002a. Lend a hand in the campaign of hope against HIV/AIDS!: An update on cabinet's statement of 17 April 2002 on fighting HIV/AIDS. DOH press release. http://www.doh.gov.za/docs/pr/2002/pr1009a.html.
——. 2002b. List of 'notifiable medical conditions.' http://www.doh.gov.za/facts/notify/2002/jan-june.html.
——. 2002c. National protocols in place for ARVs for rape survivors. Press release by Dr. Mantho Tshabalala-Msimang. http://www.doh.gov.za/docs/pr/2002/pr0529.html.
——. 2002d. Statement of cabinet on HIV/AIDS. DOH press release. http://www/doh.gov.za/docs/pr/2002/ pr0417.html.
——. 2002e. Statement by government on the Constitutional Court judgment regarding PMTCT. Press release by Dr. Mantho Tshabalala-Msimang. http://www.doh.gov.za/ docs/pr/2002/pr0705.html.
——. 2002f. Twelfth national HIV and syphilis sero-prevalence survey of women attending public antenatal clinics in South Africa 2001. DOH press release. http://www.doh.gov.za/docs/pr/2002/pr0610.html.
——. 2003. HIV prevalence in South Africa. DOH press release. http://www.doh.gov.za/docs/pr/2003/ pr0703.html.
DOH. *See* Department of National Health and Population Development; *see also (renamed in 1994)* Department of Health.
Economist. 2003a. Africa's erratic statesman, 20 December.
Economist. 2003b. Death by dithering, 9 August.
Edmunds, Marion. 1998. Zuma shuts down MCC. *Mail & guardian*, 27 March–2 April.
Ellis, Mike. 1991. AIDS – A Democratic Party response. *AIDS Analysis Africa* (southern Africa edition) 1 (5): 7.
Fleming, Alan. 1992/1993. Report on the NACOSA conference. *AIDS Analysis Africa* (southern Africa edition) 3 (4): 7–8.
——. 1993. South Africa and AIDS: Seven years wasted. *AIDS Analysis Africa* (southern Africa edition) 3 (7): 6.
Galloway, Michelle Rotchford. 2003. Treat us now! A right to treatment a right to life: Thousands march for AIDS treatment. *MRC AIDS Bulletin* 12 (1): 16–18.
Gevisser, Mark. 1992a. Getting to grips with the reality of AIDS. *Weekly Mail*, 23–29 December.

——. 1992b. Sinners – or the victims of not-so-subtle discrimination? *Weekly Mail*, 6–12 March.
——. 1992c. Where Codesa fails, AIDS wins. *Weekly Mail*, 21–27 August.
——. 1993. Sex in the schoolroom–but it's safer. *Review/Education*. Occasional supplement of *Weekly Mail* 2 (3): 1–2.
——. 1994a. Finally, the state gets serious about Aids. *Weekly Mail & Guardian*, 22–28 July.
——. 1994b. Prisoners of pain seek recognition. *Weekly Mail & Guardian*, 2–8 December.
——. 1997. The commissar of condoms. *Mail & Guardian*, 21–27 June.
Gevisser, Mark, and Paul Stober. 1992. 'Codesa' fails the Aids test. *Weekly Mail*, 30 October–5 November.
Gledhill, Lynda. 1998a. Virodene may activate the virus. *Mail & Guardian*, 2–26 March.
——. 1998b. Zuma axes another disagreeable health body. *Mail & Guardian*, 3–8 April.
Gouws, Amanda, and James L. Gibson. 2001. The study of political tolerance in the South African context. *Social Dynamics* 27 (2): 109–33.
Grundlingh, Louis. 1999. HIV/AIDS in South Africa: A case of failed responses because of stigmatization, discrimination and morality, 1983–1994. *New Contree* 46 (November): 55–81.
——. 2001a. Early attitudes and responses to HIV/AIDS in South Africa as reflected in newspapers, 1983–1988. *Journal for Contemporary History* 26 (1): 86–103.
——. 2001b. Government responses to HIV/AIDS in South Africa as reported in the media, 1983–1994. *South African Historical Journal* 45 (November): 124–53.
Hambridge, Maria. 1995. AIDS and the Reconstruction and Development Programme. *AIDS Analysis Africa* (southern Africa edition) 5 (5): 3.
Hawker, Geoffrey. 2000. Political leadership in the ANC: The South African provinces 1994–1999. *Journal of Modern African Studies* 38 (4): 631–58.
Houston, Gregory, and Yvonne Muthien. 2000. South Africa: A transformative state? In *Democracy in governance review: Mandela's legacy 1994–1999*, ed. Yvonne G. Muthien, Meshack M. Khosa, and Bernard M. Magubane, 37–67. Pretoria: Human Sciences Research Council.
Joint United Nations Program on HIV/AIDS (UNAIDS). 2002. *AIDS epidemic update: December 2002*. Geneva: UNAIDS.
——. 2004. *Report on the global AIDS epidemic*. http://www.unaids.org/bangkok2004.html.
Kaplan, Robert. 2001. The aversion project: Psychiatric abuses in the South African defence force during the apartheid era. *South African Medical Journal* 91 (3): 216–17.
Kindra, Jaspreet. 2003. Aids: Ministers revolt. *Mail & Guardian*, 15–21 August.
Letters to the editor. 2001. *South African Medical Journal* 91 (8): 617–18.
Lodge, Tom. 1999. *South African politics since 1994*. Cape Town: David Philip.
——. 2002. *Politics in South Africa: From Mandela to Mbeki*. Cape Town: David Philip.
Maharaj, Norman. 1996. Letter to editor. *Mail & Guardian*, 23–29 February.
Mail & Guardian. 2003. Don't crow too soon over nevirapine. 1–7 August.
Makgoba, Malegapuru W. 2000. HIV/AIDS: The peril of pseudoscience. *Science*, 19 May.
Maurice, Portia. 1992. Dilemma of a misdiagnosis. *Weekly Mail*, 7–13 August.

McCulloch, Jock. 2002. *Asbestos blues: The story of South Africa's asbestos miners and their legal battles with the mining companies*. Bloomington, IN: Indiana Univ. Press.

Medicines Control Council (MCC). 2003. Press release: Nevirapine – MCC resolution. http://www.mccza.com.

Medical Research Council (MRC). 1988. *Medical Research Council annual report 1987*. Tygerberg: MRC.

——. 1989. *Medical Research Council annual report 1988*. Tygerberg: MRC.

——. 1990. Minister outlines future health policy. *MRC News* 21 (3): 4.

——. 1991. Community health research valuable for SA health policy making. *MRC News* 22 (2): 3–4.

——. 1992. *Medical Research Council annual report 1991*. Tygerberg: MRC.

——. 1994. *1993 annual report*. Tygerberg: MRC.

——. 1995. *Medical Research Council annual report 1994/5*. Tygerberg: MRC.

——. 1999. *Medical Research Council annual report 1998/99*.Tygerberg: MRC.

——. 2000. *Medical Research Council annual report 1999/2000*. Tygerberg: MRC.

——. 2002. Statistics South Africa: Causes of death in South Africa 1997–2001 – Advance release of recorded causes of death. Press release. http://www.mrc.ac.za/researchreports/statsa.htm.

Mvoko, Vuyo. 1996. Aids play sparks crisis for Zuma. *Mail & Guardian*, 16–22 February.

Mvoko,Vuyo, and Justin Pearce. 1996. Health minister defends Aids musical. *Mail & Guardian*, 9–15 February.

Nattrass, Nicoli, and Jeremy Seekings. 2001. 'Two nations'? Race and economic inequality in South Africa today. *Daedalus* 130 (1): 56–57.

Nicodemus, Aaron. 1999a. Ministry refuses anti-HIV drug discount. *Mail & Guardian*, 7–13 May.

——. 1999b. Truth and lies about AZT. *Mail & Guardian*, 26 November–2 December.

Packard, Randall M. 1989. *White plague, black labor: Tuberculosis and the political economy of health and disease in South Africa*. Berkeley: Univ. of California Press.

Perlman, John. 1988. The fine line between knowledge and terror. *Weekly Mail*, 15–22 December.

——. 1989. Aids is moving fast – but can the health authorities keep up? *Weekly Mail*, 29 September-5 October.

Phillips, Howard. 2001. AIDS in the center of South Africa's epidemic history: Preliminary historical thoughts. *South African Historical Journal* 45 (November): 11–26.

Powell, Ivor. 2000. Uproar over Aids council. *Mail & Guardian*, 28 January–3 February.

Presidential AIDS Panel. 2001. Presidential AIDS advisory panel report: A synthesis report of the deliberations by the panel of experts invited by the President of the Republic of South Africa, the Honourable Mr Thabo Mbeki. http://www.doh.gov.za/docs/ index.html.

Price, Max. 1986. Health care as an instrument of apartheid policy in South Africa. *Health Policy and Planning* 1 (2): 158–70.

Pudifin, Dennis, and Isobel Windsor. 1990. Regional focus: AIDS in Natal. *AIDS Analysis Africa* (southern Africa edition) 1 (2): 4–5.

Rossouw, Rehana. 1996. Zuma's revenge. *Mail & Guardian*, 26 July–1 August.

Sanderson, Warren. 2001. The mixed blessing of anti-retroviral therapy. *AIDS Analysis Africa* (southern Africa edition) 12 (1): 12.
Shell, Robert, Andrew McKenzie, Anjali Vaidya, Farshid Meidany, and Prabha Rama. n.d. A second generation HIV/AIDS surveillance protocol based on unlinked anonymized testing of trauma patients at selected hospitals in southern Africa. Unpublished manuscript.
South African Institute of Race Relations (SAIRR). 1993. *Race relations survey 1992/93*. Johannesburg: SAIRR.
——. 1994. *Race relations survey 1993/94*. Johannesburg: SAIRR.
——. 1996. *South Africa survey 1995/96*. Johannesburg: SAIRR.
——. 1997. *South Africa survey 1996/1997*. Johannesburg: SAIRR.
——. 1998. *South Africa survey 1997/1998*. Johannesburg: SAIRR.
——. 2000. *South Africa survey 1999/2000*. Johannesburg: SAIRR.
——. 2001. *South Africa survey 2000/2001*. Johannesburg: SAIRR.
Southall, Roger. 1998. The centralization and fragmentation of South Africa's dominant party system. *African Affairs* 97 (389): 443–69.
Statistics South Africa. 2002. Causes of death in South Africa 1997–2001: Advance release of recorded causes of death. http://www.mrc.ac.za/researchreports/statsa.htm.
Terreblanche, Sampie. 2002. *A history of inequality in South Africa, 1652–2002*. Pietermaritzburg: Univ. of Natal Press.
Thom, Anso. 2002. TAC reviews disobedience campaign. http://www.health-e.org.za.
——. 2003. Shambles at Aids baby treatment sites. *Mail & Guardian*, 27 June–3 July.
Thomas, Liz, and Jenny Howard. 1998. AIDS and development planning. In *Implications of AIDS for demography and policy in southern Africa*, ed. Alan Whiteside, 95–114. Pietermaritzburg: Univ. of Natal Press.
Treatment Action Campaign (TAC). 2002. Memorandum to SANAC calling for the transformation of SANAC and a national treatment plan. Press release. http://www.tac.org.za/newsletter/2002/ns07_10_2002.txt.
——. 2003a. Leaking details of report is a moral obligation–not 'mischief' and 'theatrics.' Press release. http://www.tac.org.za/newsletter/2003.
——. 2003b. TAC welcomes cabinet adoption of treatment plan. Press release. http://www.tac.org.za/newsletter/2003.
——. 2004. First monitoring report of the antiretroviral treatment rollout. http://www.tac.org.za.
Tucker, Tim. 2001. A race against time. *MRC News* 32 (5): 5.
Van der Vliet, Virginia. 2001. AIDS: Losing the 'new struggle'? *Daedalus* 130 (1): 151–84.
Van Niekerk, Philip. 1988. Mines' Aids crisis deepens. *Weekly Mail*, 8–14 April.
Van Niftrik, Jack. 1990/1991. The pandemic and the press. *AIDS Analysis Africa* (southern Africa edition) 1 (4): 1.
——. 1992/1993. The bumblers play on – a decade of debacle. *AIDS Analysis Africa* (southern Africa edition) 3 (4): 1.
——. 1993. Opinion: Finally, the courage of cutting the crap. *AIDS Analysis Africa* (southern Africa edition) 3 (6): 4.
Van Zyl, Mikki, Jeanelle de Gruchy, Sheila Lapinsky, Simon Lewin, and Graeme Reid. 1999. *The aversion project: Human rights abuses of gays and lesbians in the*

South African defence force by health workers during the apartheid era. Cape Town: Coalition for Lesbian and Gay Equality, Gay and Lesbian Archives, Health and Human Rights Project, Center for Epidemiological Research in Southern Africa, and South African Medical Research Council.

Whiteside, Alan, and Jack van Niftrik. 1990. AIDS in South Africa: Government and ANC response. *AIDS Analysis Africa* (southern Africa edition) 1 (2): 1.

Whiteside, Alan, and Clem Sunter. 2000. *AIDS and the challenge for South Africa.* Cape Town: Tafelberg and Human & Rousseau.

Zwi, Anthony, and Deborah Bachmayer. 1990. HIV and AIDS in South Africa: What is an appropriate public health response? *Health Policy and Planning* 5 (4): 316–26.

Chapter 8

Personalist Regimes and the Insecurity Dilemma: Prioritizing AIDS as a National Security Threat in Uganda

Robert L. Ostergard, Jr. and Crystal Barcelo

Most research on HIV/AIDS and state security in Africa has had a unidirectional approach.[1] That is, it has examined how HIV/AIDS affects the national and international security of African states. While this perspective elucidates *how* the virus may threaten state security and contribute to state failure, this approach only explains part of the story. In contrast, this chapter investigates how security threats impact the ability of Africa's weak states to fight HIV/AIDS. For instance, it was only after lengthy wars that Sierra Leone and Liberia began to evaluate the extent of HIV prevalence among their populations.[2] During the conflict, the state and rebel groups mobilized resources for combat, not for HIV prevention and treatment programs. Because of the focus on war, the magnitude of the epidemic bypassed policymakers; even international AIDS organizations avoided working in Liberia and Sierra Leone while war engulfed the two countries. As a result, HIV prevalence is now a concern in each country. In 2003, 5.9 per cent of Liberians between 15 and 49 years old were HIV positive (UNAIDS 2004). In Sierra Leone, the rate was estimated to be 7 per cent (UNAIDS 2002).

The cases of Liberia and Sierra Leone suggest that state responses to HIV/AIDS must be situated in a larger framework of a state's concerns and priorities about security. When the state faces multiple security threats, how does it determine which threats must be confronted immediately? Given limited resources, how do African leaders decide how to use state resources to fight threats? These questions are not easy to answer because each state's security concerns can vary based on several factors. The mixture of priorities has led policy makers and scholars to expand the security concept to include areas outside the traditional security concerns of state control, population protection, and territorial integrity. The revised 'human security' concept includes individual-level concerns such as health, education, crime, and employment. In 1994, the United Nations Development Program argued that security should focus not solely on states, but also on individuals. Using this definition, HIV/AIDS, with its impact on individuals, families, and communities, is certainly a threat to human security. While this definitional expansion highlights the complexity of security, it has been criticized for being too broad. If all human problems are security threats, then what prevents state and nonstate actors from complacency in addressing them (Ostergard 2002; Paris 2001)?

This chapter maintains that both traditional and human security theorists have overlooked the role of a state's leadership, institutions, and decision-making processes in setting security priorities. In Africa, the state's patrimonial and personalist nature cannot be ignored in analyzing decisions about security threats. Because of limited checks on executive power and weak civil society organizations, African political leaders have much power in policy making. They build support through patronage networks, not legal-rational institutions (Migdal 1988, 206–37; Bratton and van de Walle 1997; Mazrui and Tidy 1984; Reno 1998). This tendency for politics to revolve around particular individuals means that the role of these individuals in agenda setting and issue prioritizing is crucial for maintaining a cohesive, collective response to any security threat. Leaders who want to stay in power must attend to immediate threats; these threats receive priority in an environment with scarce resources. An important factor in the success of some African states in combating HIV/AIDS has been that leaders have prioritized the epidemic as an immediate threat and mobilized resources, institutions, and citizens to fight the disease. The case study of Uganda provided below illustrates the crucial role of leadership in reframing AIDS as a security threat. It also, however, demonstrates the complex role of state and international resources in addressing that security priority.

Leadership Perceptions and the Security Threshold

State leaders must deal with three questions about any potential security threat: (1) Does the problem pose an actual threat to the state? (2) What is the time frame involved in the threat? Is it an immediate or future threat? (3) What must be done to counter the threat? For example, must the state acquire financial resources or build institutional capacity? In some part, the answers to these questions hinge on the individual or collective perceptions of the state's leaders. In cases such as an invasion, social unrest, or revolution, little information is needed to understand and give priority to these immediate threats. For problems that are not so obvious or that pose a long-term threat to the state, leadership perceptions are fundamental for determining state responses.

Jervis (1978) argues that states seek to advance their own security by creating a relative environment of insecurity for themselves and other states. This 'security dilemma' assumes that one state can counter the actions of the other, thus preventing the other from acting aggressively. The concept of the security dilemma is rooted in the cold war, during which the United States and the Soviet Union sought to balance the power of the other. However, while there may be similarities in the types of threats that states face, it is incorrect to assume that all states can react equally to security concerns. Not all states have the same level of political or economic development. Instead, Job (1992) maintains that developing states face an *insecurity* dilemma that prevents them from addressing threats. The insecurity dilemma differs from Jervis' concept in four critical areas. First, developing states usually have no single nation or socially cohesive society. This fact makes it more difficult to mobilize societal responses to a threat and may actually contribute to instability through secession movements or ethnic uprisings. Second, the lack of a single nation undermines regime support from a large portion of the population. In Africa, this means that rulers have often resorted to force and/or patronage to build networks of support for the state. Third, the state lacks the institutional capacity to maintain internal order. The lack of well-armed and professional militaries and police forces makes it more difficult to combat social instability and crime; this fact further hampers state legitimacy. Fourth, for many developing states, the prevailing security threats tend to be more domestically oriented than externally motivated. Civil wars, insurgency movements, and ethnic or religious uprisings are more apparent in developing regions than wars between states (Job 1992, 17–18).

An integration of the concepts of human security and the insecurity dilemma elucidates why security priorities vary across states. Viewing issues through the lens of human security may motivate states to respond to individual-level social problems. Yet, whether a human security threat receives high priority depends on how state leaders order their priorities, and most leaders are primarily concerned with the survival of the state and its institutions. Human security threats affect different facets of security and leaders may deal with these issues using different strategies and in longer time periods. For example, rebellion poses an immediate threat to regimes; education and crime are long-term governing problems. While education and crime may impact stability and economic security in the future, they pose little immediate threat to the state. The insecurity dilemma of developing states explains why some issues may become security crises in poor countries but not in wealthy countries. For example, health care and disease are public policy issues in advanced industrial countries, but they may pose real threats to the security of developing states. This is because wealthier states have the resources of tax revenues, health-care infrastructure, and medical personnel to address such issues before they threaten social, economic, and political institutions.

There are two factors that shape how state leaders prioritize and respond to security threats. The first is the target threatened: territorial integrity, governing institutions and infrastructure, and/or population. Threats to territory and governing institutions have usually been considered traditional security threats, while threats to the population often have fallen into the human security category. However, this dichotomy between traditional and human security is too neat since all security issues eventually affect human beings. It is more effective to analyze threats on a continuum between traditional or human security issues. Such a continuum also acknowledges that the salience of a particular security issue may change over a given time period. The second factor is the time frame in which the state perceives it must respond. While all security threats are a concern to political leaders, all threats are not equal at any given moment in time. Traditional security issues tend to be short-term crises that require immediate attention; human security issues tend to be long-term problems of governance. We use these two criteria – type of security target and time frame – to place security issues on a continuum from 'hard' to 'soft.' In this chapter, hard issues represent the most direct and immediate threats to the state; soft issues are either threats that are indirect or distant in the future. Table 8.1 presents some examples of these issue types.

Table 8.1 Security targets and time frame

Security target	Security threat time frame	Type of security issue	Example of threat
Territory	Immediate or short-term	Traditional security (hard)	War, secessionist civil wars
Institutions	Immediate or short-term	Traditional security (hard)	Coups d'etat, civil wars, revolutions
Population	Medium to long-term	Human security (soft)	Epidemics, famine, migrations, poverty
–	Immediate or short-term	Traditional security (hard)	International wars, revolutions, civil wars

Threats to territorial integrity or governing institutions are often the most critical or immediate issues that leaders face in dealing with national security. Threats to the security of the state's population can come from a host of sources. The most critical or immediate threat for the state is when the population is under direct military attack. Less clear is how state leaders prioritize threats to the population that cross other areas of public policy. For example, over time epidemics or an influx of refugees from a neighboring state can become critical issues. Since HIV/AIDS is a soft security issue, it is important for the study of African state responses to the disease to question when soft issues become critical enough to cause the state to respond. The softer an issue is, the less likely it is that state leaders will react. However, security threats and state responses to those threats are not static. Over time, the threat may worsen, forcing leaders to deem the security issue sufficient enough to warrant a response. At any given moment, leaders may perceive an issue as soft at time t; they then may reconsider that judgment at time t+1. Conversely, hard issues require a rapid response from state leaders. As leaders address the issues, these concerns may become less immediate and they may move to the soft end of the issue continuum. For instance, the state may control a secessionist rebellion that threatens territorial integrity through military force, decentralized political institutions, and/or patronage resources directed to the region. Though the rebellion against the state may not disappear, the secessionist goal may become less likely to succeed. State responses to the crisis may 'soften' the issue over time.

Two factors that cannot be generalized in determining where threats appear on the continuum between hard and soft issues are leadership perceptions of the threat and the leadership's ability to convince other governing elites and the population that the issue is a threat. In African states, presidents usually set the agenda for dealing with security concerns. But the president's ability to convince others that an issue is a threat may be more difficult if the president lacks support or legitimacy across a fragmented population. The president's claim of a security threat may face challenges from various ethnic, religious, socioeconomic, racial, or regional groups (Job 1992). Further, the parochial interests of population segments affected by the threat may shape the leader's security perceptions. In the case of AIDS, for example, the president may perceive the issue to be a critical security threat that must be addressed immediately, but traditional leaders may view the disease to be a concern for only select groups in society.

Huntington (1997) provides an example of how public perceptions of security threats and national identity shape foreign policy. The end of the cold war and the demise of the Soviet Union, as well as the shift in social and demographic patterns in the US population, have caused Americans to lose their sense of unity against a common enemy.[3] As a result, ethnic, commercial, and transnational interests have become the dominant elements in America's post-cold war foreign policy. No single entity exists for the entire population to focus on as a threat to security; hence other, more parochial interests have emerged within the diverse segments of the population. Without a common external 'other' that the population can identify, the national interest disintegrates into sub-national interests.

When the population or the very existence of the state may be threatened, it is relatively easy for a president to build a consensus among political leaders and the population that the threat is immediate and must be addressed. Agreement about policy responses will be more likely. For example, soon after 11 September, US President George W. Bush had little difficulty gaining public support for attacking the Taliban in Afghanistan or passing legislation to facilitate gathering anti-terrorist intelligence information. However, when other governing elites and the population perceive an issue to be less immediate or critical, the president will find consensus building difficult, hampering state action against the perceived threat. When the president does not perceive an issue to be a security threat and does not address it, pressure from civil society organizations or other government officials may cause the leader to respond. However, for this to occur civil society must have the resources and ability to influence state actions and there must be other political officials with enough power and institutional resources to challenge the president. These two criteria are often absent in the African context.

Policy reactions to AIDS in the United States illustrate the role of population perception in defining and addressing this soft security threat. In the early 1980s when the first AIDS cases emerged, the HIV virus became primarily associated with two groups: homosexuals and Haitian immigrants. Though Haitians were initially stigmatized, as it became apparent that the disease crossed nationality lines, this association faded. However, this was not true for gays, and AIDS became known primarily as a gay disease. The labeling emerged during a period when the American political climate turned distinctly toward a conservative agenda that emphasized 'family values' as necessary components of society's foundation. The US media continued to associate HIV/AIDS with the gay community until other societal groups such as women, children, hemophiliacs, and the recipients of blood transfusions were affected. The media then created a two-tier structure of victims – the 'innocent' victims who had contracted the disease through nonsexual contact, and the 'guilty' victims who had contracted the disease through homosexual activity or intravenous drug usage (Bastos 1999, 24–25). This media portrayal of people with HIV/AIDS influenced public perceptions of those with the disease. At first, these perceptions led to a lack of urgency in coping with the disease. The early association of HIV/AIDS with the politically unpopular gay community caused government officials to approach early calls for policy action with indifference or hostility. However, when hemophiliacs and blood recipients were affected, government and nongovernmental actors such as the Red Cross were more likely to respond with stricter regulations for blood supply safety (Siplon 2002).

Public perceptions that the disease affected people who were somehow guilty, coupled with changes in western strategic interests, also shaped policy responses to the emerging AIDS epidemic in Africa. For the United States and Western Europe the proportion of the population affected by the disease was relatively small and politically controversial. In Africa the proportion of the population affected was significantly higher. AIDS was pegged to politically unfavorable groups in the West, a fact which prevented both western and African governments from reacting early to the global spread of the disease. The end of the cold war further marginalized Africa in US foreign policy and in the international community and consequently marginalized Africa's social problems, not the least of which was AIDS. The spread of HIV/AIDS in Africa was not a direct security threat to the West in any sense of the word. For Africa, AIDS was becoming a critical security issue, reflected by the extent of the epidemic on the continent. However, because AIDS was perceived negatively by the public, and because most African leaders did not perceive the disease to be a security threat, many African presidents ignored AIDS. Only 15 years after the first AIDS cases emerged on the continent did African and western leaders seriously begin to reconsider the immediacy of this soft security threat. This changed perspective was apparent in the 2000

United Nations Security Council session which focused on HIV/AIDS as a security threat (United Nations 2000).

Leaders must confront two obstacles when building consensus to address security threats. First, states may face multiple security issues that are perceived simultaneously as immediate threats. If so, state officials must prioritize these issues. Of course, different segments in society may view security threats differently, a fact that complicates the policy-making process. Second, state capacity affects how, or if, states can respond to threats. No state has unlimited resources to respond to security threats; thus, decision makers must convince other leaders and the population that a particular security threat is severe enough to warrant the allocation of state resources. To address a threat, the state will need either to increase its capacity or to rearrange its funding priorities. Without agreement on both the need to respond to the threat and the allocation of resources, state officials may insufficiently (if at all) address a particular threat. The case of Uganda presented below illustrates how one African state has met the needs for state capacity in combating AIDS, while also tackling other security threats.

The African Context

The postcolonial history of many African states demonstrates that forging a national consensus on issues of security can be a daunting task. When the former colonial powers left Africa after World War II, they assumed that liberal democracy and its institutions would be sufficient to control problems the new African governments encountered. The former colonial powers bequeathed to the continent government institutions which lacked sufficient mechanisms of representation for the diverse social, political, and ethnic composition of African states (Davidson 1994; Mazrui 1986). During the postcolonial period, African leaders often have confronted the major obstacle of group versus national identity when forging a consensus on solutions to problems. The insecurity dilemma of African states highlights the problem of creating a national identity that supersedes the commanding strength of regional, religious, and ethnic identities among Africa's peoples. Africa's indigenous groups often identify more with their ethnic or clan affiliation than with their own state; conversely, the African state and particular leaders have struggled to identify with all of the societal groups that they are supposed to represent. Such a problem has the potential to undermine consensus building on national and international policy issues that states confront.

Western political philosophers have been concerned with the problem of pluralism in society for centuries. Burke detailed the importance of a people's tradition when he provided a scathing critique of the French Revolution of 1789. For him, the idea of a state did not start with simple geography; rather it began with its people, the nation. When people confronted difficulties with their rulers, they then could build on this foundation of history and experience to formulate a new political system. Burke believed it was a tragic discarding of the French forefathers when the revolutionaries rebuked the culture and traditions that had been established prior to 1789 (Burke 1782; Burke and Pocock 1987; Mazrui 1963). An analogy can be made with Africa. The division of Africa into modern states separated many of those peoples or nations into different territories. In essence, the modern state in Africa began antithetical to Burke's logic, with geography or territory being the primary basis for the state, rather than the nation and its culture and heritage. When colonial powers created states in Africa, they erected boundaries that often arbitrarily divided ethnic groups and placed them together even though they had little, if any, common culture or heritage. One consequence of this arrangement has been that the dominant threats to national security in post-colonial Africa have been internal instead of external. Uganda provides an example of how domestic security issues shape the state's ability to confront HIV/AIDS.

The Case of Uganda

Uganda illustrates the importance of decision makers in promoting AIDS as a security threat and defining state responses to be in the national interest. The first cases of AIDS appeared in Uganda in 1982, though the asymptomatic period between HIV infection and the first signs of AIDS makes it likely that the epidemic began in the late 1970s. Geographically, the Ugandan epidemic emerged in the southern region of Buganda. Under Idi Amin's regime from 1971 to 1979 economic policies and political tyranny drove the Ugandan economy into collapse and promoted an illicit black market centered on the highway that runs from Mombasa, Kenya to Kampala and through the Buganda region; the highway also links Uganda to Sudan, Rwanda, and Burundi. The route was lined with illicit or unregulated services, such as hotels, restaurants, and brothels that catered to truck drivers. When the Tanzanian military invaded Uganda in 1979 to oust Amin, the Buganda area, and particularly the Rakai district, became a central point of operations for the Tanzanian forces. Hooper (1987) argues that this invasion was an important turning point that created conditions for the spread of the virus.

The Tanzanian military installed the former Ugandan leader Milton Obote as president. But Obote, who had first ruled from 1966 until 1971, merely continued the negative economic policies and repression that had led to the country's downward political spiral under Amin. Obote's lack of control over the country led him to rely increasingly on the brutal actions of the military to retain power. Khadiagala (1993) reports that military crimes during this period may have surpassed those under Amin's dictatorship, and included the massacre of thousands of people in the Luwero triangle north of Kampala. Opposition to Obote began to build across Uganda and propelled the upstart of guerilla movements. When the military split along traditional ethnic cleavages, the dominant factions ousted Obote in 1985 and opposition groups vied for control of the country.

Despite attempts on the part of Kenya's President Daniel arap Moi to broker a peace agreement between warring factions, Yoweri Museveni and his National Resistance Army (NRA) marched into Kampala in January 1986 (Khadiagala 1993). But peace was not forthcoming, as domestic opposition forces took up arms against the new National Resistance Movement (NRM) government and external foes lined up against Museveni's government. The lack of national identity to trump ethnic affiliations created conditions of internal insecurity. Museveni, himself a member of the Bahima upper caste of the Bayakole of southwestern Uganda, now faced opposition from northern Acholi supporters of Obote and a growing movement of supporters of Idi Amin in the West Nile region. Museveni faced an insecurity dilemma. In order to build consensus on state security actions, Museveni would have to create institutions that crossed these ethnic lines. The development of the movement system, instead of multiparty competition, has sought to unify the country; voters confirmed support for the movement system in a national referendum in 2000.

Externally, tensions rose between Uganda and its neighbors. Moi's attempt to mediate between the competing factions in Uganda led to strains in the personal relations between Moi and Museveni, resulting in several border skirmishes between Kenya and Uganda in the late 1980s (Khadiagala 1993, 243–44). Disagreements with Sudan over accusations that Uganda militarily supported rebel groups in southern Sudan also surfaced. Finally, in the 1990s, Uganda's involvement in the invasion of Rwanda by the Tutsi-dominated Rwandan Patriotic Front and its direct military intervention in the multistate war in the Democratic Republic of the Congo added to the regional security issues that Uganda faced. Since coming to power, Museveni has not faced a shortage of immediate or hard security issues that needed attention.

By the late 1980s, the extent and nature of the looming HIV/AIDS epidemic became apparent when the disease challenged one of Museveni's security priorities – the restructuring and transformation of the NRA from a guerilla group to a national army. In 1987 Museveni sent Ugandan army officers to Cuba for training. Before the training began, the Cuban government tested the officers for HIV; the results showed that many of the Ugandan officers were HIV positive. Cuban President Fidel Castro informed Museveni of the problem directly (Garbus and Marseille 2003, 11–12). While Museveni had recognized the epidemic as a serious issue when he came to power, it appears that he did not realize the actual severity of the problem until his conversation with Castro. After the NRM solidified control over government in 1986, Museveni had established an HIV/AIDS control program, the Ugandan National AIDS Control Project (NACP), which was under the auspices of the ministry of health. The program focused on the basic issues associated with HIV prevention, such as blood safety, education, and communication. Concurrent control programs were established in 12 ministries.

It could be argued that Museveni's perception of AIDS as a security issue stems from the Castro conversation; at that point, Museveni saw how AIDS directly affected the country's ability to respond to hard security issues through its impact on military preparedness. Since the country faced several hard security threats in the late 1980s, and since Museveni's hold on power was somewhat tenuous, it is understandable how the effect of AIDS on the military could shape the president's perceptions of the disease. The institutions developed to combat AIDS were also important, but because of the underdevelopment of civil society and political institutions in Uganda, Museveni's personal zeal for addressing the disease and mobilizing a response to AIDS was crucial. Policy analysts credit Museveni with being one of the first African leaders to speak openly and candidly about AIDS (Barnett and Whiteside 2002; Price-Smith 2002; Garbus and Marseille 2003, 88). He encouraged frank discussion of the disease and assembled leaders and organizations that would be crucial in mobilizing a national response. In doing so, he tried to create a common public perception about the security threat of AIDS, something crucial for developing and sustaining a policy response to the disease. The very fact that an African leader at this time was addressing the epidemic in such a forthright manner helped to convince people that HIV was a significant problem. It is important to realize, though, that Uganda's political climate made it easy for Museveni to provide this leadership. He firmly controlled the military and there were no organized opposition parties or press; Museveni could shape the national agenda. At the same time, Museveni was responsible for bringing Uganda's epidemic to the world's attention. In 1986, the Uganda Minister of Health announced at the World Health Assembly that HIV was a major problem in Uganda and asked for assistance in dealing with the epidemic.

Despite the initial forthright response from the country's leadership, problems emerged in the first attempts to curtail the epidemic under the NACP. In its first four years, the program succeeded in raising the awareness of the problem in Uganda, but the overall response was relatively weak on the part of the public and private sectors because they tended to perceive AIDS exclusively as a health problem (Uganda AIDS Commission 1993). In response, in 1992 the government adopted the Multisectoral Approach for the Control of AIDS (MACA). The Ugandan AIDS Commission, a body established by the legislature and placed within the office of the president, coordinates MACA policies. As a high-level political institution, MACA and Museveni have been able to create a common message about AIDS. Museveni has stressed that Ugandans, from those in the highest levels of government to small communities, have a responsibility to be engaged in AIDS prevention. The approach has five specific goals: (1) to stop the spread of HIV infection; (2) to mitigate the adverse health and socioeconomic impact of the epidemic; (3) to strengthen the national capacity to respond to the epidemic; (4) to establish a national information base on HIV/AIDS; and (5) to strengthen the national capacity to undertake research relevant to HIV/AIDS (Uganda AIDS Commission 1993). In 1997, the central government adopted a policy of decentralization and encouraged local governments to adopt development and HIV/AIDS programs specific to their needs (Garbus and Marseille 2003). Since the adoption of the program, most researchers agree that the incidence of HIV prevalence in Uganda has declined, though the amount of that decline is disputed (Parkhurst 2002). UNAIDS (2004) reported a prevalence rate of 4.1 per cent in 2003.

It is essential to analyze the Ugandan case in light of the theoretical precepts about security outlined in this chapter. Though western donors and nongovernmental organizations (NGOs) have touted Uganda as the quintessential example of how governments need to approach the epidemic, the country's path to success is not so clear-cut. Given the initial opposition to the new government and its subsequent involvement in regional conflicts, the government's ability to address new security concerns was quite limited, especially in terms of the state's capacity to carry out new AIDS policies. It is easy to increase the rhetoric about needing to do something about the epidemic; ultimately though, the state must support that rhetoric with the allocation of financial resources. How did Uganda deal with the HIV/AIDS threat while also attending to its other security issues?

To begin, it is important to note that after independence Uganda had one of the best health-care systems in Africa (Wiebe and Dodge 1987, 101; Joseph 1999). In the years immediately following independence, local governments had access to resources and carried out the provision of basic social services such as roadwork, water supply, agricultural extension, the management of natural resources, and basic health and educational services (Joseph 1999, 285). The central government allocated responsibilities to local governments, which fostered an effective and efficient public sector since local governments are closer to citizens and know their needs. The years of political, economic, and social turmoil that ensued after independence devastated this arrangement. As a result, the burden of service provision was placed on numerous humanitarian-based voluntary organizations. This arrangement allowed the government to disengage from the public sector, even after Museveni came to power and the Ugandan economy and society began to rebuild after years of war.

Since 1986, Uganda has experienced remarkable economic growth because of the implementation of neoliberal policies advocated by the World Bank and the International Monetary Fund. The government's commitment to public education and health services, however, has continued to remain shallow. The state has continued to rely on the profusion of NGOs and intergovernmental organizations (IGOs) to fill the gap in state capacity. Nonstate actors have taken over state responsibilities, a fact which has increased the state's legitimacy. For instance, the United Nations Development Program indicates that public education expenditures were 3.5 per cent of gross domestic product (GDP) between 1985 and 1987, but they decreased to 2.6 per cent between 1995 and 1997. They decreased again to 2.3 per cent between 1998 and 2000, but rose to 2.5 per cent in 2001. In the late 1990s, the country's spending on public health was only 1.5 per cent of GDP (UNDP 2002, 2003, 2004).

It is possible to speculate about why the state has receded from providing public services to its people. One reason may be that the government perceives the social service policies of NGOs and IGOs as an extension of state public policy. Another reason may be that during a period of financial austerity, states have courted NGOs and IGOs, because these services are important to citizens but the state lacks resources to provide them (van de Walle 2001). Whatever the reason, the result is that in Uganda health care and education from NGOs and IGOs are more efficient than the same government-provided services; the government has not had to build state capacity to meet the needs of its people (Nabuguzi 1994). Also, IGO and NGO involvement enables the government to divert funds from state social service programs to the military.

In the early 1990s, government expenditures for the military were estimated to be 3 per cent of GDP. By 2001, that number had declined to 2.1 per cent. Yet, in comparison to spending on public health, military spending remains high. These levels of spending indicate that the epidemic still has not reached the same perceived level of threat to national security as other traditional threats (UNDP 2003). Government spending on the military has supported troops fighting rebels in the northern and western regions of Uganda and troops involved in the war in the Democratic Republic of the Congo. Moreover, in January 2004, the Ugandan government announced a new increase in military expenditures in an attempt to defeat the Lord's Resistance Army in the north (*Monitor*, 18 April 2004). It is estimated that this conflict has cost the Ugandan economy $1.33 billion over the last 16 years (Garbus and Marseille 2003). In making calculations about whether to address the soft security threat of AIDS, the Ugandan government has not had to concern itself with diverting funds from other security priorities.

The failure of the state to deliver services drives the growth of the voluntary sector, which is primarily dependent on external financial assistance. The growth in the number of NGOs and their funding has been staggering. More than 25 per cent of all official aid to Uganda since 1990 has been funneled through NGOs, accounting for approximately $125 million per year (Dicklitch 1998, 120). For the year 2003, Uganda received over $70 million in humanitarian assistance from the United States. This aid was channeled to NGOs and IGOs that assisted primarily with social service provision. In addition, according to the United Nations, external donations to Uganda for the year 2003 were over $100 million, with most of this money being spent on humanitarian and social service assistance through NGOs and IGOs (UNDP 2003). In the specific policy area of AIDS, the level of foreign support between 1989 and 1998 was quite substantial. According to the United States

Agency for International Development, over $180 million was given to Uganda, which represented about 70 per cent of the total expenditures in the government's battle against HIV/AIDS (Garbus and Marseille 2003). In 2003, the Global Fund to Fight AIDS, Tuberculosis, and Malaria approved $36 million over a three-year period to combat the epidemic, bringing the total allocated by the Global Fund to Uganda to approximately $96.7 million (Wendo 2003).

Conclusion

What the Ugandan case shows is the personalist nature of the security agenda in African states. Museveni's leadership was an important factor in pushing the HIV/AIDS epidemic to the forefront of the government's agenda. His rhetoric and the institutional structures he created to address AIDS demonstrate that the government perceived at least some level of threat from this soft security issue. However, the epidemic has not reached the level of threat to cause Museveni and the NRM government to reprioritize resources from the immediate threats of internal rebellions and regional conflicts. It could be argued that Museveni still sees the epidemic as a medium to long-term threat to the stability of the state. For Museveni to draw attention to the epidemic while not compromising his focus on hard security issues, he needed to expand the state's capacity to cope with both AIDS and more immediate threats. The only possible way to do this was to rely on the international community for assistance.

The fact that Museveni most likely could not have achieved success against AIDS without external assistance raises concerns for the international community. Clearly, weak states need help if they are to launch a full program against the epidemic. Weak states that face strong insecurity dilemmas will be forced to choose between the immediate threats that domestic instability poses or the medium and long-term security threat of the epidemic. On the other hand, the international community faces a dilemma, because assistance given to NGOs and IGOs to provide relief from the epidemic may potentially disrupt the building of civil society to address social problems and may prevent the state from making hard choices about developing state capacity.

Because the state is able to abrogate responsibility for providing needed human services by relying on external assistance during crises such as epidemics, citizens become dependent on donors instead of the state. Yet, this trend raises issues about transparency and accountability, since NGOs and IGOs are rarely accountable to the clients they serve. The costs of maintaining state functions in the traditional areas of security while tackling the increasing costs associated with the soft security issue of AIDS will most likely cause states to exceed their available resources and to become even more dependent on foreign assistance.

Notes

1 For example, see Price-Smith (2002) and Elbe (2002).
2 Liberia has experienced war intermittently between 1989 and 2003; Sierra Leone's war lasted from roughly 1991 to 2003.
3 Some might argue the attacks of 11 September have created a new common enemy of terrorism.

References

Barnett, Tony, and Alan Whiteside. 2002. *AIDS in the twenty-first century: Disease and globalisation*. Basingstoke: Palgrave Macmillian.

Bastos, Cristiana. 1999. *Global responses to AIDS: Science in emergency*. Bloomington: Indiana Univ. Press.

Bratton, Michael, and Nicolas van de Walle. 1997. *Democratic experiments in Africa: Regime transitions in comparative perspective*. Cambridge: Cambridge Univ. Press.

Burke, Edmund. 1782. Speech: On a motion made in the House of Commons, the 7th of May 1782, for a committee to inquire into the state of the representation of the Commons in Parliament.
http://www.econlib.org/library/LFBooks/Burke/brkSWv4c2.html.

Burke, Edmund, and J. G. A. Pocock. 1987. *Reflections on the revolution in France*. Indianapolis: Hackett Publishing.

Davidson, Basil. 1994. *Modern Africa: A social and political history*. London: Longman.

Dicklitch, Susan. 1998. *The elusive promise of NGOs in Africa: Lessons from Uganda*. New York: St. Martin's Press.

Elbe, Stefan. 2002. HIV/AIDS and the changing landscape of war in Africa. *International Security* 27 (2): 159–77.

Garbus, Lisa, and Elliot Marseille. 2003. *HIV/AIDS in Uganda*. San Francisco: AIDS Policy Research Center, Univ. of California.

Hooper, Edward. 1987. AIDS in Uganda. *African Affairs* 86 (345): 469–77.

Huntington, Samuel. 1997. The erosion of American national interests. *Foreign Affairs* 76 (5): 28–49.

Jervis, Robert. 1978. Cooperation under the security dilemma. *World Politics* 30 (2): 167–214.

Job, Brian. 1992. The insecurity dilemma: National, regime, and state securities in the Third World. In *The Insecurity dilemma: National security of Third World states*, ed. Brian Job, 11–35. Boulder, CO: Lynne Rienner.

Joint United Nations Program on HIV/AIDS (UNAIDS). 2002. *Sierra Leone: Epidemiological fact sheets on HIV/AIDS and sexually transmitted infections. 2002 update*.
http://www.unaids.org.

——. 2004. *Report on the global AIDS epidemic*.
http://www.unaids.org/bangkok2004.html.

Joseph, Richard. 1999. *State, conflict, and democracy in Africa*. Boulder, CO: Lynne Rienner.

Khadiagala, Gilbert. 1993. Uganda's domestic and regional security since the 1970s. *Journal of Modern African Studies* 31 (2): 231–55.
Mazrui, Ali Al'Amin. 1963. Edmund Burke and reflections on the revolution in the Congo. *Comparative Studies in Society and History* 5 (2): 121–33.
——. 1986. *The Africans: A triple heritage*. Boston: Little, Brown.
Mazrui, Ali Al'Amin, and Michael Tidy. 1984. *Nationalism and new states in Africa from about 1935 to the present*. Nairobi: Heinemann.
Migdal, Joel. 1988. *Strong societies and weak states: State-society relations and state capabilities in the Third World*. Princeton: Princeton Univ. Press.
Nabuguzi, E. G. 1994. *Structural adjustment and the informal economy in Uganda*. Copenhagen: Center for Development Research.
Ostergard, Robert. 2002. Politics in the hot zone: AIDS and national security in Africa. *Third World Quarterly* 23 (2): 333–50.
Paris, Roland. 2001. Human security: Paradigm shift or hot air? *International Security* 26 (2): 87–102.
Parkhurst, Justin. 2002. The Ugandan success story? Evidence and claims of HIV-1 prevention. *Lancet* 360 (9326): 78.
Price-Smith, Andrew. 2002. *The health of nations: Infectious disease, environmental change, and their effects on national security and development*. Cambridge: MIT Press.
Reno, William. 1998. *Warlord politics and African states*. Boulder, CO: Lynne Rienner.
Siplon, Patricia. 2002. *AIDS and the policy struggle in the United States*. Washington, DC: Georgetown Univ. Press.
Uganda AIDS Commission. 2003. The multi-sectoral approach to AIDS in Uganda: Executive summary. Kampala: Government of Uganda.
United Nations. 2000. *Security Council Resolution 1308*, 17 July. http://www.un.org.
United Nations Development Program (UNDP). 2002. *United Nations Development Programme report*. New York: Oxford Univ. Press.
——. 2003. *United Nations Development Programme report*. New York: Oxford Univ. Press.
——. 2004. *Human Development Report*. New York: Oxford Univ. Press.
van de Walle, Nicolas. 2001. *African economies and the politics of permanent crisis, 1979–1999*. Cambridge: Cambridge Univ. Press.
Wendo, Charles. 2003. Uganda and the Global Fund sign grant agreement: The government has decided how to use the Fund's money without destabilising its budgets. *Lancet* 361 (9361): 942.
Wiebe, Paul, and Cole Dodge. 1987. *Beyond crisis: Development issues in Uganda*. Kampala: Makerere Institute of Social Research, Makerere Univ.

Chapter 9

Weak and Ineffective? African States and Recent International AIDS Policies

Amy S. Patterson and David Cieminis

In the international arena, African states have traditionally been viewed to be weak.[1] Although there is great variation in African states in terms of political and historical experiences, there are commonalities among African states in the international arena. Overall, Africa lacks military might and economic power; African states are not key members of the United Nations (UN) Security Council and they have minimal representation at the World Trade Organization, the World Bank, and the International Monetary Fund. Because of underdevelopment and political instability, many African states have been viewed by their populations as illegitimate, corrupt, and inefficient (Chabal and Daloz 1999). Africa's dependence on developed countries for loans, aid, and export markets further constrains the power of African states. With the end of the cold war, African states have also suffered from a decline in foreign assistance (Lancaster 1999; Clapham 1996). The borders of African states have increasingly become porous, as states have little control over external military interventions, the actions of local and international nongovernmental organizations (NGOs), and the policy decisions of corporations (Harbeson and Rothchild 2000; Poku 2002; Barnett and Whiteside 2002).

Given these shared institutional, resource, and power limitations, how have African states acted within the international system to influence global policies on AIDS? This chapter examines the conditions that have both hampered and facilitated African state influence on recent international AIDS agreements. For the purposes of this chapter, we focus on the commonalities among African states in the global arena, though we do not deny the various political, historic, social, and economic experiences among African states. This chapter concentrates on two international actions: (1) the Declaration of Commitment on HIV/AIDS signed at the 2001 UN General Assembly Special Session (UNGASS) on HIV/AIDS; and (2) the Global Fund to Fight AIDS, Tuberculosis, and Malaria (Global Fund). First, we place the UNGASS and Global Fund in the larger context of a growing political commitment to AIDS. Second, we illustrate how aspects of the Declaration of Commitment on HIV/AIDS and the Global Fund are in tandem with the overarching policy preferences and international concerns of African states. In the third section, we demonstrate how the nature of the African state shaped its role in these recent international agreements. The chapter argues that the African state's reliance on donors, international organizations, and international NGOs hindered Africa's ability to shape the process of building these agreements. In many ways, African states were propelled to support UN-directed HIV/AIDS programs because of their need for resources. Yet, it is too simplistic to assert that African states have been weak participants in AIDS policy making. Instead, we argue that there are four variables that have shaped the nexus between the African state and the international system on the issue of AIDS: (1) the dependence of African states on donor resources; (2) the ability of African states to work with more powerful global negotiators to generate policies that benefit Africa; (3) the emergence of a moral and political dialogue pushed by international NGOs and some Western scientists supporting treatment for people living with HIV/AIDS (PLWHAs); and (4) an overarching realization of the link between global interdependence and public health.

A Growing International Commitment to AIDS

Since 2000, AIDS has been on the international policy-making agenda, with high-level discussions that illustrate a somewhat nuanced understanding of both the factors that make individuals vulnerable to HIV infection and the disease's potential impact on socioeconomic and political development. International institutions sought to develop policies on AIDS since the mid-1980s, when the World Health Organization (WHO) created its Global Program on AIDS. Since most of the early confirmed AIDS cases were in the West, there was substantial monetary support for the program from Western countries. By the early 1990s, however, this support ebbed when it became apparent that AIDS was not going to become a major heterosexual epidemic in the West (*Washington Post*, 5 July 2000; Will 1991; Gordenker et al. 1995). With a few notable exceptions such as Uganda and Senegal, African states played a minimal role in these initial UN programs and many leaders denied the existence of the disease in their countries (Fortin 1987; Batsell 2000; Lanegran and Hyden 1993; Singer 1998; Daly 2001).

Formed in 1996 to coordinate UN actions on AIDS, the Joint United Nations Program on HIV/AIDS (UNAIDS) has sought to build political support for the fight against AIDS and has encouraged political leaders to openly discuss the disease. Recent actions illustrate the success of UNAIDS in increasing political commitment to the disease (Poku 2002). In January 2000, the UN Security Council discussed AIDS, the first time a health issue had been debated as a security threat. In June 2001, the UN held the three-day UNGASS to discuss the pandemic. At the end of the session, all member-states signed the Declaration of Commitment on HIV/AIDS that outlines specific goals in the fight against AIDS. While nonbinding, the declaration serves as a blueprint for action by international organizations, national governments, and NGOs. The 2002 International Conference on HIV/AIDS in Barcelona hosted the first-ever panel of political leaders who discussed the pandemic (*Washington Post*, 14 July 2002).[2] In another politically symbolic example, 18 African first ladies met in July 2002 to form an organization to combat AIDS (UNAIDS 2002a). And US President George W. Bush used the high-profile venue of his 2003 State of the Union address to propose an increase in US funding for AIDS programs in 14 countries.

We examine the Declaration of Commitment on HIV/AIDS, and the Global Fund that emerged from it, because of the unique nature of these actions. All member-states of the UN signed the declaration without reservation. This contrasts greatly with other special sessions or UN-sponsored conferences, where signatories often express reservations to final declarations.[3] Because states are signatories, there is an implication that states will at least tacitly begin to implement some of the declaration's policies. The presence of presidents, prime ministers, foreign ministers, and health ministers at the UNGASS illustrates the magnitude of the pandemic and a heightened political awareness of AIDS. Additionally, the declaration was unlike other agreements for UN special sessions, in that there was no preliminary agreement to the document by states before the session. Finally, the Global Fund is the first attempt to incorporate state and private actors into international cooperation on AIDS. It is also the first attempt to develop a financial mechanism to address the action items outlined in the declaration (UNAIDS official, interview with author, 15 October 2002). The universal, state-centered, and political nature of these two cases provides an opportunity to examine the role of African states in these international actions.

African States, the Declaration of Commitment on HIV/AIDS, and the Global Fund

This section concentrates on three themes apparent in the declaration and the structure of the Global Fund that reflect the interests of African states: (1) human rights and the dual strategy of prevention and treatment; (2) state-centered political leadership; and (3) the role of donors in the fight against AIDS.

Human Rights and the Dual Strategy of Prevention and Treatment

The declaration recognizes that 'the full realization of human rights and fundamental freedoms for all is an essential element in a global response to the HIV/AIDS pandemic' (UNGASS 2001a, no. 16). The document outlines two aspects of human rights: nondiscrimination of PLWHAs and access to health care. While the right to nondiscrimination received widespread support among UN member-states, it was the inclusion of language on a right to health care for PLWHAs that was more controversial (UNAIDS official, interview with author, 15 October 2002).[4] The declaration states that access to medication 'in the context of pandemics such as HIV/AIDS is one of the fundamental elements to achieve progressively the full realization of the right of everyone to the enjoyment of the highest attainable standard of physical and mental health' (UNGASS 2001a, no. 15).

Numerous African delegates asserted that health care for PLWHAs is a basic human right. Former Kenyan President Daniel arap Moi said, 'the sick must not be deprived of the most basic human right – the right to life' (Kenya 2001). The prime minister of Lesotho reiterated this point. 'It is a basic human right of both the infected and the affected to have access to quality care and support' (Lesotho 2001). In contrast, the United States lobbied against defining health care and treatment for PLWHAs as a basic human right (United States 2001; Siplon 2002). In response to a UN draft document on AIDS, the United States said that 'for legal and constitutional reasons, the United States cannot accept a rights-based approach to HIV/AIDS' (Booker and Minter 2001). Before the UNGASS, the United States was the only member-state to abstain on a UN Human Rights Commission statement on access to medication to treat HIV/AIDS, because of concerns that it threatened the intellectual property rights of drug companies (Halbert 2002).

The declaration's call for treatment for PLWHAs logically follows from its statement that health care is a human right. For the first time in any international agreement on HIV/AIDS, the declaration says that 'care, support, and treatment are fundamental elements in an effective response' (UNGASS 2001a, nos. 55–57). The declaration calls for access to antiretroviral drugs (ARVs) and highlights the need to lower the cost of these medicines for the majority of individuals with AIDS in the developing world (UNGASS 2001a, nos. 15, 24). Delegates from several African countries strongly supported this aspect of the declaration (Ghana 2001; Nigeria 2001; Rwanda 2001; Burkina Faso 2001; Tanzania 2001; Burundi 2001; Botswana 2001; Kenya 2001). The minister of health and child services of Zimbabwe said, 'While [anti-retrovirals] are denied to us, the message of prevention is inadequately supported' (Zimbabwe 2001). In contrast, some delegates from industrialized countries such as the United Kingdom, Germany, and Denmark argued for devoting precious resources to prevention (Denmark 2001; United Kingdom 2001; Germany 2001). The focus on prevention over treatment was most apparent in the address by US Secretary of State Colin Powell, who said, 'Unless a strong emphasis is put on prevention, prevention and more prevention, this pandemic will continue to rage out of control' (United States 2001).

The Global Fund strives to empower states to implement the declaration's dual strategy (Global Fund 2002a). In its first three rounds of grants in April 2002, January 2003, and October 2003, the Global Fund allocated over $2.1 billion over two years to 224 programs in 121 countries. In terms of grant distribution, 46 per cent of the money went for ARVs and other drugs for opportunistic infections, while 25 per cent was allocated for human resources projects and 15 per cent, for physical infrastructure (Global Fund 2003b). Dr.

Chrispus Kiyonga, chairman of the Global Fund from 2001 to 2003, stated, 'The first round of grants reflects the Global Fund's strong commitment to a comprehensive approach to fighting HIV/AIDS ... that balances prevention and treatment' (Global Fund 2002a).

State-centered Political Leadership

Another key aspect of the declaration is its focus on political leadership. The importance of leadership is symbolized by the fact that the topic is discussed first in the declaration's operative clauses. 'Strong leadership at all levels of society is essential for an effective response to the epidemic' (UNGASS 2001a, nos. 37–46). At the UNGASS, both African and non-African countries highlighted the themes of leadership and accountability (Benin 2001; Burkina Faso 2001; Senegal 2001; Zambia 2001; Kenya 2001; Lesotho 2001; Burundi 2001). The open discussion of political leadership was possible because African states were willing to address their responsibilities in relation to HIV/AIDS (*New York Times*, 28 June 2001). Because African states are almost one-third of UN members, it would have been diplomatically difficult for the UNGASS to emphasize political leadership without Africa's agreement.

Although the document outlines several levels of leadership, it focuses on how 'leadership by governments' is essential and should be '*complemented* by the participation of civil society, the business community, and the private sector' (UNGASS 2001a, nos. 37–46; emphasis added). UNGASS delegates recommended that 'each developing country needs to lead its own effort against HIV/AIDS ... External partners need either to provide flexible programme support or to support individual projects only to the extent consistent with country strategies' (Roundtable Four 2001).

This state-centric understanding of political leadership is manifested in the grant criteria and procedures of the Global Fund. The postcolonial African state has typically tried to direct and control the development process. African state officials have perceived that the recent trend whereby donors channel funding to NGOs instead of the state has undermined state authority (Ndegwa 1996). The language of the Global Fund reflects an awareness of these concerns about African state sovereignty. 'The Fund will base its work on programs that reflect national ownership and respect country-led formulation and implementation processes.' The Global Fund attempts to distance itself from being an intrusive international organization by stating that it is 'a financial instrument, not an implementing entity' (Global Fund 2002a).

The Global Fund's procedures for distributing money through a Country Coordination Mechanism (CCM) illustrate the importance of state leadership. Before applying to the Global Fund, each state must form a CCM, or a coordinating body composed of representatives from government, NGOs, multilateral and bilateral donors, and the private sector (Global Fund 2002a). While the CCM is supposed to be a public-private partnership, senior government officials tend to chair most CCMs and thus, control their agendas. As of June

2003, only 44 per cent of the members of all CCMs submitting proposals in the second round of grants were nongovernmental representatives (Global Fund 2003a).[5] Because the CCM is responsible for drawing up proposals to submit to the Global Fund and for distributing grants, the government has a considerable amount of control over these external resources.

While this funding procedure ensures that HIV/AIDS policies have high-level political support, an example from South Africa illustrates the limitations of this model. In June 2002, the South African national government attempted to block the distribution of a grant to the KwaZulu-Natal Provincial Coordinating Mechanism, saying that the province did not go through the correct channels of the nation's CCM, the South African AIDS Council. This created uproar among Global Fund members who had praised KwaZulu-Natal's proposal for its focus on both treatment and prevention. UNAIDS Director Peter Piot noted that governments that block funding to treatment projects may need to be bypassed in the future (South African Press Association, 12 July 2002). After much debate, the leaders of KwaZulu-Natal yielded to the national government and agreed that 'all the resources that have been awarded to South Africa by the Global Fund would be pooled together under the SANAC umbrella and coordinating framework' (*BBC News*, 16 July 2002). This example demonstrates a paradox. While strong African state institutions are needed to coordinate HIV/AIDS policies, struggles over power and resources between the African central state and decentralized state institutions can negatively impact these policies. The tensions between levels of government over funding and policy direction may also limit the ability of decentralized institutions to reflect the policy input and innovations of local communities. Given the fact that many African states have at one point tried to co-opt, repress, or control civil society organizations (Rothchild and Chazan 1988; Harbeson, Rothchild, and Chazan 1994), the CCM structure may simply bolster the power and resources of the state without fostering transparency, accountability, and participation in policy making.

State control over resources from the Global Fund is also reflected in the difficulty that NGOs face in receiving grants. Although NGOs are eligible to submit proposals directly to the Global Fund, 'the proposal must demonstrate clearly why it could not be considered under the CCM process at the country level' (Global Fund 2002a). Placing the burden of proof on NGOs makes it harder for them to receive a grant. In the second and third rounds, 29 per cent of *funding* went to NGOs; in the fourth round this number was 25 per cent. Yet, the list of funded proposals reveals that few of the total number of direct grant recipients were NGOs (Global Fund 2002c, 2003c, 2003e, 2004). Much of this funding was under the control of a CCM, which in its proposal outlined specific NGOs to which it would distribute funds. For example, Kenya's successful proposal in the second round detailed how some of the grant money would be channeled to the NGOs of World Vision Kenya, CARE Kenya, and Medécins Sans Frontières (Doctors without Borders), all international NGOs with branches in Kenya (Government of Kenya 2002).

Four of 55 funded proposals in the first round, and two of 98 funded proposals in the second round, were directly from NGOs. These NGOs included Catholic Relief Services in Madagascar, Population Services International in Madagascar, the Kenya Network of Women with AIDS, Sanaa Art Promotions in Kenya, and Lutheran World Federation. However, these numbers contrast with the amounts allocated to governments: 54 per cent of funds in the second round, 50 per cent of funds in the third round, and 51 per cent of funds in the fourth round (Global Fund 2003a, 2003b, 2003c, 2004). Again, the Kenya proposal illustrates this point. Of the $129 million allocated to Kenya over a five-year period for HIV/AIDS programs, 79 per cent is estimated to go to government, 11 per cent to NGOs, 2 per cent to the private sector, 4 per cent to organizations of PLWHAs, 2 per cent to faith-based organizations, and 1 per cent to academic institutions (Government of Kenya 2002). Though Kenya is only one of 48 African states that received funding in the second round of grants, it is not alone in the high percentage of the grant money going to government. Over 50 per cent of money for HIV/AIDS programs in Benin, Botswana, Burkina Faso, Kenya, Liberia, Lesotho, Namibia, South Africa, Swaziland, and Tanzania is budgeted to go to those country's governments (Global Fund 2003c). Although clearly some states require funding to develop government health-care infrastructure, these percentages do illustrate that states thus far have benefited more from Global Fund resources than NGOs have.

A final aspect of the Global Fund that reinforces African state sovereignty is that, unlike bilateral donors or the World Bank, the Global Fund does not require a state to meet political or human rights conditions to receive a grant. For example, the government of Robert Mugabe in Zimbabwe, which has been criticized for its human rights abuses, received $10 million in the first round (Global Fund 2002c). Several African delegates at the UNGASS appealed to donor countries to 'remove subjective criteria aimed at influencing future initiatives' (Zambia 2001). Other African states 'warned against the Fund being used to impose conditions on developing nations' (UNGASS 2001b). Both the declaration and the Global Fund strive to protect state sovereignty by acknowledging the role of the central state in combating AIDS, by empowering the state with resources, by institutionalizing that power through the CCM, and by ignoring political conditions when making funding decisions. However, in August 2004, the Global Fund refused to give more resources to Zimbabwe, partially because of the high level of corruption, political violence, and state inefficiency in that country (*New York Times*, 12 August 2004). It is uncertain if such political considerations will be crucial for the Global Fund's decisions for other countries, or if Zimbabwe in 2004 is an exceptional case.

The Role of Donors in the Fight Against AIDS

The declaration and the Global Fund emphasize that donors must directly or indirectly provide resources to the most affected states in order to fight AIDS.

The declaration calls for more bilateral and international aid to combat AIDS and cancellation of debt for countries in the Heavily Indebted Poor Countries initiative.[6] These statements reflect the concern of the UNGASS delegates from developing countries, especially Ghana, Nigeria, Mozambique, Burkina Faso, and Tanzania (Ghana 2001; Nigeria 2001; Mozambique 2001; Burkina Faso 2001; Tanzania 2001). The declaration also encourages developed nations to devote 0.7 per cent of their gross national product to official development assistance (UNGASS 2001a, nos. 79–93). The inclusion of this goal demonstrates the concern of some African leaders that donors will provide money to fight AIDS at the expense of other development assistance programs (Mozambique 2001; Burkina Faso 2001).

While the declaration calls on donors to provide resources, the structure of the Board of Directors for the Global Fund seeks to provide equal representation of donor and recipient countries. The Global Fund allocates seven seats on the board to representatives from industrialized countries and seven seats to individuals from developing countries, with one additional seat to a representative from Africa. This voting structure allows developing countries to have an equal say in the direction and approval of proposals and prevents donor countries from vetoing proposals. In addition, two NGO representatives, one from a developing country and one from a developed country, and two private-sector representatives are included on the board (Global Fund 2002b). Until 2004, one of the private-sector members was the Gates Foundation, which has contributed millions of dollars to improving health care and fighting AIDS in Africa and India. This sympathetic member gave African states an ally during the initial years of the Global Fund. The appointment of Dr. Chrispus Kiyonga from Uganda to be the first chair of the board also acknowledged the importance of Africa in the AIDS fight.

As of September 2004, representation of developing and donor countries was roughly equivalent on the Technical Review Panel of the Global Fund, a group composed of experts who review submitted proposals and make recommendations to the board for funding decisions. (The by-laws for the Global Fund do not require regional representation on the panel.) Of the panel's 26 members, 10 were from developing countries, 14 were from industrialized countries, and two were from former communist countries (Global Fund 2003d). The independence of the Global Fund from the UN and the World Bank further reflects the focus on equal decision-making power between donors and developing states. Donor countries 'feared having the UN and World Health Organization in charge because of those groups' reputations for bureaucratic inefficiency' (*Los Angeles Times*, 21 June 2001). Developing countries did not want the World Bank to have a voting seat on the board, because of the World Bank's history with structural adjustment programs and its weighted vote system that favors developed countries over developing countries (Nigeria 2001; Ghana 2001). In a compromise, donors agreed to give the World Bank a nonvoting seat on the board. In return, African states allowed the Global Fund to be independent from the UN.

Representatives from the WHO and UNAIDS also serve as nonvoting members of the board (Global Fund 2002b).

While the decision-making processes of the Global Fund represent the voices of developing countries, it is important to acknowledge the Global Fund's limitations as a source of revenue in the fight against AIDS. While one of its assets is its independence, this fact also means that the Global Fund is dependent on the generosity of donor countries and private individuals. It has received $3.5 billion in pledges through 2004, roughly the amount needed for new grants during the same time period. However, the Global Fund will need an additional $1.5 billion for the renewal of existing rounds by 2005 (Global Fund 2004). Though the United States pledged approximately $1.6 billion for the period between 2001and 2008, this amount clearly will not be sufficient without additional resources from other industrialized countries. Furthermore, through the 2003 President's Emergency Plan for AIDS Relief, the United States Congress limited US contributions to the Global Fund to no more than 33 per cent of total resources (*Washington Post*, 19 August, 2004). The lack of resources illustrates one of the obstacles to meeting the objectives outlined in the declaration. Further, this situation demonstrates Africa's dependence on donors, since 61 per cent of grants in the four rounds have gone to sub-Saharan Africa (Global Fund 2003b, 2004).

The African State and International Policies on AIDS

Given their limited resources, underdeveloped institutions, and overall weakness in the global arena, what role did African states play in achieving the above policies and Global Fund structures? Throughout the process of developing the declaration and the Global Fund, were African states proactive or reactive? In this section, we will illustrate that the role of African states was complex. Dependence on international organizations and donor resources hampered Africa's ability to *lead* this consensus-building process. However, Africa's linkages to more powerful global negotiators and the emergence of a moral and political consensus in support of treatment for PLWHAs permitted African states to gain some of their objectives. The nature of the AIDS epidemic in a global environment further enabled African states to reach some of their goals.

African States and Dependence on International Organizations and Donor Resources

Although African states are the most negatively affected by HIV/AIDS, they were more reactive than proactive in the process of building support for the Declaration of Commitment on HIV/AIDS and the Global Fund. This fact was apparent in two ways. First, African states did not lead the consensus-building process for these international agreements. Instead, it was experts at

UNAIDS that played this key negotiating role (UNAIDS official, interview with author, 15 October 2002). UNAIDS wanted to gain global support for fighting AIDS, before calling for a UN special session on the topic. This bottom-up consensus-building process began with the International Partnership against AIDS in Africa, which was first discussed with African health ministers, World Bank officials, and UNAIDS staff in 1998. Before this program, discussions about formulating and implementing AIDS policies had been on a bilateral basis, between a particular African leader and either the World Bank or UNAIDS. Goals and objectives from the 1998 meeting were solidified in 1999 in a document sent to the UN Secretary General's office. In November 1999, bilateral donors, UN agencies, foundations, African national governments, and civil society organizations met to agree to these objectives. The Secretary General chaired this meeting, lending the weight of his office to the African partnership. The partnership eventually led to the 2001 African Summit on HIV/AIDS and Other Related Infectious Diseases in Abuja, Nigeria.

Because African states lack resources, expertise, and large UN missions, it is doubtful that they could have played a leadership role throughout the pre-UNGASS consensus-building period. UNAIDS has over 100 professional staff members with technical and policy-making experience; UNAIDS had the knowledge, information, and institutional resources to build international support for the goals in the declaration. At the UNGASS, UNAIDS officials built consensus with member-states and explained aspects of the declaration to representatives (Official at Swedish UN mission, correspondence with author, 1 October 2002). In fact, UNAIDS controlled this process so effectively that when Ukraine introduced a resolution to address HIV/AIDS during the 2000 session of the General Assembly, UNAIDS officials worked to get it off the agenda. Staff at UNAIDS believed that the time was not yet right for such a universal statement (UNAIDS official, interview with author, 15 October 2002).

The 2001 Abuja meeting, and donor conditions that preceded it, illustrate a second way that African states were followers, not leaders, in this period before the UNGASS. At Abuja, African leaders made their political commitment to HIV/AIDS explicit; this was a necessary step before any international agreement on AIDS could emerge. African leaders promised to 'place the fight against HIV/AIDS at the forefront' and 'to commit ourselves to take personal responsibility and provide leadership [on HIV/AIDS]'. These leaders vowed to end the stigma against PLWHAs and to involve PLWHAs in policy making. As evidence of their commitment, African leaders pledged to devote 15 per cent of their national budgets to improving health care (*Africa Recovery*, June 2001).

For many donors, this statement from African leaders, and especially the pledge of 15 per cent of state revenue for health, gave Africa a new level of legitimacy in global discussions on HIV/AIDS. After years of denial, it appeared that African officials were finally willing to take a leadership role on

AIDS (US delegation member to the UNGASS, interview with author, 21 October 2002). As part of the UNAIDS strategy, the statement at Abuja put pressure on donors to provide a stronger financial commitment to HIV/AIDS, since poor African countries were willing to pledge a sizeable portion of government budgets to public health. Yet, it is important to realize that because of their resource dependence, African states had little choice but to agree to the ideas outlined at Abuja. By 2000, it was apparent that AIDS could very well ravage African societies, economies, and communities. It was also evident that because of their economic problems and increased dependence on foreign aid, African countries would be unable to address the epidemic without international assistance. Though foreign aid to Africa had declined by one-fourth by the late 1990s, the percentage of African gross domestic product that came from foreign aid had increased to roughly 12 per cent in 2000 (van de Walle 2001; UNDP 2004). Given the fact that many donor countries (especially the US) perceived that African states lacked transparency and efficiency in the management of foreign aid (Lancaster 1999), African leaders needed to illustrate their commitment to AIDS through high-level and well-publicized actions.

African states also reacted to discussions among multilateral and bilateral donors about the rising cost of addressing HIV/AIDS. For example, a 1993 study calculated that it would cost $2.5 billion per year, about 20 times that year's global AIDS budget, to prevent half of the 20 million new infections projected by 2000 (*Washington Post*, 5 July 2000). Yet, spending by UNAIDS and bilateral donors had held relatively constant since the early 1990s. Given these financial demands, UNAIDS officials and donors began to question how they could divert existing resources to address these needs. Since African leaders in several of the most affected states had been unwilling to either admit the existence of the disease in their populations or to cooperate with donors, lack of political commitment became a justification for diverting resources from Africa to other regions. In response to the possibility of losing needed resources, individual African leaders began to admit the presence of AIDS and privately agree with UNAIDS officials to more aggressively combat the disease. These national actions were necessary steps before the pledges at Abuja could emerge (UNAIDS official, interview with author, 15 October 2002).

Although the Abuja statements were a pragmatic reaction to the international donor environment, it is important to realize that publicly addressing AIDS can be politically costly for leaders. Unlike many other public health messages such as childhood immunization programs, HIV/AIDS messages are hampered by the stigma attached to the disease. The difficulty of addressing the intimate behaviors associated with HIV prevention was apparent at the UNGASS, when many Muslim countries did not want to include language about homosexuality, drug abuse, or prostitution in the declaration (*New York Times*, 26 June 2001). Even in Uganda, which has had a very proactive, state-sponsored HIV prevention program since 1986, the

HIV status of presidential candidates in the 2000 election became a highly contentious political question (Ostergard 2002).

In sum, Africa's overall weakness in the international community, especially its dependence on international resources, meant that African states did not lead the process of building support for the declaration and the Global Fund. Rather, African states provided necessary public commitment to fight the disease at a key point in the process. While African states did not initiate this process, their actions were essential for enabling the international community to reach consensus on these two international AIDS policies. However, limited state resources also meant that African states had little choice but to make the difficult political commitment to address HIV/AIDS.

African States and Linkages to Powerful Negotiators

At the UNGASS, delegations from individual African countries such as Senegal, South Africa, Zambia, and Nigeria were articulate and well-prepared. Senegal and Nigeria captured the attention of other delegates, because their presidents have taken a keen interest in AIDS. President Olusegun Obasanjo of Nigeria was the de facto spokesperson for African states because he had overseen the Abuja conference. Because South Africa and Zambia have high HIV prevalence rates (21 per cent and 16.5 per cent in 2003, respectively), they had a level of legitimacy in the debate that made other UNGASS delegates pay attention to them (UNAIDS 2004; UNAIDS official, interview with author, 15 October 2002; Official at Swedish UN mission, correspondence with author, 1 October 2002).

However, as a *regional* bloc, African states did not play a visible and active role at the special session. Because of capacity and resource constraints, African missions to the UN often lack the staff to do in-depth research on issues, to negotiate on several fronts, and to be fully prepared for international conferences (Representative of Ghana NGO, correspondence with author, 27 November 2002). Africa also has traditionally faced language and regional divisions in multilateral diplomacy. At the UNGASS, African states were willing to let other states, particularly those in Latin America, argue for inclusion of one of their priorities, the dual strategy of prevention and treatment (UNAIDS official, interview with author, 15 October 2002). While not the region with the most AIDS cases, Latin America had legitimacy in this debate because of the region's successful treatment programs, especially in Brazil. Since 1996, Brazil has provided generic ARVs to over 100,000 HIV-positive citizens, a strategy country officials claim has reduced the number of annual AIDS deaths by one-third (UNAIDS 2002b). The Brazilian success shaped the discussion of treatment and access to ARVs (Official at Swedish UN mission, correspondence with author, 1 October 2002).

Additionally, African states have benefited from the strong global leadership that Secretary General Kofi Annan has provided on the HIV/AIDS issue. Although Jonathan Mann and Peter Piot also played crucial roles in the development of international AIDS policies, the Secretary General specifically energized support for the declaration and the Global Fund. Along with UNAIDS staff, he understood the political necessity of gaining universal support for a declaration on HIV/AIDS. Without wide support, such a statement would ostracize Africa, since it is the region most affected by the disease. In some ways, the Secretary General had a natural interest in the topic, since he is from Ghana. More importantly, because of his public position, he was constantly surrounded by representatives of the public and private sectors who wanted to address the pandemic (UNAIDS official, interview with author, 15 October 2002).

Leaders often use their public positions to advance negotiations on global agreements (Gordenker et al. 1995; Young and Osherenko 1993, 234). At the 2000 meeting of the African Development Forum in Addis Ababa, the Secretary General urged African states to address HIV/AIDS, saying that the 'leadership we need in Africa cannot come from outside, but rather must flow from within' (*Africa Recovery*, January 2001). He argued that political commitment to the disease among African leaders could be a means by which to gain Western confidence for future development, trade, and investment initiatives (*New York Times*, 28 June 2001). After Abuja, the Secretary General galvanized support for the dual strategy of prevention and treatment and prioritized a policy of 'ensuring that care and treatment is [*sic*] within the reach of all.' He called for spending almost half of the Global Fund resources on treatment (*Newsday*, 24 June 2001).

Before the UNGASS, the Secretary General contributed to the momentum for a universal statement by calling for the Global Fund to help finance the declaration's objectives. Based on 2000 discussions with industrialized countries and the European Union Commission, he issued a call for the creation of the Global Fund in April 2001. As part of this process, the Secretary General met with US President Bush and US Secretary of State Colin Powell before the conference to gain support for the Global Fund (White House 2001). Demonstrating entrepreneurial leadership, Secretary General Annan gained support for the fund from Western European countries, even though many had publicly voiced concerns about the fund (United Kingdom 2001; Germany 2001; Denmark 2001). According to a European delegate, 'At a private meeting of EU representatives in New York leading up to this conference [UNGASS], there was almost unanimous opposition to Kofi Annan's idea for a global fund' (*Vancouver Sun*, 27 June 2001). Yet, by the end of the UNGASS, Western European states signed the declaration with its operative clauses instituting the fund. And since then, most of these states have given millions of dollars to the Global Fund (Global Fund 2002a).

Because of their limited international power and lack of diplomatic resources, it is doubtful that African states could have attained international policies such as the Global Fund and support for treatment for PLWHAs without linkages to Latin American negotiators or the leadership of Secretary General Annan. While pushing developing states to confront the disease openly, he called on developed states to provide needed resources. In strong, unanimous affirmation of his actions on HIV/AIDS, member-states elected Kofi Annan to a second five-year term as Secretary General at the beginning of the UNGASS (Weissman 2001). And the Secretary General's central role in forging international agreements to combat HIV/AIDS was cited as one reason that he and the UN received the Nobel Peace Prize in 2001.

African States and the Emergence of Support for Treatment

Another factor that increased the likelihood that African goals on treatment would be incorporated into the Declaration of Commitment on HIV/AIDS and the Global Fund was growing political support for access to ARV treatment for PLWHAs in the developing world. Since the 2000 International Conference on HIV/AIDS in Durban, South Africa, NGOs have increasingly called for the international community to make ARVs more accessible and affordable in poor countries. Médecins Sans Frontières, AIDS Coalition to Unleash Power (ACT UP), the Treatment Action Campaign, and Health Gap, as well as some public health officials and scholars, argued for the necessity of treatment for PLWHAs. Before the UNGASS, Médecins Sans Frontières demonstrated that HIV prevention is more difficult if people are unwilling to be tested, and people will not get tested if no treatment for AIDS is available. Treatment will help break the stigma that accompanies AIDS (*Newsday*, 24 June 2001; MSF 2001). Health Gap used epidemiological studies to argue that treatment using ARVs can be one prevention strategy, since ARVs lower the number of HIV cells in the body and make a person less contagious (*New York Times*, 16 July 2002; Gray et al. 2001).[7] Health Gap founder Alan Berkman (2001) also asserted that the most effective advocates for prevention are HIV-positive individuals; lengthening their lives will help societies to fight AIDS. Other nonstate actors pointed out that in southern African countries where AIDS will greatly reduce life expectancy, companies such as Debswana and Anglo-American Mining have realized the economic necessity of extending the lives of their HIV-positive workers by providing access to ARVs (*Africa News*, 31 January 2002). At the UNGASS, a variety of nonstate actors effectively articulated the economic, social, humanitarian, and public health reasons to provide treatment to all PLWHAs.

Additionally, African states have benefited from new programs to demonstrate the feasibility of administering ARV treatment in poor countries. In 2000, Botswana gained $100 million in grants from the Gates Foundation and Merck Pharmaceutical Company to provide ARVs to its HIV-positive population. In 2001, over 100 public health and development scholars at Harvard University designed a plan to treat one million Africans with ARVs using community-based health workers who would encourage participants to follow the drug regimen and thus, lower the likelihood that resistant HIV strains would emerge (*Africa Recovery*, June 2001; See also Journalists Against AIDS 2002). Brazil's aforementioned successful ARV program, the large corporate commitment in Botswana, and the Harvard statement bolstered the call for ARV treatment in the declaration.

There are two noticeable aspects of the emergence of support for widespread access to ARVs. First, the argument for treatment was not initially made by African states as the most AIDS-affected countries, but rather, by Western NGOs and scientists. Organizations such as ACT UP, Médecins Sans Frontières, and Health Gap have used access to media, well-organized lobbying, and scientific studies to articulate their arguments for the dual strategy of prevention and treatment. The resources and personnel of these organizations have enabled them to shape the dialogue on treatment and their linkages to international organizations such as UNAIDS have further enabled them to lobby for treatment policies (Söderholm 1997). Yet, because these groups advocate many of the policies that African states support, Africa as a region has benefited from their involvement.

Second, though scientific knowledge often plays a key role in international agreements on technical issues such as health or the environment (Underdal 1989; Young 1989; Cooper 1989), it must be acknowledged that as of 2004, many questions still remain about treatment in developing countries. There is continued concern that patients in countries without well-developed health-care systems will be unable to adhere to the ARV regimen (*Washington Post*, 24 June 2001). Though regimens have become simpler since 2002, resistance or toxic side effects such as liver damage and kidney failure still can occur. Poorer nations may not have the drugs to treat these side effects. There also has been fear that if people discontinue treatment because of cost or side effects, more virulent and resistant strains of HIV will emerge.[8] A 2003 study illustrated that drug resistance could increase because of lack of regulation of ARVs prescribed by private health-care providers in developing countries (Brugha 2003). Some scholars also worry about diverting resources from prevention activities, since these are the only certain way to reduce HIV infections and are more cost effective than treatment (*New York Times*, 5 July 2002; *Washington Post*, 27 December 2000; Potts and Walsh 2003). In addition to these scientific and logistical concerns, there is the question of equity in access to treatment. Even with grants from the Global Fund, it is questionable whether all HIV-positive Africans will have access to ARVs, especially those in rural areas who may lack access to health-care services. In such a case, who decides who has access? Will the voices of all citizens be heard in such a debate?

Though these concerns are very real, they have been overtaken by the human rights argument that ARVs can and should be provided.[9] Since the UNGASS, it has become more *politically* difficult for policy makers to deny ARV access to millions of HIV-positive individuals as part of a comprehensive policy on HIV/AIDS. At the 2002 International Conference on HIV/AIDS in Barcelona, there was overwhelming agreement among the 17,000 participants that neither prevention nor treatment alone is sufficient in the fight against HIV/AIDS (*New York Times*, 16 July 2002). And the theme of the 2004 International Conference on HIV/AIDS in Bangkok was 'Access for All', signaling that the question was not whether to provide ARVs but how to do so fairly. The fact that the Global Fund has provided grants for treatment programs has helped to further legitimate the feasibility of treatment. John Ruxin, director of the Access Project for the Global Fund, said in 2002, '[The Global Fund grants are] absolutely unprecedented, because up until now international donor funds have not gone to put any human being on anti-retrovirals. The attitude until now is that it's too expensive and too difficult to do' (*Boston Globe*, 26 April 2002). The political and moral message that treatment cannot be denied to millions of HIV-positive individuals was apparent in President Bush's 2003 State of the Union address, when he said, 'In an age of miraculous medicines, no person should have to hear [that treatment is unavailable]. ... Seldom has history offered a greater opportunity to do so much for so many. ... This nation can lead the world in sparing innocent people from a plague of nature' (White House 2003).[10] Likewise, the WHO announced in late 2003 a goal of delivering ARVs to three million AIDS patients by the end of 2005 (*New York Times*, 1 December 2003). Though African states often lack resources and institutional capacity, they have benefited from the arguments, studies, and actions of Western NGOs, scholars, and corporate decision makers. The growing political acceptance of the need for treatment helped African states to achieve several of their goals in the Declaration of Commitment on HIV/AIDS and the Global Fund.

African States, the AIDS Pandemic, and Global Interdependence

HIV/AIDS exists within a context of interdependent states and is the first pandemic of globalization (Barnett and Whiteside 2002). The end of the cold war, rapid communication and transportation networks, increased migration, and the emergence of a liberal trade regime have heightened interdependence among states (Keohane and Nye 1977). This interdependence increases the ability of infectious diseases to negatively impact economic development, national and international security, and human rights (Garrett 1994; CIA 2000; ICG 2001). The World Bank reported that in 1990, preventable infections caused 34 per cent of global deaths while war caused only .64 per cent. The emergence and rapid spread of infectious diseases such as AIDS, severe acute respiratory syndrome, the West Nile virus, and tuberculosis have made all societies susceptible (Price-Smith 2001). As Secretary Powell said at the UNGASS, 'We are all vulnerable – big nations and small, the wealthy and the poor' (United States 2001).

Of course, an individual's vulnerability to HIV infection varies greatly across national, gender, age, and class lines. Yet, because of interdependence, all states and citizens are to an extent susceptible to the disease's negative impact on security and socioeconomic development. That is, even though over 90 per cent of HIV-positive individuals live in the developing world, the pandemic can still affect industrialized countries because of trade networks, the reliance of multinational corporations on labor in poor countries, and migration. The nature of the disease itself heightens its potentially pernicious effects. Unlike other infectious diseases such as smallpox, measles, cholera, and malaria that disproportionately affect children and the elderly, AIDS attacks individuals in their most productive years. And the long asymptomatic phase between HIV infection and AIDS makes prevention and impact mitigation programs more difficult, especially in countries such as China and India where the disease is only beginning to emerge (ICG 2001).

The increasing awareness of global health interdependence and the nature of AIDS itself have contributed to the international community's willingness to address the pandemic through specific actions such as the declaration and the Global Fund. As a resource-poor region which, for the most part, has only recently become willing to politically commit to the disease, Africa has not led in these efforts. Yet, because of interdependence, the region cannot be ignored. As Mark Malloch-Brown of the UN Development Program said, '[The AIDS issue] is forcing the West to engage with Africa, not just on the old basis of "You've got problems, we want to help", but out of a much more fundamental sense of self-interest, of a global war where – like it or not – the front-line generals are African leaders' (*New York Times*, 28 June 2001).

Conclusion

This chapter has illustrated that central aspects of the Declaration of Commitment on HIV/AIDS and the Global Fund reflect African preferences for AIDS policies. The right to health care, the dual strategy of prevention and treatment, a state-centric understanding of political leadership, and the role of donors as resource providers with equal decision-making powers are policy themes that African states supported. These policy statements emerged despite Africa's limited resources, its lack of diplomatic sway, and its weak international position. Rather, because of the actions of UNAIDS, the articulate lobbying of Latin American allies and the UN Secretary General, new political support for treatment, and global interdependence, African states benefited from the objectives in the declaration and the formation of the Global Fund.

Throughout the process of building support for the declaration and the Global Fund, it is possible to see the complex nature of the African state. First, the African state is often porous and easily affected by the actions of other states, international organizations, corporations, and NGOs. Instead of leading, African states reacted to the UNAIDS-directed process of building consensus for a universal AIDS agreement, especially when it became apparent that needed development resources might be lost. Policies on AIDS in Africa have also been shaped by private foundations and corporate decisions to provide ARVs to workers. Second, the African state's lack of resources is also evident, as dependence on donors necessitated that African leaders at the Abuja conference make the politically difficult decision to publicly address AIDS. Third, because of their international weakness, African states have been sensitive about preserving their central role in the development process and controlling NGOs and foreign donors (Patterson 2000; Bates 1981; Harbeson, Rothchild, and Chazan 1994; Kasfir 1998). The structure of the Global Fund and the state-centric view of political leadership outlined in the declaration illustrate this concern.

The AIDS crisis brings to light a paradox about the nature of the African state. African states have often been described as patrimonial, as evidenced 'by a lack of institutionalization, a general disregard for the rules of the formal political and economic sectors, and a universal resort to personal(ized) and vertical solutions to societal problems' (Chabal and Daloz 1999, xix). Though patrimonialism varies throughout Africa, state officials in such systems need access to material resources to address socioeconomic problems, garner societal support, and maintain power. Yet structural adjustment policies, and their accompanying budget cuts, have strained state resources. Might programmatic aid for HIV/AIDS simply become another means by which African state officials gain resources for patronage? As Batsell demonstrates in this volume, the AIDS issue may be ripe for political manipulation by some African state leaders. Again, an examination of grants to African states from the Global Fund illustrates the millions of new dollars to be allocated to *government* agencies and programs (Global Fund 2002c, 2003c, 2003e). Yet, and here is the paradox, most African states need these resources to build the state capacity that is essential to address the long-term impact of the disease. And, as their actions through the 1990s illustrate, most bilateral and multilateral donors will not provide funding for AIDS without African state officials calling attention to the disease and without African states developing high-level government administrative bodies to address AIDS. Can international programs, such as grants from the Global Fund, both provide necessary resources to fight AIDS and ensure transparency and accountability? Can global AIDS policies empower African states to combat the pandemic, while limiting unnecessary demands on African states? Scholars examining the politics of AIDS in Africa must continue to ask such questions.

Notes

1 Earlier versions of this chapter were presented at the annual meeting of the African Studies Association, Washington, DC, 5–8 December 2002 and for the African Studies Program at Michigan State University, Lansing, MI, 13 March 2003. We are grateful for numerous constructive comments in both venues. Partial funding for this research was provided by Calvin College and the McGregor Scholars Program.

2 William Clinton (former president of the United States) and Nelson Mandela (former president of South Africa) participated in this panel, as did current or former officials from Canada, Mozambique, St Kitts, India, Rwanda, Tanzania, and Portugal. See International

AIDS Trust at http: //www.internationalaidstrust.org. In contrast, when a similar panel was organized for political leaders at the 2004 International AIDS Conference, it had to be cancelled because of a lack of participation (*New York Times*, 12 July 2004).

3 For example, many states expressed reservations to the final agreement at the 1994 International Conference on Population and Development in Cairo.

4 The Secretary General said about nondiscrimination, 'In the ruthless world of AIDS, there is no us and them' (Secretary General 2001a). African and Western states reiterated this norm, arguing against immigration limits for HIV-positive individuals and for policies to protect PLWHAs in the workplace (Ghana 2001; Mozambique 2001; Lesotho 2001; Namibia 2001; Iceland 2001; United States 2001; Uganda 2001).

5 In November 2003, the Global Fund reported that this percentage increased to 66 per cent (Global Fund 2003b). However, these percentages are only an average; it is possible that some countries have thoroughly incorporated nonstate actors into their CCMs, while others have not.

6 The World Bank and International Monetary Fund launched this initiative in 1996 to reduce the debt stock of 42 countries. To qualify, a country's debt repayments must comprise a large proportion of its gross domestic product. As of April 2004, Benin, Bolivia, Burkina Faso, Cameroon, Chad, Côte d'Ivoire, the Democratic Republic of Congo, Ethiopia, the Gambia, Ghana, Guinea, Guinea-Bissau, Guyana, Honduras, Madagascar, Malawi, Mali, Mauritania, Mozambique, Nicaragua, Niger, Rwanda, São Tomé and Principe, Senegal, Sierra Leone, Tanzania, Uganda, and Zambia are either receiving or negotiating debt reduction. For more information, see http://www.worldbank.org/hipc/progress-to-date/progress-to-date.html.

7 Treatment advocates realize that health officials must include prevention messages with any treatment programs. Further, it is too early to translate the results from these small-scale studies about HIV transmission to larger populations, though some simulations suggest a significant reduction in HIV-positive cases (Berkman 2001).

8 These fears are not unfounded. In August 2002, scientists announced that HIV is becoming more resistant to ARVs. Growing resistance makes it more difficult to use these drugs effectively in developing nations and increases treatment costs since new drugs must constantly be developed (National Public Radio, 7 August 2002).

9 To clarify our argument: it is not that we do not support treatment programs. Rather, we are interested in the various ways that treatment has been framed in policy discussions about AIDS.

10 It should be noted that the NGO Debt, AIDS, Trade and Africa headed by U2 singer Bono lobbied the Bush administration to include treatment in its AIDS proposal (*New York Times*, 30 January 2003).

References

Barnett, Tony, and Alan Whiteside. 2002. *AIDS in the twenty-first century: Disease and globalisation*. Basingstoke: Palgrave Macmillan.

Bates, Robert. 1981. *Markets and states in tropical Africa*. Los Angeles: Univ. of California Press.

Batsell, Jake. 2000. AIDS, politics, and NGOs in Zimbabwe. Paper presented at the annual conference of the African Studies Association, Nashville.

Benin. 2001. Statement to the United Nations General Assembly Special Session on HIV/AIDS.
http://www.un.org/ga/aids/statements/docs/beninF.html.

Berkman, Alan. 2001. Confronting global AIDS: Prevention and treatment. *American Journal of Public Health* 91 (9): 1348–49.

Booker, Salih, and William Minter. 2001. Global apartheid. *The Nation*. http://www.thenation.com/doc/mhtml?i=20010709&s=booker.
Botswana. 2001. Statement to the United Nations General Assembly Special Session on HIV/AIDS. http://www.un.org/ga/aids/statements/docs/botswanaE.html.
Brugha, Ruairi. 2003. Antiretroviral treatment in developing countries: The peril of neglecting private providers. *British Medical Journal* 326: 1382–84.
Burkina Faso. 2001. Statement to the United Nations General Assembly Special Session on HIV/AIDS. http://www.un.org/ga/aids/statements/docs/bfF.html.
Burundi. 2001. Statement to the United Nations General Assembly Special Session on HIV/AIDS. http://www.un.org/ga/aids/statements/docs/burundiF.html.
Central Intelligence Agency (CIA). 2000. *The global infectious disease threat and its implications for the United States*. http://www.cia.gov/publications.nie/report/nie99–17d.html.
Chabal, Patrick, and Jean-Pascal Daloz. 1999. *Africa works*. Bloomington: Indiana Univ. Press.
Clapham, Christopher. 1996. *Africa and the international system*. New York: Cambridge Univ. Press.
Cooper, Richard. 1989. International cooperation in public health as a prologue to macroeconomic cooperation. In *Can nations agree*? ed. Richard Cooper, Barry Eichengreen, C. Randall Henning, Gerald Holtham, and Robert Putnam, 178–254. Washington, DC: Brookings Institute.
Daly, John. 2001. AIDS in Swaziland: The battle from within. *African Studies Review* 44 (1): 21–35.
Denmark. 2001. Statement to the United Nations General Assembly Special Session on HIV/AIDS. http://www.un.org/ga/aids/statements/docs/denmarkE.html.
Fortin, Alfred. 1987. The politics of AIDS in Kenya. *Third World Quarterly* 9 (3): 906–19.
Garrett, Laurie. 1994. *The coming plague: Newly emerging diseases in a world out of balance*. New York: Penguin.
Germany. 2001. Statement to the United Nations General Assembly Special Session on HIV/AIDS. http://www.un.org/ga/aids/statements/docs/germanyE.html.
Ghana. 2001. Statement to the United Nations General Assembly Special Session on HIV/AIDS. http://www.un.org/ga/aids/statements/docs/ghanaE.html.
Global Fund. 2002a. Background. http://www.theglobalfund.org/en/.
——. 2002b. The by-laws of the Global Fund to Fight AIDS, Tuberculosis, and Malaria. http://www.theglobalfund.org/en/files/publicdoc/bylaws_uk.pdf.
——. 2002c. First round approved proposals. http://www.theglobalfund.org/search/default.aspx?lang=en.
——. 2003a. *Progress report – June*. http://www.theglobalfund.org/files/progressreport030611.pdf.
——. 2003b. *Progress report – November*.

http://www.theglobalfund.org/en/files/progressreport.pdf.
——. 2003c. Second round approved proposals. http://www.theglobalfund.org/search/default.aspx?lang=en.
——. 2003d. Technical review panel. http://www.theglobalfund.org/en/about/technical.
——. 2003e. Third round approved proposals. http://www.theglobalfund.org/search/default.aspx?lang=en.
——. 2004. *Progress report – August.* http://www.theglobalfund.org/en/files/progressreport.pdf.

Gordenker, Leon, Roger Coate, Christer Jönsson, and Peter Söderholm. 1995. *International cooperation in response to AIDS.* New York: Pinter Press.

Government of Kenya. 2002. National proposal to the Global Fund, round II. http://www.theglobalfundatm.org/search/portfolio.aspx?land=en&countryID=KEN.

Gray, Ronald H., Maria J. Wawer, Ron Brookmeyer, Nelson K. Sewankambo, David Serwadda, Fred Wabwire-Mangen, Tom Lutalo, Xianbin Li, Thomas van Cott, Thomas C. Quinn, and the Rakai Project Team. 2001. Probability of HIV-1 transmission per coital act in monogamous, heterosexual, HIV-1-discordant couples in Rakai, Uganda. *Lancet* 357: 1149–53.

Halbert, Debora. 2002. Moralized discourses: South Africa's intellectual property fight for access to AIDS drugs. Paper presented at the Ohio University conference on HIV/AIDS and the African child, Athens, OH.

Harbeson, John, Donald Rothchild, and Naomi Chazan, eds. 1994. *Civil society and the state in Africa.* Boulder, CO: Lynne Rienner.

Harbeson, John, and Donald Rothchild, eds. 2000. *Africa in world politics.* 3rd ed. Boulder, CO: Westview Press.

Iceland. 2001. Statement to the United Nations General Assembly Special Session on HIV/AIDS. http://www.un.org/ga/aids/statements/docs/icelandE.html.

International Crisis Group (ICG). 2001. *HIV/AIDS as a security issue.* http://www.crisis.org/projects/issues/hiv_aids/reports/A400321_19062001.pdf.

Joint United Nations Program on HIV/AIDS (UNAIDS). 2002a. African first ladies launch historic organization to fight HIV/AIDS. http://www.unaids.org/whatsnew/press/eng/pressarc01/Firstladies_160702.html.
——. 2002b. *Fighting AIDS: A new global resolve.* http://www.unaids.org/barcelona/presskit/barcelona%20report/chapter1. html.
——. 2004. *Report on the global AIDS epidemic.* http://www.unaids.org/bangkok2004.html.

Journalists Against AIDS. 2002. ARV treatment can work in poor communities. http://www.nigeria-aids.org/MsgRead.cfm?ID=821.

Kasfir, Nelson, ed. 1998. *Civil society and democracy in Africa: Critical perspectives.* London: Frank Cass.

Kenya. 2001. Statement to the United Nations General Assembly Special Session on HIV/AIDS. http://www.un.org/ga/aids/statements/docs/kenyaE.html.

Keohane, Robert, and Joseph Nye. 1977. *Power and interdependence.* Boston: Little Brown.

Lancaster, Carol. 1999. *Aid to Africa: So much to do, so little done.* Chicago: Univ. of Chicago Press.

Lanegran, Kim, and Goran Hyden. 1993. Mapping the politics of AIDS: Illustrations from East Africa. *Population and Environment* 14 (3): 245–63.

Lesotho. 2001. Statement to the United Nations General Assembly Special Session on HIV/AIDS.
http://www.un.org/ga/aids/statements/docs/lesothoE.html.

Médecins Sans Frontières (MSF). 2001. Press release.
http://www.un.org/News/briefings/docs/2001/msfpc.doc.htm.

Mozambique. 2001. Statement to the United Nations General Assembly Special Session on HIV/AIDS.
http://www.un.org/ga/aids/statements/docs/mozambiqueE.html.

Namibia. 2001. Statement to the United Nations General Assembly Special Session on HIV/AIDS.
http://www.un.org/ga/aids/statements/docs/namibiaE.html.

Ndegwa, Stephen. 1996. *The two faces of civil society: NGOs and politics in Africa.* Westport, CT: Kumarian Press.

Nigeria. 2001. Statement to the United Nations General Assembly Special Session on HIV/AIDS.
http://www.un.org/ga/aids/statements/docs/nigeriaE.html.

Ostergard, Robert. 2002. Politics in the hot zone: AIDS and national security in Africa. *Third World Quarterly* 23 (2): 333–50.

Patterson, Amy S. 2000. Decentralization in Senegal: Reordering authority or reinventing past reforms? In *Re-distribution of authority: A cross-regional perspective*, ed. Jeanie Bukowski and Swarna Rajagopalan, 125–44. Westport, CT: Praeger.

Poku, Nana. 2002. The global AIDS fund: Context and opportunity. *Third World Quarterly* 23 (2): 283–98.

Potts, Malcolm, and Julia Walsh. 2003. Tackling India's HIV epidemic: Lessons from Africa. *British Medical Journal* 326: 1389–92.

Price-Smith, Andrew. 2001. *Plagues and politics: Infectious disease and international policy.* Basingstoke: Palgrave Macmillan Press.

Rothchild, Donald, and Naomi Chazan, eds. 1988. *The precarious balance: State and society in Africa.* Boulder, CO: Westview Press.

Roundtable Four. 2001. International funding and cooperation.
http://www.unaids.org/whatsnew/others/un_special/roundtables/041435_en.doc.

Rwanda. 2001. Statement to the United Nations General Assembly Special Session on HIV/AIDS.
http://www.un.org/ga/aids/statements/docs/rwandaE.html.

Secretary General. 2001. Statement to the United Nations General Assembly Special Session on HIV/AIDS.
http://www.un.org/News/Press/docs/2001/ga9883.doc.htm.

Senegal. 2001. Statement to the United Nations General Assembly Special Session on HIV/AIDS.
http://www.un.org/ga/aids/statements/docs/senegalF.html.

Singer, Merrill, ed. 1998. *The political economy of AIDS.* Amityville, NY: Baywood Publishing.

Siplon, Patricia. 2002. *AIDS and the policy struggle in the United States.* Washington, DC: Georgetown Univ. Press.

Söderholm, Peter. 1997. *Global governance of AIDS: Partnerships with civil society.* Lund, Sweden: Lund Univ. Press.

Tanzania. 2001. Statement to the United Nations General Assembly Special Session on HIV/AIDS.
http://www.un.org/ga/aids/statements/docs/tanzaniaE.html.

Uganda. 2001. Statement to the United Nations General Assembly Special Session on HIV/AIDS.
http://www.un.org/ga/aids/statements/docs/ugandaE.html.

Underdal, Arild. 1989. The politics of science in international resource management: A summary. In *International resource management: The role of science and politics*, ed. Steinar Andresen and Willy Ostreng, 253–67. New York: Belhaven Press.

United Kingdom. 2001. Statement to the United Nations General Assembly Special Session on HIV/AIDS.
http://www.un.org/ga/aids/statements/docs/uk.html.

United Nations Development Program (UNDP). 2004. *Human Development Report*. New York: Oxford Univ. Press.

United Nations General Assembly Special Session (UNGASS). 2001a. *Declaration of commitment on HIV/AIDS*.
http://www.unaids.org/whatsnew/orthers/un_special/ARES26–2_en.pdf.

——. 2001b. Press release for 8th and 9th meetings.
http://www.un.org/News/Pres/docs/2001/ga9888.doc.htm.

United States. 2001. Statement to the United Nations General Assembly Special Session on HIV/AIDS.
http://www.un.org/ga/aids/statements/docs/usaE.html.

van de Walle, Nicolas. 2001. *African economies and the politics of permanent crisis, 1979–1999*. New York: Cambridge Univ. Press.

Weissman, Robert. 2001. The AIDS fund fight. *The Nation*.
http://www.thenation.com/doc/mhtml?i=20010709&s=weissman.

White House. 2001. Remarks by the president during announcement of proposal for the Global Fund to Fight AIDS, Tuberculosis, and Malaria.
http://www.whitehouse.gov/news/releases/2001/05/print/200105211–1.html.

——. 2003. State of the union address.
http://www.whitehouse.gov/news/releases/2003/01/20030128–19.html.

Will, Kurt Dieter. 1991. The global politics of AIDS: The World Health Organization and the international regime for AIDS. PhD diss., Univ. of South Carolina.

Young, Oran. 1989. Science and social institutions: Lessons for international resource regimes. In *International resource management: The role of science and politics*, ed. Steinar Andresen and Willy Ostreng, 7–24. New York: Belhaven Press.

Young, Oran, and Gaile Osherenko, eds. 1993. *Polar politics: Creating international environmental regimes*. Ithaca: Cornell Univ. Press.

Zambia. 2001. Statement to the United Nations General Assembly Special Session on HIV/AIDS.
http://www.un.org/ga/aids/statements/docs/zambiaE.html.

Zimbabwe. 2001. Statement to the United Nations General Assembly Special Session on HIV/AIDS.
http://www.un.org/ga/aids/statements/docs/zimbabweE.html.

Chapter 10

AIDS, Pharmaceutical Patents and the African State: Reorienting the Global Governance of Intellectual Property

Debora Halbert and Christopher May

Although AIDS is only one of many deadly diseases that affect Africa, it has become emblematic of the difficulties that surround global health crises when political and economic interests of different groups clash. The plight of Africa today is an indicator of what can be expected worldwide if HIV/AIDS remains widely untreated. The famine, collapse of family and community institutions, and decline in socioeconomic development that have emerged in Africa suggest the disruptive potential of AIDS. These effects will become increasingly globalized (*Newsday*, 15 October 2002). Given the enormous threat posed by HIV/AIDS, there is wide agreement that HIV/AIDS in Africa must be addressed and action must be taken; but the agreement ends there.

Until quite recently, education and prevention were emphasized as the only workable strategies available for Africa to combat the epidemic. Most African states lacked the resources to provide effective treatment to people living with HIV/AIDS. Also, there was a distinct lack of international leadership exemplified by the early unwillingness of the United States and the European Union (EU) to fund treatment programs. Yet, as the chapter by Patterson and Cieminis illustrates, several factors changed this view of access to treatment in Africa, including the watershed legal case in South Africa. In 1998, major domestic and international pharmaceutical companies sued the South African government over the South African Medicines Act of 1997, which enabled the government to engage in compulsory licensing of medication in a health emergency. Compulsory licensing allows a country to require a patent owner to provide a license to manufacture a product at a negotiated price. Without compulsory licensing, the patent owner retains a strict monopoly over the product until the patent expires and can charge monopoly prices. To complicate matters, South Africa interpreted the Medicines Act to fall under the parameters of the Trade-Related Aspects of Intellectual Property Rights (TRIPS) Agreement that all members of the World Trade Organization (WTO) signed. Article 8 of the TRIPS Agreement allows for compulsory licensing in health emergencies and public health situations, but this interpretation was strongly resisted by the United States, acting on behalf of the pharmaceutical industry. The case highlighted the politics of access to AIDS medication and the role of pharmaceutical companies in pricing medicines out of the reach of poor South Africans.

Additionally, even as the South African legislature was passing legislation to provide South Africans better access to treatment, the executive was rejecting treatment for rape victims and for prevention of mother-to-child transmission. On becoming president in 1999, Thabo Mkeki argued that antiretroviral (ARV) drugs were dangerous to citizens' health. As the actions of the South African government illustrate, the African state has not always behaved as a unified actor when dealing with the issue of AIDS treatment, or more broadly, HIV/AIDS. In the case of South Africa, only when AIDS activists working internationally revealed the role of the multinational pharmaceutical industry in curtailing poor patients' access to AIDS medication and put pressure on President Mbeki, did the state and the international community begin to rethink the issue of treatment (Halbert 2002).

Since the South African lawsuit, there have been significant concessions on access to AIDS medication, the creation of alternative generic options, and the use of compulsory licenses and parallel imports to combat the AIDS pandemic. Parallel imports allow a country to seek the best prices for a drug internationally and import those medicines available at the lowest price. Since pharmaceutical companies set different prices for medicines in various countries, parallel importation makes it possible to buy drugs at lower prices than in the home country. The South African case energized AIDS activists, and later African states, as they campaigned for access to medication. Some African states such as Uganda and Kenya, as well as other states throughout the developing world, also have begun to resist the global trade regime that has hindered access to AIDS medication. As a result, compulsory licensing and parallel importation were revisited in the 2001 WTO meetings in Doha, Qatar and the 2003 WTO negotiations that occurred before the Cancún Ministerial Conference.

The TRIPS Agreement has language amenable to the creation of compulsory licenses if there is a public health crisis, language that has now been interpreted as providing the necessary legal framework for access to AIDS medications. Thus, at the 2001 meetings, the WTO issued the Doha Declaration on TRIPS and Public Health *reasserting* the rights of developing countries to use parallel importation and compulsory licensing to provide AIDS medication in times of health threats. Even given this reassertion of already-existing rights, and the general belief that Doha raised important health concerns for developing countries, the legal gains made during these negotiations have yet to be translated into access to medication.

Despite many new government and nongovernmental organization (NGO) programs, AIDS treatment in Africa is still limited by the high price of AIDS medication, the availability of drugs, the funding to pay for these drugs, and the restrictions placed on distribution. Efforts to increase accessibility to medication continue to be frustrated and only a fraction of those with the disease are being treated (Nerozzi 2002, 613). It is estimated that of the over 25 million people infected with HIV/AIDS in Africa, only about 50,000 are receiving treatment (Copson 2003, 10; UNAIDS 2004). Even after the Doha declaration, international negotiators continue to debate the scope of patent protection. The US government continues to emphasize intellectual property rights (IPRs) in negotiations over access to medication. Even with creative programs to increase the number of Africans receiving AIDS treatment, the supply of medicines remains limited by a discourse on IPRs that ignores the vast global social inequalities between members of the WTO.

In this chapter, we first examine the construction and logic of intellectual property rights as protected by the TRIPS Agreement. Second, we investigate the status of access to medication after the Doha declaration and we question the impact of the 2003 WTO agreement on cross-border trade in generic pharmaceuticals. In the final section, we offer some hopeful observations about the struggle to provide treatment to Africans with HIV/AIDS. We believe that with effort, the current struggle between IPRs and access to medicine will ultimately be resolved in favor of widened access to treatment. International laws, including international trade agreements, function only when they are broadly legitimate and require minimal sanctions to enforce them. Legitimate agreements assume the goodwill of states that see some benefit coming from their adherence to these agreements. The chapter argues that in the case of the WTO, the AIDS crisis has fundamentally weakened the legitimacy of the TRIPS Agreement. We emphasize that the lack of universal acceptance of absolute protection of IPRs has enabled a new view of health care as a human right to emerge. The chapter asserts that the Doha declaration, the 2003 WTO agreements, and the actions of African states and NGOs have contributed to a gradual reorientation of policy towards intellectual property *users*.

The Global Governance of Intellectual Property Rights

Since 1995, IPRs have been subject to the TRIPS Agreement overseen by the WTO. A large number of multinational corporations interested in protecting their IPRs played a significant role in the negotiations that led to the inclusion of the TRIPS Agreement in the Uruguay Round negotiations of the General Agreement on Tariffs and Trade. These corporations drafted most of the documents that became the successful position advocated by the US trade representative (USTR) (May 2000, 82–84; Sell 2003). The United States and the EU wished to locate IPRs in an agreement because this would enable countries to use the coercive tool of trade sanctions to force adherence to IPRs (Braithwaite and Drahos 2000, 61–64). Stronger protection internationally of IPRs would translate into even greater profits for pharmaceuticals, software, and entertainment products. Including IPRs in trade-related talks was part of a general strategy by the United States and the EU to force developing countries to adopt multilateral agreements which they had previously resisted (Steinberg 2002). In contrast, developing nations did not want to include IPRs into the framework of the WTO. They preferred for the World Intellectual Property Organization to remain in charge of intellectual property considerations, since the organization offered the developing world a better opportunity to vote as a bloc. By requiring that countries sign the TRIPS Agreement to be a member of the WTO, the United States and the EU undermined the ability of developing nations to resist intellectual property arguments.

To encourage developing countries to accept the TRIPS Agreement, the USTR threatened bilateral trade sanctions and promised to open US markets to goods from the developing world. The USTR can use the Special 301 section of the Omnibus Trade and Tariff Act of 1988 to impose trade sanctions on countries charged with violating US intellectual property rights. While negotiating the TRIPS Agreement, the US government used Special 301 to 'persuade' developing countries to agree with the US position. For example, the Indian pharmaceutical industry was targeted in an effort to change India's position on the TRIPS Agreement (Matthews 2002, 31). The threat of trade sanctions was combined with the promise to open up agricultural markets and to abolish the multilateral Multi-Fiber Agreement, which since 1974 had allowed developed countries to use quotas to limit imports of textiles and clothing from developing countries. Thus, developing countries were led to believe that in exchange for their support for the TRIPS Agreement they would be given greater access to US and EU markets.

During negotiations for the TRIPS Agreement, developing countries generally lacked the legal expertise and human resources to fully resist extensive bilateral pressure. These limitations were particularly apparent for sub-Saharan African states. Power imbalances and 'negotiating fatigue' among the officials from developing countries led them to finally accept the agreement (Braithwaite and Drahos 2000, 197). Resistance was led by India and Brazil, but for the most part, poor states did not have the negotiating power or the expertise to influence IPR-related talks. The combination of political pressure and weakened resistance resulting from inadequate diplomatic resources for the complex negotiations ensured that when the developing countries joined the WTO they had to accede to the TRIPS Agreement as well (Matthews 2002).

Most African states joined the WTO in 1995, with Ethiopia and Algeria retaining observer status. Of the 49 countries considered to be least developed by the United Nations (UN), 30 have become members of the WTO. They include Angola, Chad, Democratic Republic of the Congo, Gambia, Malawi, Rwanda, Senegal, Sierra Leone, Uganda, and Zambia (WTO 2003b). The agreement to become members rested on the hope of free trade for African export markets. Since African states are not intellectual-property producers, but intellectual-property consumers, the potential risks of the TRIPS Agreement may not have been apparent. Additionally, the agreement was signed before most of the powerful ARV combination therapies were developed and used extensively in developed countries. Since 1996, when these treatment regimens became widely available, the number of people with HIV/AIDS dying in industrialized countries has declined greatly. African states could not have predicted the emergence and success of these drug regimens when they signed the TRIPS Agreement, nor the way patent law would be used to prohibit access to life-saving medications. Furthermore, even if AIDS drugs had been more available in 1995, it is not necessarily true that African states would have actively lobbied for their exclusion from the TRIPS Agreement, at least on the basis of access to medication. In 1995, few African state leaders had acknowledged the presence of AIDS in their countries or the potential devastating impact of the disease; many African state leaders still had invested little political capital into addressing HIV/AIDS.

Even with the recent extension from 2006 to 2016 of the deadline for compliance for the least developed countries, the fact that many developing countries must now comply with the TRIPS Agreement requires significant costs to all African states. Poor countries that face pressing health, development, and social-welfare needs now must devote resources to creating a legal structure to protect IPRs that meets the requirements of the TRIPS Agreement. For WTO members to be compliant with the TRIPS Agreement, their domestic laws on intellectual property must support the protections and rights outlined in the agreement's 73 articles. Under Article 67 of the agreement, poor states receive some technical cooperation and support to establish compliance, in terms of both legislation and enforcement policies. However, these capacity-building programs focus on the replication of laws and practices followed by the developed members of the WTO.

The passage of the TRIPS Agreement represents the consolidation of a neoliberal view of the role of IPRs in international economic relations. The agreement upholds certain standards of protection for IPRs and provides legal mechanisms for their enforcement. Most importantly, the robust dispute settlement mechanism, which is a central aspect of the WTO, now encompasses international disputes over the regulation of IPRs. The extension of the protection of intellectual property to the international realm, as well as the harmonization of law to protect intellectual property across WTO members, was a major triumph for the 'US pharmaceutical, entertainments, and informatics industries that were largely responsible for getting TRIPS on the agenda' of the Uruguay Round (Hoeckman and Kostecki 1995, 156). By bringing IPRs under the purview of the WTO, the TRIPS Agreement stipulates that 'procedures shall be applied in such a manner as to avoid the creation of barriers to legitimate trade', which are central to intellectual property law (GATT 1994, 19). In other words, the lack of protection of IPRs in one country can be interpreted as a hindrance to free trade. Traditionally, trade barriers have been viewed as legal instruments such as tariffs that governments create. Under the TRIPS Agreement, it is the *absence* of laws protecting IPRs that is considered to be a barrier to trade. The argument behind the TRIPS Agreement is that the failure to protect the rights of patent owners hinders commerce because these owners cannot be certain their intellectual property will not be copied. The lack of protection constrains trade, because patent holders will not risk supplying goods to a market where cheap (and often illegal) competing products can be developed and marketed. To address these potential problems, the agreement provides conditions which national legislation must meet, in order to transparently and promptly protect the owners of IPRs.

The TRIPS Agreement mandates clear limits to the parallel importation of licensed goods from other jurisdictions. However, this is expanded to cover not only trademarked goods but also 'pirated copyright goods … [and] goods which involve other infringements of intellectual property rights' (GATT 1994, 23). In the realm of pharmaceuticals, generics are seen to be pirated goods. Crucial for the treatment of AIDS, this aspect of the TRIPS Agreement renders the importation of 'pirated' generic pharmaceuticals illegal for any WTO member, even if it has enacted the health emergency provisions of the agreement. Under these provisions, such as those in Article 8, signatories may 'adopt measures necessary to protect public health' (GATT 1994, 5).

Aside from parallel importation, the possibilities for compulsory licensing in the TRIPS Agreement appear under Article 31 (GATT 1944, 14–15). This article restricts pre-license efforts to create an agreement with the patent holder and it limits the scope of use of the compulsory license. For the purposes of this chapter, it is important to note that Article 31 limits compulsory licenses 'predominantly for the supply of the domestic market' (GATT 1994, 14; Gold and Lam 2003, 14–19). The provision limiting compulsory licenses for the supply of domestic markets did not appear in the Paris Convention, the international treaty which established international rules on patent-related issues and which has been replaced by the TRIPS Agreement (Oddi 1996, 456). The provisions under Article 5a of the Paris Convention had been revised during the 1960s to favor the sovereign right of states to appropriate intellectual property when they deemed the public interest to be served by such appropriation. Various United States-based industry organizations lobbied against this viewpoint on the basis that these rights had become too extensive (Reichman and Hasenzahl 2002, 6–8).

Ultimately, the TRIPS Agreement makes the implementation of compulsory licenses difficult despite their legitimacy under the agreement's health emergency provisions. 'Some countries that have provided for them in their legislation have faced the threat of unilateral retaliations, or the suspension of aid, by some developed countries', primarily the United States and the EU (Correa 2002, 50).[1] The US government frequently uses IPR clauses in bilateral trade agreements to curtail the use by developing nations of the health-related provisions of the TRIPS Agreement.

Even after passage of the TRIPS Agreement, the United States continues to push for more protection than is required under the agreement. The use of US law, not the multilateral TRIPS Agreement, is often referred to as 'TRIPS-plus'. These bilateral TRIPS-plus provisions expand the protection of IPRs beyond what the TRIPS Agreement mandates and explicitly bypass the accord's health emergency safeguards. The USTR uses the developing countries' need to secure entry into US markets to undermine the international agreements that the United States itself signed. The USTR Robert Zoellick stated in 2003 that one of the key negotiating aims of his office in the recently commenced negotiations toward a free-trade agreement with the Southern African Customs Union is to 'establish standards that reflect a standard of [patent] protection similar to that found in US law and then build on the foundations established in TRIPS' (Mokhiber and Weissman 2003).

Furthermore, the United States continues to utilize Special 301, despite the fact that the TRIPS Agreement is now part of the WTO. Special 301 notes that 'a country can be found to deny adequate and effective intellectual property protection *even if it is in compliance* with its obligations under the TRIPS agreement' (USTR 2003, 9; emphasis added). The USTR uses US law as a way to further limit the use of provisions of the multilateral TRIPS Agreement when they contradict the interests of US pharmaceutical companies. Until the 2003 WTO agreements, which are discussed in the next section, solutions to the AIDS crisis rooted in the TRIPS Agreement have been firmly resisted by the US government.

Access to Treatment: Private Rights versus Human Rights

Critics of the TRIPS Agreement argue that private rights are systematically privileged throughout the agreement's text. Oddi (1996, 440) asserts that the use of a natural *rights* discourse tries to establish that:

> these rights are so important that individual [WTO] member[s] welfare should not stand in the way of their being protected as an entitlement of the creators. This invokes a counter-instrumentalist policy that members, regardless of their state of industrialization, should sacrifice their national interests in favor of the posited higher order of international trade.

Such criticisms highlight the underlying assumptions built into the TRIPS Agreement. Although the agreement itself is a complex and wide-ranging set of requirements on signatories (Matthews 2002), at its core is a particular set of norms regarding the treatment of knowledge as property. These norms are based on the notion that the private ownership of knowledge is a major spur to continued economic advancement and social welfare. Supporters of the TRIPS Agreement further emphasize that the development of knowledge is an individualized endeavor and that ownership of property rights is the legitimate reward for such efforts. The end result of such a view is that knowledge and information become commodities. It is, however, important to recognize that the present governance of IPRs is not ahistorical; it reflects the innovation and technoeconomic development of particular countries. For example, France, Germany, Japan, and Switzerland extended patent protection to pharmaceuticals only until the 1960s and 1970s, by which time their industries had matured. The bargain between social costs and private rewards on which IPRs are built is historically contingent, not a reflection of timeless natural rights. Perhaps the biggest problem is the continuing discourse of *rights* when it comes to the commodification of knowledge and information. There is a need to recall that both the history and use of IPRs is predicated on the uses to which this knowledge is put. It is too often forgotten that the origins of IPRs are not in political or natural rights, but rather in the limited award of monopoly privileges, with linked duties incumbent on the rights holder (May 2000).

As we have described above, the TRIPS Agreement itself is somewhat flexible, in that it recognizes that private property rights must be balanced with the national-level public-policy goals of development and public welfare. Despite this fact, advocates of absolute protection of IPRs have often prevailed in their interpretation and enforcement of the TRIPS Agreement. Yet, an interpretation of the TRIPS Agreement that privileges the private ownership of knowledge and information is hardly universal and therefore, represents a major problem for the legitimate *global* governance of IPRs. This lack of universality means that other views of IPRs can and do exist and, in the context of access to AIDS treatment, have become more prevalent. Higgott and Ougaard (2002, 12) maintain that while a 'thick interconnectedness' between 'political structures, agents and processes with transnational properties' characterizes the contemporary global polity, these structures and agents are only linked by a 'thin community that transcends the territorial state'. Through the widened reach of branded products and the increasingly global use of information and communications technologies, the *globalized* interconnectivity of knowledge commodification has become more pronounced, reflecting this thick interconnectedness. However, there remains only a thin community that recognizes the social values and costs of various actions and practices within this nascent global community and specifically, its economic dimension.

AIDS has become an important political issue that challenges the legitimacy of the TRIPS Agreement. Because of limited access to patented medicines and the privileging of IPRs over public health, developing countries have begun to question the legitimacy of the TRIPS Agreement. For example, at the 2001 United Nations General Assembly Special Session on HIV/AIDS, President Daniel arap Moi of Kenya said, 'The time has come when we are compelled to make a decision between the human lives and the right of commercial interest. Human life must surely come before anything else' (Kenya 2001). The political justifications that have previously been used to underpin IPRs do not have sufficient purchase in the current global situation of socioeconomic inequality. What has emerged is the recognition that there is a considerable tension between the logic of the TRIPS Agreement and the Universal Declaration of Human Rights. The declaration seeks to ensure everyone the right to enjoy the benefits of cultural life and scientific development and asserts a right to health and a standard of living adequate for a person's health and well-being. While allowing for the enjoyment of private benefits from innovative and creative activity, the declaration implies that it is global societal benefits that should be given priority (Cullet 2003, 152).[2] The human-rights agenda raises three issues that relate to access to AIDS medicines in Africa. First, AIDS-related medicines should be available to all; this currently is compromised by the unevenness of wealth across the continent. Second, there should be physical accessibility to medicines; they must be available locally, not simply because of their general existence. Third, medicines should be affordable. Given the market orientation of the modern world, any human right to medicine is crucially dependent on price, especially because complex treatment regimens are under patent protection (Sun 2003, 113).

These concerns about access to AIDS medications led the UN Commission on Human Rights to pass a resolution acknowledging that access to AIDS-related medicines was 'one fundamental element for achieving progressively the full realization of the right of everyone to the enjoyment of the highest attainable standard of physical and mental health' (Ferreira 2002, 1163). The resolution calls on states to ensure their populations have access to such medicines. The availability of AIDS medicines that prolong the lives of those infected is an issue of human rights and social justice. However, supporters of the TRIPS Agreement have been mostly concerned with ensuring the maximum reward for property owners. For them, social justice is understood as efficiency that encourages innovation, rather than as equal diffusion of such innovations.

The Doha Conference: Piecemeal Solutions?

Given the controversy surrounding access to AIDS medication and the emerging problems with the TRIPS Agreement, the trade negotiations in Doha were intended to initiate a new trade round. According to negotiators from developed states, the round would have a development focus. The previous negotiations that led to the adoption of the TRIPS Agreement had involved considerable deal making, but had resulted in few benefits to developing countries (Drahos 2002). While the developed countries have demanded rapid implementation of the TRIPS Agreement, the implementation of promises to open markets to agricultural goods and textiles from poor countries has been slow. In a letter to the *Financial Times* (London) on 8 December 1999, Rubens Ricupero, the Secretary General of the UN Conference on Trade and Development, summarized the injustice of this situation:

> Over half a century after the birth of the GATT [General Agreement on Tariffs and Trade], a few industrialized countries continue to drag their feet on liberalizing

> their textiles and clothing industries, claiming they need still more time for their economies to adjust. Meanwhile, they insist that weak developing countries swallow the bitter medicine of adjustment to agreements on issues such as TRIPS as quickly as possible – preferably in under five years. What is sauce for the goose is sauce for the gander. All the rest is rank hypocrisy.[3]

Much the same could be said of agriculture. In light of this disquiet, and after considerable negotiation, WTO members agreed to the Doha Declaration on TRIPS and Public Health in November 2001.

Some hailed the Doha declaration as proof that the WTO could respond to its poorer members' problems (Vandoren 2002). Yet, despite extensive and difficult negotiations, the declaration only restated in more lengthy terms the provisions that were already included in Article 8 of the TRIPS Agreement. The declaration contends that its signatories 'reaffirm the right of WTO Members to use, to the full, the provisions in the TRIPS agreement, which provide flexibility to [deal with health crises]' (WTO 2001, par. 4). However, significant problems with access to AIDS treatment remain.

One problem is that compulsory licensing is only allowed on the basis of a national emergency and for production of pharmaceuticals for a domestic market. While Article 31(k) allows exportation of medicines where a patent holder has adopted anticompetitive practices, this leaves the importation into a country with a compulsory license outside any explicit provision of the agreement.[4] While this domestic-production provision benefits countries with high HIV prevalence rates that want to produce AIDS pharmaceuticals for their citizens, countries must have the manufacturing capacity to produce such medicines. Most developing countries, and particularly those in sub-Saharan Africa, lack this production capacity and must rely on the international trade in pharmaceuticals. Countries that might produce AIDS medicines cheaper than brand-name products through compulsory licensing cannot export such medicines to countries in need of them.

A further problem arises for developing countries that must import AIDS medicines if they cannot produce these pharmaceuticals themselves: not only must the country importing medicines declare a health emergency, but the country producing them must also. (The health emergency then becomes justification for the compulsory license that enables the country to produce the pharmaceutical.) If the potential exporter of a medicine is not suffering from a similar health crisis, then no compulsory license can be given under the TRIPS Agreement. If no license can be given, then the importing country may still have no supplier other than the patent holder. In that case, there will be no price reduction for the pharmaceutical, since the patent holder can effectively set the price. The only other option for the importing country is to depend on generic suppliers which are not WTO-member countries. Since the WTO has 148 members, this option is not very feasible.

A final set of problems that the Doha declaration does not effectively address is the fact that some developing countries cannot take advantage of compulsory licensing because they have signed TRIPS-plus agreements with the United States. If they have not signed such agreements, they still have to consider the possibility of the USTR discounting their health crises and putting economic pressure on them to import from patent holders. For example, in 2000, with support from developed countries, GlaxoSmithKline threatened to sue the government of Ghana for importing ARVs from Cipla, an Indian producer. The Ghanaian distributor halted the program and, as of late 2003, the only comprehensive treatment program available in Ghana was through the US Agency for International Development (Thomas 2002; Patterson 2003).

Therefore, the Doha declaration provides only limited solutions within the context of the TRIPS Agreement for the poorest sub-Saharan African countries with high HIV prevalence rates. Those countries without domestic manufacturing ability face the same situation as before the declaration. They are still unable to import medicines legally, since compulsory licenses are limited to domestic markets, and they lack the capacity to produce these pharmaceuticals domestically. While some of these difficulties are recognized in Paragraph 6 of the declaration, the document merely 'instruct[s] the Council for TRIPS to find an expeditious solution to this problem and to report to the General Council before the end of 2002' (WTO 2001, par. 4). This report has been undermined by the USTR, which has aggressively sought to protect the patents of pharmaceutical companies. But, without action on the report, the declaration remains empty rhetoric. As we discuss in the next section, the 2003 WTO agreement sought to address some of these problems.

In response to the limits of the Doha declaration, some policy makers and AIDS activists have urged states to extend their sovereign rights within the TRIPS Agreement and to take full advantage of Article 30, which says:

> Members may provide limited exceptions to the exclusive rights conferred by patent, provided that such exceptions do not unreasonably conflict with the normal exploitation of the patent, and do not unreasonably prejudice the legitimate interests of the patent owner, taking account of the legitimate interests of third parties (GATT 1994, 14).

For sub-Saharan African states suffering from AIDS, the legitimate interest of their citizens (i.e., third parties) is continued good health. A broad interpretation of Article 30 is one way to make AIDS medicines more available while still complying with the TRIPS Agreement (Abbott 2002). The main advantage this interpretation has over the use of compulsory licensing in Article 31 is that under Article 30, a clear blanket exemption to patent protection can be established in domestic law. Under Article 31, this exemption is subject to case-by-case litigation, a scenario which could limit the ability of developing countries to access AIDS medications from nonpatent holders. Aside from arguing for the abolition of Article 31(f), Article 30 may provide the best solution within the agreement's framework.

Following this logic, on 23 October 2002 the European Parliament adopted Amendment 196 to the European Medicines Directive, which states, 'Manufacturing shall be allowed if the medicinal product is intended for export to a third country that has issued a compulsory license for that product, or where a patent is not in force and if there is a request to that effect of the competent health authorities of that third country' (Sun 2003, 127).

The problem of compulsory licensing and international trade in pharmaceuticals was a major area of discussion at a 2002 workshop organized by the Quaker United Nations Office and the Norwegian Ministry of Foreign Affairs. At the conference, delegates explicitly recognized the role of compulsory licensing in the balance between private property rights and public interests such as health (Quaker United Nations Office 2002, 17). A number of delegates from African states and NGOs stressed that issuing patents is a public-policy decision. If patents become an obstacle to a specific policy aim such as public health, and if a system of compulsory licensing cannot be made to work, then further actions need to be taken. The problem has been that the TRIPS Agreement emphasizes the role of policy in supporting innovation instead of the role of policy in promoting the public good. The latter types of government actions have historically blocked the private holding of patents.

To briefly summarize, while initially persuaded to sign the TRIPS Agreement as part of becoming members of the WTO, African states, which now face pressure to provide treatment for their citizens with HIV/AIDS, have begun to question the legitimacy of the agreement and, more generally, the WTO. The emerging language of health care as a human right has provided AIDS activists and African states suffering from overwhelming HIV prevalence rates with a compelling issue with which to rethink the TRIPS Agreement. In the Doha negotiations, African states and numerous other developing countries began to reassert the need to balance private rights with public goods such as health, but there is still significant work to be done. In the next section, we will investigate how access to treatment has evolved since the Doha negotiations.

Access to AIDS Treatment in Africa after Doha

Despite the rhetorical gains and new international commitment to providing treatment, there are still some significant issues to work out after Doha. As mentioned in the previous section, the Doha declaration did little to change access to medication in the short term because the TRIPS Agreement privileges the rights of patent *owners* (Correa 2003). Nonstate actors, states, and international organizations have responded to the limitations of Doha in a variety of ways. In doing so, they have challenged the absolute rights of patent owners and have provided more options for patent users to gain access to medications.

First, WTO members sought to address some of the problems with compulsory licensing, specifically the inability of generic manufacturers to export their medicines to poor countries that lack manufacturing capacity. On 23 August 2003, the WTO members agreed to allow companies that produce generic versions of patented pharmaceuticals, including active ingredients of pharmaceuticals and diagnostic kits, to export these products to eligible importing countries. The decision was issued as a waiver to Article 31, which states that generic drugs manufactured under compulsory license must be produced primarily for domestic consumption (Scherer and Watal 2001, 29). The 2003 accord is intended to last until the TRIPS Agreement is amended. Before the 2003 accord, the United States had supported the position of the pharmaceutical industry and had resisted an agreement that would allow generics to be imported (Irwin, Millen, and Fallows 2003, 128–29). The United States agreed to the accord, on the condition that the statement set out measures to ensure that countries will not use it to make commercial profits instead of meeting public health needs (*New York Times*, 31 August 2003; Moran 2003; *Financial Times* [London], 1 September 2003). On that issue, 23 industrialized countries voluntarily announced that they will not use the system to import, and 11 other countries agreed that they will only use the system in extreme health emergencies (WTO 2003a).

Although this action attempts to deal with the shortcomings of the TRIPS Agreement, it also has several limitations (Roman 2003). The accord requires an annual renewal process, a fact which makes it somewhat temporary in its legal status. According to AIDS activists, the provision that the system should not be used to advance commercial objectives creates uncertainty for the businesses that produce generics. The definition of an 'eligible' country under the accord is nebulous, a fact that opens the door for additional lobbying by the United States and the EU to limit access of generics to particular countries. The agreement also adds several regulations on the business practices of generic producers (MSF 2003a). In a larger sense, the difficult and lengthy process of negotiating such an agreement attests to the political challenges of circumscribing the widest interpretation of IPRs from the TRIPS Agreement.

India, Brazil, and Thailand have generic drug industries that will be able to export drugs to African states without domestic production capabilities under the new agreement. However, countries such as India and Brazil are in the first round of developing countries that will have to comply with the TRIPS Agreement by 2005.[5] As a result, without additional action on the part of the WTO, it is unclear if generic manufacturers in these countries will be allowed to manufacture generic medicines after 2005 (*Guardian*, 18 February 2003). Even if they continue to manufacture generics, the complex and bureaucratic compulsory licensing scheme will continue to make access to medication a struggle for many. In response to criticisms that generic producers could not easily receive licenses from the United States for use in US-funded AIDS relief programs, the Food and Drug Administration announced an expedited review process in early 2004. It is too early to tell if this process will make generics more available.

Despite the problems of the 2003 WTO accord, some states and NGOs have responded to the potential opportunities it provides. In late 2003, the Canadian government introduced legislation that would allow drug manufactures to export low-cost generics to the world's poorest countries (Canada.com, 7 November 2003). Additionally, the William Clinton Presidential Foundation announced in October 2003 that it had negotiated an agreement with three Indian producers and one South African company to provide one combination of AIDS medicines for roughly $139 per year. Since the pharmaceuticals will be used in the foundation's programs in several countries, the agreement assures demand for the product and enables the producers to offer lower prices because of economies of scale (*Hindu Business Line*, 22 November 2003; William Clinton Foundation 2003).

A second response to the Doha declaration has been that the major pharmaceutical companies began cutting prices on their brand-name AIDS medications, partially to avoid the threat of generic manufacturers' competition and partly to combat the bad publicity they have received over the high price of AIDS medicines. For example, GlaxoSmithKline reduced the price of Combivir, a drug the World Health Organization (WHO) recommends for treatment, to 90¢ per day in April 2003. However, these prices are only available to NGOs, the Global Fund to Fight AIDS, Tuberculosis and Malaria, governments in sub-Saharan Africa, and an additional 10 countries (Baker 2003).[6] As the program of GlaxoSmithKline illustrates, even with price reductions, the major pharmaceutical companies tend to provide medicine only under certain conditions. In many cases, they continue to price their products so that only the wealthiest members of the developing world can take advantage of them (Nerrozi 2002, 631). Some AIDS activists maintain that price reductions are motivated by a desire to control markets, more than a desire to provide access to medication (Baker 2003). Providing cheaper medicines allows the pharmaceutical companies to keep out generic products, which might be cheaper than brand-name drugs with the discounted price.

Third, there has been a heightened realization of the role of generics in the fight against HIV/AIDS. The issue of generic drugs remains a complex problem, despite the 2003 accord. The continued failure of the WTO to comprehensively address the cross-border supply of generics during health emergencies means that many individuals and agencies dedicated to treatment have resorted to civil disobedience to provide needed medications. For example, Médecins Sans Frontières (Doctors without Borders) has imported and distributed more medicine than would otherwise have been possible by using generics like those produced by Cipla. Based on the Doha declaration and the Kenyan Industrial Property Act of 2001, Médecins Sans Frontières has provided treatment to 'up to four times as many patients as before' (MSF 2002, 8). In January 2002, Médecins Sans Frontières and the Treatment Action Campaign began importing generics from Brazil into South

Africa. As a result of their civil disobedience, 85 people have begun to receive therapy at costs significantly lower than would be possible with brand-name drugs (CNN.com, 29 January 2002). Additionally, some doctors in Africa and throughout the developing world are relying on leftover drugs shipped to them by American patients (*New York Times*, 22 July 2003).

Scherer and Watal (2001, 5–6) maintain that access to generic drugs is essential for combating HIV/AIDS throughout Africa because generic competition decreases the price of all AIDS drugs. While the industries' price reductions close the gap between generic prices and brand-name prices, it is still cheaper to buy generic drugs where they are available. At the discounted price of 90¢ per day, a year's supply of Combivir costs $328.50; generic alternatives cost approximately $209 per year. Generic substitutes have lowered the costs of the most common ARV combination of stavudine (d4T) + lamivudine (3TC) + nevirapine (NVP) from $10,000 per year to $209 per year (MSF 2002, 2).[7]

Brazil illustrates the successful use of generic medicines in the fight against HIV/AIDS. Brazil has been able to reduce its death rate from AIDS and curb its HIV infection rates through a commitment to education, prevention, and free treatment programs for all infected patients. As part of its commitment to solving the HIV/AIDS crisis, Brazil has engaged in aggressive negotiations for access to affordable medicine when it cannot produce its own (Galvão 2002). Brazil demonstrates that through a state commitment to systematic testing, counseling, and free treatment for people with AIDS a poor country can fight the disease. Brazil also has expressed interest in providing AIDS medication to Mozambique (*Africa News*, 3 May 2003).

A fourth response to the Doha declaration has been for some African countries to begin to develop their own pharmaceutical companies, although importation remains crucial for the majority of African states (*Financial Times* [London], 1 September 2003). Namibia and Burundi have announced that they will begin to manufacture generic AIDS medication locally in an effort to further reduce the price of medicine (UN Integrated Regional Information Networks, 11 June 2003; *BBC News*, 10 February 2003). Ethiopia began manufacturing AIDS drugs in April of 2003 (UN Integrated Regional Information Networks, 15 April 2003). Additionally, Pharmacia Corporation said that it planned to transfer licenses for the AIDS drug Rescriptor to the Dutch non-profit organization International Dispensary Association, a move which will allow generic producers to provide affordable versions of the drug throughout sub-Saharan Africa (US Department of State 2003). However, when Pfizer purchased Pharmacia in late 2003, this agreement was revoked (*Wall Street Journal*, 12 November 2003). Uganda began importing generic drugs from Cipla after the Doha declaration. The cost of ARV treatment has decreased from around $600 per month to $30 per month, and the government provides drugs to 10,000 of the estimated 30,000 Ugandans receiving treatment (*Africa News*, 24 February 2003). The Kampala-based Quality Chemicals Company announced in January 2004 that it would begin producing ARVs for 50¢ per day before the end of the year (UN Integrated Regional Information Network, 5 January 2004). These national drug production programs must be viewed in the larger context of greater political commitment to AIDS among African states. For example, as of 2002, over 40 countries in sub-Saharan Africa had established national strategies to fight AIDS, a threefold increase over two years before, and 19 countries had National AIDS Councils (UNAIDS 2002, 3).

Additionally, some industrialized states and international organizations have developed new programs to provide more AIDS medications to poor countries. Internationally, as the chapter by Patterson and Cieminis illustrates, in 2001, the member-states of the UN developed the Global Fund to Fight AIDS, Tuberculosis and Malaria (Global Fund). Of grants allocated in its first two rounds, 65 per cent of money was designated for HIV/AIDS and 46 per cent, for medicines and commodities (Global Fund 2003). Furthermore, the funds used for medicines were used to purchase generics, when available. In 2003, the WHO launched its '3 by 5' program that aims to provide three million people with HIV/AIDS in developing countries with treatment by 2005. As part of the program, the WHO has endorsed the use of a generic three-drug combination pill that can be taken twice a day. This important program is partially made possible because the current chief of the WHO, Dr. Lee Jong-wook, has framed the AIDS crisis as a 'global health emergency' (*San Francisco Chronicle*, 2 December 2003).

At the national level, the US government has sought to develop its own program on treatment. President George W. Bush promised $15 billion to fight HIV/AIDS in poor countries in his 2003 State of the Union address. Although the proposal raised attention to the need for affordable treatment, AIDS activists have criticized the plan because of the president's limited political commitment to appropriations (Africa Action 2003; Global AIDS Alliance 2003; Health Gap Global Access Project 2003). The *Wall Street Journal* reported on 10 December 2003 that President Bush did not ask congress for significant increases in AIDS funding for 2004, a departure from his initial promise. While the original proposal provided funding for the Global Fund, overall the US approach is problematic because it tends to bypass international organizations that may more efficiently serve as a common source for AIDS funding (*Guardian*, 2 December 2003; *Boston Globe*, 11 July 2003). Instead, the United States has focused on creating a program headed by an ambassador-level official who will report directly to the secretary of state. In a move that many AIDS activists criticized, former Eli Lilly and Company executive Randall Tobias was chosen to lead the new AIDS program (Lobe 2003). Furthermore, the US government has seemed determined to use funds only for brand-name AIDS drugs, not generics, despite the fact that recipient governments would prefer to purchase generic ARVs (*New York Times*, 14 July 2004).

In addition to the reconfiguration on the international scene and the growing acceptance of generic drugs, AIDS activists must continue to exert effort to ensure that funding promises are kept and the United States and the EU do not prevent additional generic drugs from reaching Africa. Ultimately, while an improvement, current policy responses to AIDS have remained somewhat piecemeal because of the problems that remain with the TRIPS Agreement. Temporarily reduced prices, drug donations, and limited programming by the developed world must be supplemented by more universal, comprehensive AIDS policies that seriously reconsider the relationship of patent rights to health-care rights. As we outline in the conclusion, we believe that even with these challenges, it is possible to increase access to AIDS medication.

Hope for the Future?

Despite a preference for the TRIPS Agreement and TRIPS-plus negotiations on the part of developed countries, a general acceptance of treatment as an important response to HIV/AIDS now exists. In only a few short years, dedicated AIDS activists and health care professionals have successfully called attention to the systemic problems of world trade as related to intellectual property. Indeed, the moral arguments about AIDS treatment are very different from those which existed in 1998 when the pharmaceutical companies sued South Africa, or a decade ago when the developed countries pushed through the TRIPS Agreement. While the Doha declaration was somewhat limited, it did establish that health care and issues of human rights need to be considered within the intellectual property framework. Furthermore, the 2003 WTO agreement has established the acceptability of cross-border trade in generics within certain constraints. Access to treatment is slowly becoming a reality in Africa and it can be hoped that the language of health care as a human right will continue to expand from HIV/AIDS to include all life-threatening diseases.[8]

National solutions and civil disobedience over access to AIDS medicines have challenged the pharmaceutical industry to rethink its global markets. For example, providing different levels of protection for IPRs in developed and developing states has received more attention. On 18 February 2003, the *Guardian* reported that Jean Pierre Garnier, chief executive officer of GlaxoSmithKline, said:

> In the poorest countries of the world – and there is a list prepared by the WHO – they should be able to disregard patents. That's what I'm for, in all the diseases that constitute healthcare crises for those countries. So it's HIV, and malaria and TB and infectious diseases and so forth. What I don't agree is that patents would be disregarded in China, in India and so forth and those companies would be able to prosper by pirating our discoveries made in Europe and the US and therefore we'd be shut out of 80 per cent of the world population. That is not fair.

While this statement does not fully endorse the end of patents or differential protection for pharmaceutical products in developing countries, it reveals the shifts that the industry has been forced to contemplate.

Recently, other solutions to the problems that the TRIPS Agreement presents have received more attention. Differential pricing has been discussed among developing and developed states, as well as being supported by the WHO in collaboration with the WTO (United Kingdom 2002; WHO and WTO 2001). Legal scholars also have developed a number of suggestions for multilateral solutions within the continuing framework of the TRIPS Agreement. For example, Lanjouw (2002) links securing property rights in developed countries with freedom for generic manufacture in developing countries. Although these ideas have yet to reach fruition, a clear political momentum toward some new settlement seems to be emerging (Attaran 2002; Bourgeois and Burns 2002). Such solutions, however, demand sufficient political will. If it can be mustered, then workable political solutions to the problems of access to AIDS treatment are possible.

In the struggle to provide access to medication, it is clear that a nascent global civil society can support and encourage national resistance to any international settlement on IPRs that ignores social costs. Higgot and Ougaard (2002) assert that the global polity remains underdeveloped relative to the interconnectedness of global economic relations. However, an increasing public awareness of the plight of Africans with AIDS has led to expanded political pressure on countries that prioritize IPRs over humanitarian needs. Resistance need not necessarily be 'anti-TRIPS,' but it should recognize the possibility of maintaining national policies to deal with health emergencies through compulsory licensing and other patent-related measures. Given the growing strength of the generic sector outside the developed countries, there is a real opportunity to challenge a globalized legal settlement that has become increasingly problematic and illegitimate. African states are not impotent in this struggle. Unlike their acceptance of the TRIPS Agreement in 1995, they forcefully lobbied for the Doha declaration and the 2003 WTO decision. In fact, South Africa and Kenya were among only five WTO members negotiating for the 2003 accord (MSF 2003b). Likewise, the actions of African states to import generics, to develop their own manufacturing facilities, and to more vocally demand access to treatment have shaped the political and moral discussion of AIDS medicines.

Few African states want to dispense with IPRs completely. However, they, like the United States or EU countries, do demand the ability to protect their citizens' lives. For intellectual property law to remain legitimate, it needs to change to meet these demands. It is our belief that while progress may be slow, we are seeing the gradual shift in response to the AIDS crisis. Certainly, considerable resistance to widespread generic production continues. However, even in the last year, the terrain of the argument has shifted and clear possibilities have emerged for widening access to crucial medicines on the African continent. Africans may still be dying of treatable diseases, and this remains unacceptable, but no longer does the future look quite as hopeless as it once did.

Notes

1 Despite this position, in developed countries the social costs that may result from the exploitation of IPRs have historically been mediated through national legislation for compulsory licensing. Developed countries regard compulsory licenses to be legitimate when patents do not work in the jurisdiction in which they have been registered and when patents create high prices that restrict socially desirable usage. After September 11, when terrorist use of anthrax appeared to threaten US citizens, the US government quickly threatened the makers of the antibiotic Cipro with the possibility of abrogating their patents in order to ensure an available drug supply (Singh 2002). At the same time, the Canadian government considered enacting a compulsory license and utilized this threat to obtain a deep price discount for needed drugs. The threat of compulsory licensing prompted several commentators to question why the TRIPS Agreement was applicable to Africa, where millions of people with AIDS have no access to medicines, but not to the United States and Canada, where few individuals had died from anthrax.

2 While many states have signed the Universal Declaration of Human Rights and the TRIPS Agreement, it is unclear how binding any human-rights document is on corporations, as opposed to states. Ferreira (2002) argues forcefully that the pharmaceutical corporations *do* have human-rights obligations, although this is by no means an uncontested position.

3 See also Dasgupta and Debroy 2002.

4 Eppich (2002, 311) notes that this might allow a domestic manufacturer to reach significant economies of scale (and therefore, reduce its price) by expanding the market share in transitional and non-WTO economies.

5 Under the Doha declaration, the least developed countries can now defer enforcing patent protection until 2016 (MSF 2002, 3).

6 GSK did not identify the additional 10 countries in its press release, but said that the program will affect a total of 63 countries (GlaxoSmithKline 2003).

7 Generic manufacturers can produce an efficient single pill by combining different patented drugs that could not normally be combined. Cipla has produced a single pill of patented medicines from GlaxoSmithKline and Boehringer Ingelheim. The single dose pill makes it easier for people to take the medicine. While there is little evidence supporting the assumption that combination treatment programs are difficult for Africans to follow, the single pill can further improve adherence to treatment regimens. African patients have followed combination or sequenced self-dosage regimens as diligently as western patients. Indeed, 80–85 per cent of African patients take their combination programs as prescribed, compared to 60 per cent of patients in the developed world (*Economist* 2003).

8 The United States already plans to fight the expansion of access to medication beyond AIDS, tuberculosis, and malaria. US negotiators responded to the request for compulsory licenses to counter significant health problems in developing countries by developing an 'approved disease list' to be used when determining if a public health crisis is significant enough to warrant compulsory licensing. Moran (2003) finds that aside from HIV/AIDS, tuberculosis, and malaria, the list does not include diseases commonly causing deaths in Africa. Furthermore, the diseases on the list for which African states may override patents are ones for which there is either no treatment available or the available treatments are not patented.

References

Abbott, Frederick. 2002. Legal options for implementing Paragraph 6 of the Ministerial Declaration on the TRIPS Agreement and Public Health. Summary of presentation at meeting of Quaker United Nations Office and Norway Ministry of Foreign Affairs. Utstein Monastery, Norway. http://www.geneva.quno.info/pdf/Legal%20Options%20Abbott.pdf.

Africa Action. 2003. Grim reapers gather at White House. *Africa Policy E-journal*. http://www.africaaction.org.

Attaran, Amir. 2002. The Doha Declaration on the TRIPS Agreement and Public Health, access to pharmaceuticals, and options under WTO law. *Fordham Intellectual Property, Media and Entertainment Law Journal* 12 (3): 859–85.

Baker, Brook K. 2003. The real politics of GSK's price cut. *Africa Policy E-journal*. http://www.africaaction.org/docs03/acc0304b.htm.

Bourgeois, Jacques H. J., and Thaddeus J. Burns. 2002. Implementing Paragraph 6 of the Doha Declaration on TRIPS and Public Health: The waiver solution. *Journal of World Intellectual Property* 5 (6): 835–64.

Braithwaite, John, and Peter Drahos. 2000. *Global business regulation* Cambridge: Cambridge Univ. Press.

Copson, Raymond W. 2003. AIDS in Africa. Issue briefing for congress. Washington, DC: Congressional Research Service.

Correa, Carlos. 2002. Pro-competitive measure under TRIPS to promote technology diffusion in developing countries. In *Global intellectual property rights: Knowledge, access and development,* ed. Peter Drahos and Ruth Mayne, 40–57. Basingstoke: Palgrave Macmillan.

——. 2003. Introduction: TRIPS and access to drugs: Toward a solution for developing countries without manufacturing capacity? *Emory International Law Review* 17: 389–406.

Cullet, Philippe. 2003. Patents and medicines: The relationship between TRIPS and the human right to health. *International Affairs* 79 (1): 139–60.

Dasgupta, A., and B. Debroy, eds. 2002. *Salvaging the WTO's future: Doha and beyond*. Delhi: Konark Publishing.

Drahos, Peter. 2002. Developing countries and intellectual property standard-setting. *Journal of World Intellectual Property* 5 (5): 765–89.

Economist. 2003. Trick or treatment. 19 July.

Eppich, Christopher K. 2002. Patenting dilemma: Drugs for profit versus drugs for health. *Santa Clara Law Review* 43 (1): 289–318.

Ferreira, Lissett. 2002. Access to affordable HIV/AIDS drugs: The human rights obligations of multinational pharmaceutical corporations. *Fordham Law Review* 71 (3): 1133–79.

Galvão, Jane. 2002. Access to anti-retroviral drugs in Brazil. *Lancet* 360: 1862–65.

General Agreement on Tariffs and Trade (GATT). 1994. *Final act embodying the results of the Uruguay Round of Multilateral Trade Negotiations*. Geneva: GATT.

GlaxoSmithKline (GSK). 2003. GSK again reduces its not-for-profit price of HIV/AIDS medicines for the developing world. Press release. http://www.gsk.com/media/archive.htm.

Global AIDS Alliance. 2003. President Bush's record on the global AIDS epidemic. http://www.globalaidsalliance.org/policyupdate.html.

Global Fund to Fight AIDS, Tuberculosis, and Malaria. 2003. Where is the Global Fund money going? http://www.theglobalfundatm.org/en/.

Gold, E. Richard, and Daniel K. Lam. 2003. Balancing trade in patents: Public noncommercial use and compulsory licensing. *Journal of World Intellectual Property* 6 (1): 5–31.

Halbert, Debora. 2002. Moralized discourses: South Africa's intellectual property fight for access to AIDS medication. *Seattle Journal for Social Justice* 1 (2): 257–95.

Health Gap Global Access Project. 2003. The U.S. global AIDS bill is not a cheque: Myths and facts about the U.S. $15 billion and the Global Fund to Fight AIDS, TB and Malaria. Press release. http://www.healthgap.org/press_releases/03/052703_HGAP_PS_WHA_GWB_G8_fund.html.

Higgott, Richard, and Morten Ougaard. 2002. Introduction: Beyond system and society – Towards a global polity. In *Towards a global polity*, ed. Morten Ougaard and Richard Higgott, 1–20. London: Routledge.

Hoeckman, B. M., and M. M. Kostecki. 1995. *The political economy of the world trading system: From GATT to WTO*. Oxford: Oxford Univ. Press.

Irwin, Alexander, Joyce Millen, and Dorothy Fallows. 2003. *Global AIDS: Myths and facts, tools for fighting the AIDS pandemic*. Cambridge: South End Press.

Joint United Nations Program on HIV/AIDS (UNAIDS). 2002. *AIDS epidemic update*. http://www.who.int/hiv/pub/epidemiology/epi2002/en/.

——. 2004. *Update on the global AIDS epidemic*. http://www.unaids.org/bangkok2004.html.

Kenya. 2001. Statement to the United Nations General Assembly Special Session on HIV/AIDS. http://www.un.org/ga/aids/statements/docs/kenyaE.html.

Lanjouw, Jean O. 2002. A new global patent regime for diseases: US and international legal issues. *Harvard Journal of Law and Technology* 16 (1): 85–124.

Lobe, Jim. 2003. AIDS appointee shows that business still rules the roost. *Africa Policy E-journal*. http://www.africaaction.org/docs03/doha0307.htm.

Matthews, Duncan. 2002. *Globalising intellectual property rights: The TRIPS Agreement*. London: Routledge.

May, Christopher. 2000. *A global political economy of intellectual property rights: The new enclosures?* London: Routledge.

Médecins Sans Frontières (MSF). 2002. Equitable access: Scaling up HIV/AIDS treatment in developing countries. http://www.msf.org/content/page.cfm?articleid=3B6E5EC7-A242–4212–9B8ED0135636229F.

——. 2003a. Joint NGO statement on TRIPS and public health WTO deal on medicines: A 'gift' bound in red tape. http://www.accessmed-msf.org/prod/publications.asp?scntid=1292003916443&contentype.

——. 2003b. US seeks further restrictions on generic medicines for developing countries. http://www.accessmed-msf.org/prod/publications.asp?scntid=25820031117538&contenttype.

Mokhiber, Russell, and Robert Weissman. 2003. The two faces of George Bush in Africa. *Focus on the Corporation Newsletter*. http://lists.essential.org/pipermail/corp-focus/2003/000156.html.

Moran, Mary. 2003. *Reneging on Doha: An MSF analysis of recent attempts to restrict developing countries' use of compulsory licensing to a set list of diseases*. http://www.cptech.org/ip/wto/p6/msf052003.pdf.

Nerozzi, Michelle M. 2002. The battle over life-saving pharmaceuticals: Are developing countries being 'TRIPped' by developed countries? *Villanova Law Review* 47: 605–41.

Oddi, Samuel. 1996. TRIPS – Natural rights and a 'polite form of economic imperialism.' *Vanderbilt Journal of Transnational Law* 29: 415–70.

Patterson, Amy. 2003. AIDS policy making in Africa: A comparison of Ghana and South Africa. Paper presented to the annual meeting of the African Studies Association, Boston.

Quaker United Nations Office. 2002. *The WTO TRIPS Agreement and the protection of public health: Implementing Paragraph 6 of the Doha declaration.* http://www.geneva.quno.info.

Reichman, Jerome H., and Catherine Hasenzahl. 2002. *Non-voluntary licensing of patented inventions*. Geneva: UN Conference on Trade and Development/International Center for Trade and Sustainable Development.

Roman, Monica. 2003. Needy nations' new drug deal. *Business Week*, 15 September.

Scherer, F. M., and Jayashree Watal. 2001. Post TRIPS options for access to patented medicines in developing countries. Commission on Macroeconomics and Health paper WG4–1. Geneva: WHO.

Sell, Susan. 2003. *Private power, public law: The globalization of intellectual property rights*. Cambridge: Cambridge Univ. Press.

Singh, Kavaljit. 2002. Anthrax, drug transnationals, and TRIPS. *Foreign policy in focus*. http://www.fpif.org/outside/commentary/2002/0204trips_body.html.

Steinberg, Richard H. 2002. In the shadow of law or power? Consensus-based bargaining in the GATT/WTO. *International Organization* 56 (2): 339–74.

Sun, Haochen. 2003. A wider access to patented drugs under the TRIPS Agreement. *Boston University International Law Journal* 21 (1): 101–36.

Thomas, Caroline. 2002. Trade policy and the politics of access to drugs. *Third World Quarterly* 23 (2): 251–64.

United Kingdom. 2002. *Policy recommendations and strategy.* Report to the prime minister from UK working group on increasing access to essential medicines in the developing world. http://www.dfid.gov.uk/Pubs/files/access_to_medicines_report28.11.pdf.

US Department of State. 2003. Pilot program to provide cheap AIDS drug to poor countries. http://usinfo.state.gov/regional/af/usafr/a3012403.htm.

US Trade Representative (USTR). 2003. *2003 Special 301report.* http://www.ustr.gov/sectors/intellectual.shtml.

Vandoren, Paul. 2002. *Médicaments sans frontières?* Clarification of the relationship between TRIPS and public health resulting from the WTO Doha Ministerial Declaration. *Journal of World Intellectual Property* 5 (1): 5–14.

William Clinton Foundation. 2003. Clinton Foundation announces agreement on major reduction in price of AIDS drugs. http://www.clintonpresidentialcenter.org/drug_announcement.html.

World Health Organization (WHO), and World Trade Organization. 2001. *Report on the workshop on differential pricing and financing of essential drugs.* http://www.who.int/medicines/library/edm_general/who-wto-hosbjor/wholereporthosbjorworkshop-fin-eng.pdf.

World Trade Organization (WTO). 2001. Declaration on the TRIPS Agreement and Public Health. Geneva: WTO.

——. 2003a. Decision removes final patent obstacle to cheap drug imports. http://www.wto.org/english/news_e/pres03?3/pr350_e.htm.

——. 2003b. Understanding the WTO: Least developed countries. http://www.wto.org/english/thewto_e/whatis_e/tif_e/org7_e.htm.

Chapter 11

Pursuing African AIDS Governance: Consolidating the Response and Preparing for the Future

Maite Irurzun-Lopez and Nana Poku

> 'Would you tell me, please, which way I ought to go from here?'
> 'That depends a good deal on where you want to get to,' said the Cat.
> 'I don't much care where. ...' said Alice.
> 'Then it doesn't matter which way you go,' said the Cat.
> '... So long as I get somewhere,' Alice added as an explanation.
> 'Oh, you're sure to do that,' said the Cat, 'if you only walk enough.'
>
> Lewis Carroll, *Alice in Wonderland*

This final chapter concentrates on defining and achieving the next steps in the fight against HIV/AIDS. It is time for those of us concerned about AIDS in Africa to be strategic in our thinking. We need to start by asking ourselves where we want African states to be in the near future. The vision presented here pictures African governments taking responsibility for tackling AIDS, with members of society acting in a nonconfrontational and coordinated manner. The response envisioned lasts as long as needed to combat AIDS, and includes processes that strengthen the state's legitimacy and developmental capacity. The suggestions outlined in this chapter aim to sustain and improve the responses to AIDS while simultaneously improving the governance capacities of the state and civil society. Particularly, the ideas presented here seek to address the aspects of the African state highlighted in this volume which directly affect the AIDS fight. In brief, African states need to pursue *AIDS governance*.

The chapter first reviews two sets of reasons for AIDS governance: (1) the resource limitations that constrain the state's response to AIDS; and (2) external factors that may influence international attention to AIDS. The chapter then recommends AIDS governance as the most suitable strategy to best consolidate the fight against AIDS. The principles of AIDS governance are a commitment to pursue long-term AIDS policies, incorporation of a gender approach into AIDS policies, inclusion of participatory and accountable decision-making processes, promotion of equity in health care, and the development of a human rights-based rationale for treatment. African governments must take these actions to consolidate the current responses to AIDS and to ensure the sustainability of these responses.

What Aspects of the State Response to AIDS Need to Change?

It is important to recognize that despite numerous deficiencies in African state responses to the epidemic, there have been many accomplishments. The first stage of the response – acknowledging the crisis – has broadly been achieved in most affected African countries. African leaders have publicly discussed the crisis that the epidemic poses and they have committed their personal leadership to fight the disease (OAU 2001; AU 2003). Additionally, most countries have developed HIV/AIDS National Strategic Plans and have set up functioning National AIDS Councils. Many countries are expanding mechanisms to fund their National Strategic Plans and to systematically monitor and evaluate them. States are working to build capacity inside and outside the health sector and to develop policies that mitigate the epidemic's impact. For example, all 29 sub-Saharan African countries surveyed by the Joint United Nations Program on HIV/AIDS (UNAIDS) in 2003 said they had adopted HIV/AIDS National Strategies (UNAIDS 2003). Using the measure of the AIDS Program Effort Index, Africa has made major advancements on the AIDS response in the areas of policy, planning, and political commitment (USAID et al. 2003).[1] Moreover, as the chapter by Halbert and May demonstrates, some African countries have committed to providing care, support, and treatment with antiretrovirals (ARVs) to people infected with HIV/AIDS. Many people five years ago would not have expected such an extensive response to AIDS.

Despite these successes, African states continue to face many challenges. These include the limited institutional capacity of the African state to follow through on its AIDS priorities and the disjointed relationship between the state and civil society which may hamper coordination, participation, and accountability in the AIDS fight. However, this chapter focuses on the worrying issue of sustaining responses to the epidemic. It questions the sustainability of funding and the continuation of ongoing and future programs. As this book's introduction illustrates, external sources heavily finance the budgets of African governments. This dependency is even more acute for AIDS budgets. Unless this situation is reversed, the success of the AIDS struggle will remain uncertain. African state officials must ask themselves first, how much they should depend on external funds and second, how they can meet the increasing demands for prevention, support, care, and especially ARV treatment without outside resources.

Three major issues suggest caution. The first is the question of what percentage of funds promised by donors will actually materialize and how quickly they will be allocated. For example, the Global Fund to Fight AIDS, Tuberculosis and Malaria (Global Fund) has suffered a continuous shortage of money since its formation in 2001. In 2003, the Global Fund lacked the necessary resources to finance its third round of proposals, and it called for an urgent injection of money from the private and public sectors. In response, civil society associations launched the 'Fund the Fund' campaign. Though the necessary resources finally were made available, the Global Fund's precarious situation raises larger questions about its long-term sustainability. The Global Fund needed $3.6 billion for the successful proposals in its fourth round in April 2004 (Global Fund 2004). Though several governments have pledged money to meet these needs, there is no guarantee that these funds will actually arrive. Will international donors continue to be generous to the Global Fund? What factors will determine their level of generosity? Because roughly 60 per cent of Global Fund money has gone to Africa, the answers to these questions are essential for determining the sustainability of African state responses to AIDS.

A second question that affects sustainability is the short duration of funding for many AIDS programs. Short- and medium-term funds do not facilitate long-term investments. Three to five years of funding is inadequate to sustain the life-long provision of ARVs for those who need the drugs (Morris 2003). It is not only grants from the Global Fund that are for less than five years, but also the majority of programs and grants from private foundations. For example, the much heralded public-private partnership between pharmaceutical companies, the Bill and Melinda Gates Foundation, and the government of Botswana will provide $100 million over a five-year period (Martin 2003). Yet, since a considerable amount of this funding will be for treatment, care, and support for those infected with or affected by AIDS, what will happen to these programs (and their beneficiaries) after the five-year funding period? It is necessary for international partners to commit resources to AIDS for the long term. Long-term funding facilitates mutual accountability between development partners. Yet, given the dependence that African states have on external resources, how can African officials demand or ensure the long-lasting support required for AIDS programs?

Third, it is important to identify and question the conditions that accompany AIDS funding. As this book's introduction illustrates, external funds are likely to be conditional on a set of policies and programs. For example, the US legislation supporting the President's Emergency Plan for AIDS Relief (PEPFAR) specifies that one-third of the money allocated for HIV prevention programs be used to promote abstinence and monogamy programs (Kaiser Family Foundation 2003). In April 2004, when the first round of funds from PEPFAR was granted, the US Global AIDS Coordinator Randall Tobias defended the use of prevention programs that emphasize sexual abstinence in countries that receive PEPFAR money (Kaiser Family Foundation 2004). In contrast, organizations such as Christian Aid have criticized severely this approach and have advocated for comprehensive prevention HIV programs. The organization argues that condoms are effective in preventing HIV infection among young people when used correctly and consistently (Garvey 2003). Furthermore, Feuer (2004) cites research that maintains that condoms are the only protection against HIV for married people or those in long-term relationships in which sexual abstinence is not feasible. These above-mentioned issues seriously challenge the sustainability of current AIDS responses in Africa. Before outlining crucial elements of AIDS governance, the chapter examines how possible changes in the international arena may shape the global commitment to help African states combat HIV/AIDS.

Expected Changes in the International Political Arena

In order to make strategic plans, it is important to identify future international changes that may shape the context in which AIDS policies operate. This section identifies four major issues that may affect Africa's position in the international political arena and speculates about how these possible scenarios may influence the fight against AIDS.

The first issue is the concentration of American and European aid initiatives in the fight against terrorism. Since 11 September 2001, the 2003 invasion of Iraq, and the Madrid bombing of 11 March 2004, an increasing portion of North American and European aid has concentrated on the fight against terrorism. The worsening of the Iraqi situation in April 2004 clouded the hope for an imminent end to that conflict. The consequences for the AIDS fight are immediate; the large amount of financial, strategic, and human resources employed in the war against Iraq are at the expense of what could have been spent on fighting poverty and AIDS. Even though AIDS is considered an international security threat – a fact that has encouraged international actors to address the disease – it may receive only secondary attention if the fight against terrorism remains the top priority for Western states.

Second, China, India, and Eastern Europe have become strategic areas for investment for the United States and West Europe. They have large economies, with markets that are expanding both in terms of production and demand. These rising powers increasingly command the attention of international trade agreements and economic cooperation, as the 1 May 2004 accession of 10 new members to the European Union illustrates. This geographical shift in the interests of the major powers may divert attention from the African continent, which has less strategic and economic importance to the West. However, HIV/AIDS is spreading very rapidly in Asia and Eastern Europe, especially in densely populated countries such as India and China. As a result, these countries threaten to become critical zones for combating AIDS. In fact, the National Intelligence Council, an organization which advises the US Central Intelligence Agency, reported that rates of HIV infection in India, China, and Russia are increasing so quickly that they pose a potential regional and international security threat (*New York Times*,

1 October 2002). These dynamics of the AIDS pandemic may justify strategic choices that divert AIDS resources from Africa to India, China, and former communist states.

Third, the last five years have witnessed an exceptional global commitment to eradicating poverty, marked by new initiatives such as the United Nations (UN) Millennium Development Goals (MDG), the International Monetary Fund's (IMF) Heavily Indebted Poor Countries Initiative, and IMF/World Bank Poverty Reduction Strategy Papers (PRSPs). These programs have prioritized human development through health and education programs. Member countries prepare PRSPs using a participatory process that involves domestic stakeholders and external development partners. The papers analyze a country's poverty situation and describe the existing poverty reduction strategy. The global momentum behind these initiatives has heightened the international attention to sub-Saharan Africa, the region in the world with the lowest human development index (HDI). According to the *Human Development Report* (UNDP 2004), the HDI for sub-Saharan Africa was 0.465 in 2002, in comparison to 0.584 for South Asia. These HDI levels mark a decline for Africa and an increase for South Asia since 2000 (UNDP 2002).[2] These global initiatives have led to numerous laudable achievements that focus strategies and structures on a pro-poor approach to development. Unfortunately, results from these efforts have proven inadequate. Progress on MDGs is slow and insufficient (United Nations 2004). PRSPs have been severely criticized for not serving their purpose and not complying with the principles of ownership and participation (Bretton Woods Project 2004). These disappointing results may discourage donors, who often require an immediate and tangible impact to justify continued program funding. A possible response from donors may be to reformulate development strategies. New development plans may be less likely than the MDGs to emphasize investments in human capital. This in turn may undermine the strategic focus on fighting AIDS and poverty together in Africa, despite the fact that the two are intricately linked.

Finally, the end of UN Secretary General Kofi Annan's second term in 2006 may indicate the end of an opportunity for fighting poverty and disease on the African continent. The tradition of rotating the geographic representation for the Secretary General means that his successor will not be an African. Because of the increasing focus on Asia, there are reasons to presume the next Secretary General will be Asian. This is not to imply that the work of the UN directly depends on the nationality of the Secretary General, but the Secretary General does highlight particular issues, as Kofi Annan has done with AIDS. The nationality of the chosen Secretary General also may reflect the priorities of key UN member-states. If so, it is not unlikely to see Kofi Annan's successor focus on issues such as trade and terrorism.

All these projected scenarios suggest that international attention will turn from Africa to Asia and Eastern Europe. This possible shift in international development priorities will jeopardize external support for existing and future programs in Africa. In practical terms, such a shift implies less foreign aid to the continent. If the future scenarios outlined in this section materialize, development programs in Africa should immediately search for ways to become self-sustainable and independent from external funding.

On the other hand, there are reasons to believe that the potential 'lost momentum for Africa' may not affect AIDS programs as much as overall development programs. First, international commitment to fight AIDS has been unprecedented; there has been strong support at high levels of government. Second, civil society, and in particular international nongovernmental organizations (NGOs), has played a key role in setting the agenda and successfully lobbying for the implementation of global policies against AIDS, as the Patterson and Cieminis' chapter illustrates. Third, there has been an extraordinarily quick mobilization and disbursement of AIDS funds, especially by the Global Fund and some private foundations. These reasons suggest that national and international support to fight AIDS has not been 'business as usual.' Rather, there is a level of genuine effort and leadership on AIDS that may be permanent. However, if the epidemics in China, India, and Eastern Europe keep growing, this financial commitment to combating AIDS in Africa may be tested.

On the one hand, the focus of development issues may shift from Africa toward Asia and Eastern Europe. On the other hand, the extraordinary global leadership against AIDS in recent years may prevent AIDS programs in Africa from being forgotten. It is possible that these projections about the future international environment may be completely wrong. However, what is important is that African states and nonstate actors plan for the future. What are expected contributions from external and internal sources? What do these contributions need to be? How can African states ensure the long-term continuity of international support for AIDS programs? Or maybe the question should be: How can African states decrease their dependence on international support and become self-sustainable?

AIDS Governance: Consolidating the Response

> There are men who fight one day, and they are good;
> Others fight for a year, and they are better;
> There are men who fight many years, and they are very good;
> But there are those who fight all their lives:
> These are the indispensable ones.
>
> Bertold Bretch, in Silvio Rodriquez's song 'Sueño con Serpientes'

Many African leaders are aware that maintenance of AIDS policies, especially treatment programs, is insecure, and that the tentative nature of AIDS programs is an immediate problem. Throughout the continent, calls to develop sustainable programs are common within ministries of health

(CHGA 2004). However, African state leaders and donors have often put off addressing the long-term viability of AIDS policies, arguing 'let's do as much as we can today and deal with tomorrow's problems when they come'. The urgency of caring for citizens today explains this desperate attitude, though it is not the most rational decision. African state leaders and donors often do not act on the idea that 'prevention is better than a cure'. There are many actions that African states can take immediately to prevent future sustainability problems. Now is the time for African states to think strategically about the medium- and long-term policies needed to fight AIDS and to pursue AIDS governance.

Through its various case studies, this book argues that the criteria of ownership, participation, and self-sustainability need to drive the responses of the African state to AIDS. Such a strategy may not include new policies or programs, but it aims to 'do things differently'. For example, as Siplon argues in her chapter, it is necessary to move away from the patriarchy embedded in African states to develop more gender-inclusive institutions. In other words, the way forward is for African states to promote AIDS governance in collaboration with nonstate actors. AIDS governance aims to consolidate AIDS policies and to improve the quality and depth of the responses in the medium and long term. To do so, African states need to pursue financial independence, promote ownership and self-sustaining approaches, act in partnership with civil society, address gender inequalities, strengthen health systems, show a firm commitment to equitable health care, and attain positive impacts for the duration of the response. These principles are not merely conceptual guidelines. Their application comes down to very concrete and practical recommendations that are feasible for African governments, as illustrated below.

- *Reducing dependency on external funding*. African states need to gradually increase contributions from domestic funding to AIDS programs and to minimize costs through innovative initiatives. They need to harness external funds toward investment rather than recurrent costs (Martin 2003). They should take full advantage of trade agreements promoting the use of generic drugs and domestic production of drugs. As the chapter by Halbert and May illustrates, the 2003 World Trade Organization accord that allows the production of genetic versions of patented pharmaceuticals and the export of those products to eligible countries may create new opportunities for African states to provide treatment to their citizens with HIV/AIDS. In doing so, African states can reduce their reliance on price agreements negotiated by international organizations and drug companies. This aspect of AIDS governance also has implications for external partners, who should adhere to their commitments for support in the medium and long term.
- *Promoting ownership and approaches based on national need.* Consolidating the response implies that African states take responsibility for strategic priorities based on their specific national contexts. Now is the

time for African stakeholders to assume leadership and responsibility in the continent's AIDS fight. Knowledge, resources, and commitment are there. Capacity building is taking place all over the continent. As mentioned above, most African countries have working National AIDS Councils that coordinate the national multisectoral response (UNAIDS 2002). Because current external support may not be available in the future, it is necessary to begin to employ the acquired capacities and lessons learned in a responsible manner. It is time to move from globally designed policies and structures toward strategies tailored to national needs. For example, the World Bank's Multi-Country AIDS Program has provided millions of dollars in loans to design high-level, multisectoral AIDS policy-making institutions. However, while these structures may work well in one country with more state capacity, they may be less effective in a country rebuilding after war or a society with deep ethnic or regional divisions. The experiences with the Country Coordinating Mechanisms (CCMs), national-level organizations established to manage Global Fund grants, also demonstrate the different ways institutions can function across the continent. Variation has been particularly evident in the CCMs' ability to achieve the participation of civil society in AIDS policy making. While some Tanzanian NGOs have felt underrepresented and have decided to bypass the CCM and apply directly to the Global Fund, NGOs in Mozambique have been more incorporated into CCM structures. Civil society participation in Mozambique was more successful because of structures of cooperation between stakeholders that previously existed (ICASO 2002). In order to develop relevant programs and institutions, African states must carry out studies to inform, design, and consolidate national programs.

- *Participation of nonstate actors*. The contributions by Siplon, Batsell, and Furlong and Ball underline how the tension between the state and civil society hinders the fight against AIDS. Though partnership has become one of the buzz words in the policy arena, partnership is only possible with a common goal or a convergence of interests among stakeholders. It is essential that the African state begin to perceive nonstate actors not as a threat to the state's legitimacy, but as an asset. Scholars and policy makers must demonstrate that empowering nonstate actors does not undermine state authority; rather, open dialogue and collaboration between nonstate actors and state officials bolsters the state's legitimacy. As the chapter by Eboko argues in reference to Cameroon, strengthening political culture is a priority for expanded responses to AIDS. Actions to address the epidemic should build on the channels of communication and decision making between state and nonstate actors.
- *Engendering the response*. As Stephen Lewis (2004), UN Special Envoy on HIV/AIDS to Africa, stressed when he highlighted the need for gender equality, 'Have I not addressed the fundamental question?' Only by seriously addressing the gender inequalities embedded in society will African

states have a chance of tackling AIDS. As Siplon discusses, there is a wide consensus that gender inequality is one of the main driving factors of the epidemic. However, this broad recognition has not led to the systematic tackling of gender inequalities in AIDS-related programs. Policy makers, scholars, and international donors need to take the gender issue seriously. First, it is necessary to provide an enabling environment within policy-making mechanisms for addressing gender inequalities and ensuring lessons about gender are learned. This is not simply a matter of writing the word 'gender' in strategic papers; this process includes mainstreaming how plans impact gender inequalities and monitoring and evaluating the outcomes of a gender-based approach. Second, it is important to broaden the scope of gender to act on the causes of gender inequalities and women's vulnerability to HIV infection. For example, domestic and international policy makers must promote economic empowerment for women, enhance female access to education, pursue women's right to control resources (particularly land), and promote legislation that penalizes rape, especially if the perpetrator is HIV positive. Third, it is an imperative that women and young girls have access to health information and care, including maternal care.

- *Strengthening health systems*. Given the weak health care systems of most African countries, it is legitimate to acknowledge the trade-off between AIDS and other health issues. Strategic investments should maximize the synergies between AIDS programs and other health programs. *New* resources allocated to AIDS should strengthen rather than undermine health systems; for example, investments in antenatal services are likely to benefit AIDS control and to reduce maternal mortality. Equally, designing the systems necessary to scale-up the distribution of ARVs for people with HIV/AIDS will benefit drug distribution for individuals with other diseases such as malaria and tuberculosis. Nonetheless, in many African countries where the high HIV prevalence is eroding state capacity, AIDS is no longer a health issue but a development one. This fact may justify giving AIDS programs priority and even diverting resources from other health and social issues.
- *Equity considerations in health services*. Health care equity is a challenging issue that decades of development programs have not managed to address fully. For example, equity in public health has been pursued ever since the Declaration of Alma-Ata in 1978.[3] Yet, the development of AIDS programs may provide a window of opportunity to achieve health care equity. Marginalized populations such as sex workers, migrant workers, homosexual men, and injecting drug users have tended to lack access to health care services; these individuals also have been identified as being particularly vulnerable to HIV infection. Programs to ensure these populations can access AIDS-related services should be a priority in all countries. In doing so, it may be possible to provide a more equitable distribution of health care services. In addition, purposely targeting

women's access to health care and improving maternal health care will contribute to a more equitable distribution of health services. Another issue is providing equitable access to treatment for those with HIV/AIDS, especially when introducing ARVs and scaling up their distribution. The social factors that prevent some individuals from accessing health care and questions about who will receive treatment must be addressed in any treatment plan. If such issues are not tackled, the inequalities in health care in Africa will be replicated in AIDS treatment.

- *Achieving impact.* As the chapter by Patterson and Cieminis demonstrates, representatives to the African Summit on HIV/AIDS and Other Related Infectious Diseases at Abuja, Nigeria and the United Nations General Assembly Special Session on HIV/AIDS pledged themselves to devoting the necessary resources and developing institutions to fight AIDS. The situation is now different from what it was in 2001 when these two meetings were held: substantial resources have been mobilized, AIDS decision-making institutions have been created, and strategic plans have been developed. African states, international donors, and AIDS activists must now move beyond merely monitoring the processes that have started to demanding results. What actually has been achieved? Are new infections being averted, particularly in newborns? Do women have more control over sexual negotiations so they can become less vulnerable to HIV infection? Has the quality of life of those infected improved? Are orphans receiving care and social support? Those involved in the fight against AIDS must implement programs based on the results they expect to achieve; new goals in the AIDS struggle must be ambitious.

To conclude, it is time for African states to pursue AIDS governance in collaboration with nonstate actors. The actions discussed in this chapter are crucial for consolidating the current response, making the response sustainable, and strengthening the governance capacity of the African state. African states must not waste the strategic opportunities that are available now. They must pursue win-win policies to strengthen the possibilities of the African state for AIDS governance.

Notes

1 The index provides a profile of national efforts to combat the AIDS epidemic. It was developed by UNAIDS, the US Agency for International Development, the World Health Organization, and the Policy Project. It first was applied to 40 countries in 2000 and then to 54 countries in 2003.

2 The HDI measures the average achievements in a country in three areas: health (life expectancy at birth), education (adult literacy rate and school enrollment ratio), and standard of living (gross domestic product per capita). The composite measurement is on a scale of 0 to 1, with a score closer to 1 indicating a higher level of human development.

3 The declaration was the outcome of the International Conference on Primary Health Care, which was held in Alma-Ata, USSR in 1978. Concerning inequality, the declaration says:

'The existing gross inequality in the health status of the people particularly between developed and developing countries as well as within countries is politically, socially and economically unacceptable and is, therefore, of common concern to all countries' (WHO 1978, par. II).

References

African Union (AU). 2003. *Decision on the progress report of the Secretary General on the follow-up on the implementation of the Abuja Declaration and Framework Plan of Action on HIV/AIDS, TB and Other Related Infectious Diseases (ORID).* Presented at the African Union summit, 10–12 July, Maputo. http://www.au2003.gov.mz/key_documentation/cmdec1.htm#658.

Bretton Woods Project. 2004. PRSPs: A continuation of structural adjustment. http://brettonwoodsproject.org/article.shtml?cmd[126]=x-126–42231.

Commission on HIV/AIDS and Governance in Africa (CHGA). 2004. Minutes of the second CHGA commissioners' meeting, 23–25 March, Maputo. Unpublished document.

Feuer, Cindra. 2004. Can PEPFAR save the most vulnerable? Paper for the American Foundation for AIDS Research (AmFAR) Treatment Insider. http://www.amfar.org/cgi-bin/iowa/td/feature/record.html?record=119.

Garvey, Mary. 2003. *Dying to learn – Young people, HIV and the churches.* Report for Christian Aid. http://www.christianaid.org.uk/indepth/310learn/dyingtolearn.pdf.

Global Fund. 2004. Progress report – April. http://www.theglobalfund.org.

International Council of AIDS Service Organizations (ICASO). 2002. Information on the Global Fund to Fight AIDS, Tuberculosis and Malaria. Global Fund update for NGOs and civil society. http://www.icaso.org.

Joint United Nations Program on HIV/AIDS (UNAIDS). 2002. *Report of the Secretary-General on Progress towards implementation of the Declaration of Commitment on HIV/AIDS.* New York: United Nations General Assembly.

——. 2003. *Follow-up to the 2001 United Nations General Assembly Special Session on HIV/AIDS.* Progress report on the global response to the HIV/AIDS epidemic. Geneva: UNAIDS.

Kaiser Family Foundation. 2003. Politics and policy: President Bush signs into law $15B international HIV/AIDS bill; Some Democrats say White House commitment 'hollow.' Daily report. http://www.kaisernetwork.org/daily_reports/rep_index.cfm?hint=1&DR_ID=17940

——. 2004. U.S. Global AIDS Coordinator Tobias defends emphasis on abstinence for prevention programs. Daily report. http://www.kaisernetwork.org/daily_reports/rep_hiv_recent_rep.cfm?dr_Date Time=04–22–04&show=yes

Lewis, Stephen. 2004. Keynote by Stephen Lewis, UN Special Envoy on HIV/AIDS in Africa, to the 'Microbicides 2004' conference in London, 30 March. http://www.stephenlewisfoundation.org.

Martin, Gayle. 2003. *A comparative analysis of the financing of HIV/AIDS programmes.* Report for the Human Sciences Research Council.

http://www.hsrcpublishers.co.za/index.html?finance.html~content.
Morris, Kelly. 2003. Paying the price of HIV/AIDS: South Africa and beyond. *Lancet: Infectious Diseases* 3 (9): 532.
Organization of African Unity (OAU). 2001. The Abuja Declaration on HIV/AIDS, Tuberculosis and Other Related Infectious Diseases. http://www.uneca.org/adf2000/Abuja%20Declaration.htm.
United Nations. 2004. Overall progress on Millennium Goals uneven at best, Secretary-General says in message to high-level Beijing conference. Press release. http://www.un.org/News/Press/docs/2004/sgsm9222.doc.htm
United Nations Development Program (UNDP). 2002. *Human development report*. New York: Oxford Univ. Press.
——. 2004. *Human development report*. New York: Oxford Univ. Press.
US Agency for International Development (USAID), UNAIDS, WHO, and the Policy Project. 2003. *The level of effort in the national response to HIV/AIDS: The AIDS Program Effort Index (API) 2003 round*. http://www.policyproject.com/pubs/monographs/API2003.pdf.
World Health Organization (WHO). 1978. Declaration of Alma-Ata. http://www.who.int/hpr/NPH/docs/declaration_almaata.pdf.

Index